THE PRESENT ILLNESS

THE PRESENT ILLNESS

American Health Care and Its Afflictions

MARTIN F. SHAPIRO, MD, PhD, MPH

JOHNS HOPKINS UNIVERSITY PRESS | *Baltimore*

© 2023 Johns Hopkins University Press
All rights reserved. Published 2023
Printed in the United States of America on acid-free paper
9 8 7 6 5 4 3 2 1

Johns Hopkins University Press
2715 North Charles Street
Baltimore, Maryland 21218
www.press.jhu.edu

Library of Congress Cataloging-in-Publication Data is available.

ISBN 978-1-4214-4565-6 (paperback)
ISBN 978-1-4214-4566-3 (ebook)

A catalog record for this book is available from the British Library.

Special discounts are available for bulk purchases of this book. For more information,
please contact Special Sales at specialsales@jh.edu.

To my parents

CONTENTS

Prologue. The Present Illness   1

1   The Best of Times? A Tale of Two Health Care Narratives   7
    Dialogue #1   18

2   A Heart in a Heartless World: What Patients Want and Need   20
    Dialogue #2   48

3   Doctors and Dollars: Antecedents, Actions, and Consequences   50
    Dialogue #3   97

4   Procedural Proficiency or Human Connection? Attitudes,
    Aptitudes, and Opportunities   98
    Dialogue #4   128

5   Idealism on Life Support: Missed Opportunities in Medical Student
    Education   130

6   Errors of (com)Mission: Misdirected Priorities in Education,
    Practice, and Research   172
    Dialogue #5   211

7   Making a Killing: Corporate Providers of Medical Care   213
    Dialogue #6   242

8   Biomedical Scientists and Their Truths: Disinterested Investigation
    or Prioritized Self-Interest?   244
    Dialogue #7   289

9   "Doing Everything for Money": The Producers of Health Care
    Products   290
    Dialogue #8   315

10 Human Rights and Wrong Turns: Some Problems with Health Care
    Financing, American Style   317

11 Protagonists, Pitfalls, and Lessons from Abroad: The Tortuous
   Path to Health Care for All   346
   Dialogue #9   382
12 Rectitude or Revenue? American Health Care in the
   Marketplace   383
   Dialogue #10   399
13 Atomization and Its Discontents: The Consciousness and
   Connectedness of Participants in Health Care   400
   Dialogue #11   420
14 Malevolent Messaging: Toxic Interactions in Health Care   421
   Dialogue #12   444
15 Healing American Health Care: To Palliate, to Cure, or Both?   446
Epilogue. Lessons Learned   462

Acknowledgments   465
Appendix. Quixotic Proposals for Treating American Health
   Care's Afflictions   467
Index   473

The Present Illness

Setting: An office in a medical school adjoining an outpatient clinic.
Situation: A student is about to present a case to her professor.

Student: I just saw a patient. This is a frustrating case. He is very sick, and
   I don't know if he will survive.
Professor: Tell me what you have learned so far.
Student: The patient has been here many times with the same complaint, but
   there does not appear to have been much improvement. He was
   brought here by concerned friends and relatives. He is not sure why he
   is here. He doesn't think anything is wrong. He was helpful with some
   parts of the history. His entourage filled in other key details.

   I took a careful history and identified four major problems. The first
   one is grandiosity or at least exaggerated sense of well-being. He feels
   like he has always been in perfect health. In fact, he insists that there is
   no one in the world that is as healthy as he is. He asked me to write and
   sign a letter saying that, but I did not.

   I consulted psychiatry, and they think that he is delusional. They also
   noted that he makes poor decisions, going on frequent spending sprees
   and buying things he doesn't need with money he doesn't have. So, his
   finances are a mess. Psych thinks that, combined with his delusions,
   this may represent mania or hypomania.
Professor: Tell me about the other problems. What is his name?
Student: He is identified as the US health care system, although it turns out
   that he may not really be a system, just a mess. His system, if we call it
   that, is at least 50% more expensive than that in any other economically
   advanced country. At the same time, there are serious inequities in the
   care that people receive in the United States, and the health outcomes

here are worse than in other countries that spend a lot less for their care.

Professor: Let's discuss these problems one at a time.

Student: Well, in the past 60 years, costs have risen at breakneck speed, and not just because the cost of living has gone up. The share of the GDP, or gross domestic product, allocated for health care increased from 5% to 18%.[1]

Professor: Spending 18% of the GDP on health care translates into Americans having to work on average more than seven hours a week to pay for it!

Student: That's an interesting way to put it.

Professor: Did you compare cost escalation in the US to that in other countries?

Student: I did. It is much greater here. Back in the 1960s, Canada and the US were spending about the same proportion of the GDP on health care. They began to diverge in the 1970s. Now the US is spending about 6% more of GDP on health care than Canada—I guess you'd say about two and a half more hours of work per week—and even more than that compared to some other countries.[2]

Professor: That's right. Tell me about the other problems.

Student: Well, the second problem is access to care. This is a big problem for African Americans, Latinos, and people who are poor. Some people have easy access to all kinds of care; others do not. Unlike all these other developed countries, tens of millions of Americans don't have any health insurance. Many more with low incomes have Medicaid, but lots of doctors won't take Medicaid because the reimbursement is low.[3]

Even when they have insurance, people of color may not receive the same treatment as whites. For example, Blacks were less likely than whites to receive surgery or chemotherapy when they had early-stage lung cancer, or to get a heart catheterization, coronary angioplasty, or bypass surgery when they presented with symptoms of concern for coronary artery disease, even though they have a higher death rate from heart problems.[4] Being poor is just as much a factor in not getting equivalent care as is race or ethnicity.

Professor: Yes, a great deal of research has been done on this issue. Efforts to alleviate the disparities have not had much effect to date.

Student: The third problem is that health outcomes are poor overall in the US, and they are worse for people of color and for the poor. Before the COVID-19 pandemic, Americans' life expectancy in 2019 was 78.5 years, while most advanced countries had life expectancies of 81 or greater. In the US, poor people die much younger. Infant mortality is twice as high among African Americans as among whites, and overall infant mortality in the US ranks 52nd in the world![5]

Professor: You've done a nice job of identifying some key issues: people spend a lot more for health care, yet many cannot get it, and the health of the population is worse. A related issue is that the United States spends less of their health resources on public health and social services than do many other countries.[6] Many systems are involved with this disorder. Do you think that there a single treatment that can address all of them effectively?

Student: Well, for sure, getting health insurance for everybody would help.

Professor: But that treatment has been tried numerous times. The "patient" was given prescriptions at least six times.[7] They never worked. Sometimes, the patient wouldn't take the treatment at all. Other times, treatment relieved some symptoms but did not solve the problem. There have been separate prescriptions in most years since 1988 to do something just about costs. They never worked very well, either. What do you think we should do?

Student: Some people feel that the medicine wasn't strong enough. How about if we try the same medicine at a stronger dose: a health reform that would cover everyone?

Professor: There are many advocates of doing that, but I am skeptical that it will achieve the intended effects.

Student: With all due respect, professor, I think that you are wrong. Providing insurance coverage is the key.

Professor: I have studied, practiced, and taught medicine over several decades. I have seen many cases where lack of insurance and discrimination were the underlying problems and others where they were not. But let's assume for the moment that you are right and I am misguided in my perceptions. I am working right now on a project through which I hope to gain an understanding of all of the "systems" involved in this patient's illness. If you are interested, you can join with me in this effort, and we will see if lack of insurance is the only disorder.

Student: I'd like to do that, but where do we start?

Professor: I have written an outline of some of the issues as an introduction to the book. After that, I intend to develop a series of chapters around these themes, focused on patients, doctors, medical educators, scientists, corporations, and so on. I have lots of personal experiences that will help to develop these ideas, but they need to be presented in the context of history and other published evidence. The last few chapters will try to tie together these diverse topics in a framework that makes sense of what's going on in health care. Take a look at it, and then let's talk again.

Student: Thanks, professor. I'll do that.

Professor: By the way, I've changed the names of almost all of the patients and most of the others whom I describe to protect their privacy.

Student: I understand.

Notes

1. In 1960, 5% of the GDP went to pay for health care in the United States. That increased to 6.9% in 1970, 8.9% in 1980, 12.1% in 1990, 13.3% in 2000, 17.4% in 2010, and 17.6% in 2019. In 2020, the first year of the COVID-19 pandemic, it jumped even higher, to 19.7%. "U.S. National Health Expenditure as a Percent of GDP from 1960 to 2020," Statista, December 2021, https://www.statista.com/statistics/184968/us -health-expenditure-as-percent-of-gdp-since-1960/.

2. From 1975 to 1980, Canada's health care costs stayed around 7% of GDP and then increased to about 8.7% in 1990, which was only about half of the increase in the US that decade. By 2000, Canada was at about 9.2%, then 11.5% by 2010. In each decade, Canada's increase in share of the GDP going to health care was about half that in the US. By 2010, the US was spending about 6% more of GDP on health care than Canada. During the past decade, Canada's numbers have stayed in the range of about 11% to 12%. As for other countries, the Organisation for Economic Co-operation and Development reports that its members (all advanced economies) most recently averaged spending 8.9% of GDP on health care. France, Germany, Japan, and Sweden all were at about the same level as Canada. Canadian Institute for Health Information, *National Health Expenditure Trends*, 1975 to 2019 (Ottawa: Canadian Institute for Health Information, 2019), 7–11, https://www.cihi.ca/sites/default/files/document/nhex -trends-narrative-report-2019-en-web.pdf; "Health Expenditure and Financing," Organisation for Economic Co-operation and Development, accessed October 22, 2021, https://stats.oecd.org/index.aspx?DataSetCode=SHA; "Total National Health

Expenditures as a Percent of Gross Domestic Product, 1970–2020," in Nisha Kurani et al., "How Has US Spending on Healthcare Changed over Time?," Peterson-KFF Health System Tracker, February 25, 2022, https://www.healthsystemtracker.org /chart-collection/u-s-spending-healthcare-changed-time/#item-start.

3. In 2019, apart from the elderly, the great majority of whom have Medicare coverage, 19% of nonelderly Hispanics and 11.4% of African Americans lacked health insurance, compared to 7.8% for whites and 7.2% for Asian Americans. As a result of this and the additional problem of out-of-pocket costs, many Americans do not go to see a doctor. That is true of 13% of whites, 17% of African Americans, 21% of Hispanics, and 10% of Asians. Nambi Ndugga and Samantha Artiga, "Disparities in Health and Health Care: 5 Key Questions and Answers," Kaiser Family Foundation, May 11, 2021, https://www.kff.org/disparities-policy/issue-brief/disparities-in-health-and -health-care-five-key-questions-and-answers/.

4. Dale Hardy et al., "Racial Disparities and Treatment Trends in a Large Cohort of Elderly Black and White Patients with Nonsmall Cell Lung Cancer," *Cancer* 115, no. 10 (May 2009): 2199–211, https://doi.org/10.1002/cncr.24248; Nancy R. Kressin and Laura A. Peterson, "Racial Differences in the Use of Invasive Cardiovascular Procedures: Review of the Literature and Prescription for Future Research," *Annals of Internal Medicine* 135, no. 5 (September 2001): 352–66, https://doi.org/10.7326/0003 -4819-135-5-200109040-00012.

5. Life expectancy in Austria, Belgium, Germany, the Netherlands, and the United Kingdom were all 81.4 years or higher; Canada, France, and Sweden were 82 years or higher; Australia, Italy, South Korea, Spain, and Switzerland were 83 years or more, and Japan was 84.3 years. In 2020, these differences were even larger because the decline in life expectancy in the US was greater than in these other countries, For Blacks, life expectancy at birth in the US was 4.1 years less than for whites in 2019 and 5.8 years less in 2020. Raba Kamal, "Life Expectancy and Healthy Life Expectancy Data by Country," World Health Organization, Global Health Observatory Data Repository, accessed September 13, 2021, https://apps.who.int/gho/data/node.main .688; Jared Ortaliza et al., "How Does U.S. Life Expectancy Compare to Other Countries?," Peterson-KFF Health System Tracker, September 28, 2021, https://www .healthsystemtracker.org/chart-collection/u-s-life-expectancy-compare-countries /#item-start. Those in the bottom 1% of income distribution die about 14 years sooner than the top 1%, and that difference increased by two years between 2001 and 2014. Nearly half of the lowest 5% of the income distribution die by age 76, compared to less than 20% of the top 5%. Raj Chetty et al., "The Association between Income and Life Expectancy in the United States," *JAMA* 315, no. 16 (April 26, 2016): 1750–66, https://doi .org/10.1001/jama.2016.4226.

While infant mortality statistics have improved for all groups, there still is a large difference between whites, with a rate of 4.6 per 1,000 live births, and Blacks, with a rate of 10.8 in 2017. "Infant Mortality Rate by Race/Ethnicity," KFF State Health Facts, accessed September 13, 2021, https://www.kff.org/other/state-indicator /infant-mortality-rate-by-race-ethnicity/?currentTimeframe=0&sortModel=%7B%2 2colId%22:%22Location%22,%22sort%22:%22asc%22%7D. Recent data indicate that the overall US infant mortality rate of 5.2/1,000 ranked behind Latvia and Slovakia, and it was higher than those in 51 other countries, including Canada (4.4), the United Kingdom (3.8), Ireland (3.5), and Japan (1.9). "Country Comparisons: Infant Mortality Rate," Central Intelligence Agency, World Factbook, accessed August 17, 2022, https://www.cia.gov/the-world-factbook/field/infant-mortality-rate/country-comparison.

6. Elizabeth H. Bradley, Heather Sipsma, and Lauren A. Taylor, "American Health Care Paradox—High Spending on Health Care and Poor Health," QJM 110, no. 2 (February 2017): 61–65, https://doi.org/10.1093/qjmed/hcw187.

7. There were health reform proposals in 1910–1912, 1927–1932, 1943–1949, 1964–1965, 1993–1994, and 2009–2010. See chapter 11 in Paul Starr, *Remedy and Reaction: The Peculiar American Struggle over Health Care Reform* (New Haven, CT: Yale University Press, 2013).

1

The Best of Times?

A Tale of Two Health Care Narratives

It is a time of scientific breakthroughs. It is a time of clinical neglect. It is an age of exploding knowledge of the mechanisms of disease. It is an age of blissful ignorance toward the chasms in health and life expectancy. It is an epoch of extraordinary profits for corporations in the health sector. It is an epoch of personal bankruptcies due to medical debts. It is a season of life-saving medical interventions. It is a season of choosing between paying for health care or for food, clothing, or housing. It is the spring of personalized medicines costing tens of thousands of dollars per person treated. It is the winter of avoidable deaths of those whose problems lack priority. We are all going to approach immortality, except for those facing premature mortality.
—With apologies to Charles Dickens

Advances in health care are among the finest accomplishments of contemporary societies. Emerging technologies have provided vastly more diagnostic information than was conceivable even half a century ago. Pharmaceutical and biological products have been developed to treat or prevent diseases that previously had wiped out millions of people. New surgical approaches and other invasive techniques have dramatically transformed the prognosis of many serious diseases. Social science and humanities research studies have pointed the way to humane, compassionate, ethical practice of medicine. The prospects for further progress appear to be limitless.

Yet health care is a crucible in which we can see how societies such as the United States fail to live up to their professed ideals. In many ways, health care is an affliction upon members of those societies as much as a source of healing, particularly (but not only) when they lack universal health insurance. Life expectancy and health have improved dramatically for those with privilege, but far less for those who lack it. Technologies, rather than human relationships, define much of medical practice. The funders and most practitioners of medical science pay relatively little attention to many major health problems that affect the poor and marginalized members of society, focusing, for the most part, on research that stands to benefit relatively few.

Health care costs in the United States have risen at a rate and to a level that almost everyone understands is not sustainable. Yet business interests—not clinical need—drive the responses to this situation at multiple levels.

The failure to enact universal insurance coverage for health care has produced a crisis in the US, the only advanced, industrialized country lacking such a program. But the dawning of this realization in many quarters has not produced a consensus on how to fix the range of problems that afflict health care today. These problems are painfully evident in the United States, which is the focus of this book, but it would be wrong to presume that other societies do not face many similar issues.

Why is it so difficult to reform health care in America? It is a series of self-evident truths that health care costs too much, that vast numbers of individuals lack health insurance, and that many lack adequate access to care as a consequence. It also is clear that health care outcomes in the United States are worse than other countries with advanced economies, and that Americans pay much more for health care that often is worse. Can't reasonable policy makers convene and solve this problem? Yet even partial solutions, such as the Affordable Care Act of 2010, meet with fierce resistance.

Polarized and vociferously expressed opinions—a vast array of them— make it difficult to disentangle the sources of the problems and their underlying nature. How can we think about addressing these issues comprehensively? In order to do so, we need to reflect upon what health and health care represent in contemporary society.

Many people tend to think about health care as a relationship between a doctor and a patient, in the context of some clinical transactions. Some, but by no means all, doctors see it this way. Other clinicians think far less about the relationship with the patient than about the disease or diseases that they are treating. Specialists' interests often do not extend much beyond the narrow range of conditions and procedures that are the focus of their specialties.

To the clinical scientist, health care may be primarily the search for the basic mechanisms triggering a disease or for a new way to treat it. To the entrepreneur or corporation, health care may be one of a range of business opportunities. To the social scientist, the societal and environmental factors that contribute to poor health, particularly in disadvantaged communities, may seem more relevant than what happens in doctors' offices or hospitals. The government official may think about health care primarily as an increasingly burdensome share of expenditures that need to be controlled. The health services researcher may look at it as a series of technical or organizational challenges to be solved in order to optimize care.

Each of these perspectives is aligned with certain values, needs, and expectations of the members of those groups. These in turn profoundly influence attitudes about the system and potential changes in it. This is painfully evident in the United States, where almost everyone agrees that health care is seriously dysfunctional.

In this book, I explore the range of influences upon all of the participants in health care. My goal is to illuminate the array of challenges that need to be addressed in the effort to create a health care environment that can meet the needs of the entire population. In doing so, I examine issues that may seem, at first glance, to be unrelated and perhaps beside the point. Shouldn't it be possible just to pass a law and fix things?

I am a physician who trained in general internal medicine in Canada and the United States. I entered university in the late 1960s. Like many of my cohort, I wanted to change the world, and I was not at all sure that medicine was the way to do that. I was sufficiently ambivalent about a medical career to seriously consider dropping out of medical school on the day that I was to start classes. Fortunately, a wise dean of students convinced me to proceed, saying that sometimes those who are most ambivalent about medical careers make the most important contributions to the field.

I knew that I wanted to work on repairing the health care system, so I pursued graduate studies in public health and history. I subsequently spent my entire career working in medical schools as a clinician, educator, and researcher on the delivery of health care. As a Canadian who came to the United States years ago, I expected that universal health insurance on a model something like that in Canada would soon be adopted. I wholeheartedly believed (and still do) that such change is urgently needed. Yet it is not forthcoming. This book is an expression of my journey through medical practice, education, and research, and as a recipient of care. In writing it, I have sought to elucidate why that change has not come.

The issues are complex, and they also are diverse. At times, I present personal experiences as illustrations of the kinds of problems that need to be addressed.

The Specialist Clinician: Attention Should Be Paid

Myer was a 59-year-old man admitted to the hospital with complications of kidney failure. A loving husband and father, he was a small businessman who worked long hours to support his family. He also had high blood pressure and elevated cholesterol, and he had had a heart attack 14 years earlier. His kidney disease was due to chronic glomerulonephritis, a degenerative condition that often leads to the need for dialysis or transplant. As his kidney disease advanced, he became profoundly weak. He needed to work to support his family, and he did so as long as he could, even crawling up the stairs at his job because he was so exhausted. It was inevitable that he would need dialysis, but the kidney specialist wanted to delay it as long as possible. The doctor was focused on the blood tests of kidney function, which he felt were not yet bad enough to start those treatments.

The doctor ignored the entreaties of the patient and of his wife and daughter, and expressed the opinion that Myer was exaggerating his symptoms. When the evidence that Myer's disease was advanced became impossible to ignore (vomiting dried blood and hallucinating), he already was profoundly ill. Dialysis was started when he was admitted to the hospital, but he developed pneumonia, a common complication of severe kidney failure. The doctor prescribed antibiotic pills for the pneumonia. A couple of days later, Myer complained that his breathing was getting much worse. His wife shared this complaint with the doctor, but the doctor insisted that her husband was improving and did not need any additional treatment. Myer died later the same day.

As Arthur Miller might say, attention should have been paid to this man. There were a number of errors in this case that contributed to his death, but the main one was that the doctor focused upon the patient's biochemical profile and not on the person in front of him.

I was a third-year medical student at the time in a city more than 1,000 miles away. When my uncle telephoned me with the news that this man—my father—had died, my life was changed. Like many who have lost a loved one, I desperately wanted to undo the events leading to his death. As a medical student, I wondered if I could have intervened had I been there. Of course, nothing would have brought my father back, but there was something that I could do as a future physician. I vowed not to be a doctor like the one who had ignored my father's experience. I would treat the patient, and not just the disease, and focus upon patients as whole human beings in the context of their lives.

The Academic Hospital: Go Off and Die

Luis was a 23-year-old man from Central America with a mild learning disability who lived with his parents. He also had congenital immune deficiency, requiring immunoglobulin infusions since birth to prevent life-threatening infections. Early on, he developed hepatitis C virus infection from an infusion. When Luis was 7 years old, his parents moved to the United States, and he came to our teaching hospital for his care. We took care of him for 15 years.

During this time, his hepatitis C progressed and he developed end-stage liver disease. He was evaluated by the liver transplant service, which declined to put him on the transplant waiting list. They said that Luis had no insight about his illness, and because both his parents worked, he did not take his medicines consistently. They believed that if he were the recipient of a transplant, he would not reliably take the medicines needed to prevent transplant rejection.

I was supervising a hospital ward team at the time of his admission. My residents and I sat down with the family to discuss his situation in Spanish. It turned out that Luis had never missed a single dose of medicine. Because of his illness and disability, his loving parents had chosen to work different shifts, so he was never alone if he needed a medicine or became ill. Also, Luis did understand his illness and the importance of taking his medicines. At his bedside, we could not help but notice the family dynamics. Luis's parents' faces were "radiant with joy," and they displayed unequivocal commitment to the well-being of their ailing child.[1] He was a wonderful patient with parents who were totally devoted to keeping him well. Without a transplant, he was going to die.

We shared this information with the liver team. They pointed out that Luis was an undocumented immigrant and that while coverage had been arranged for his routine care, he did not have insurance to pay for the transplant. I discussed the case with the liver transplant surgeon, noting that he had been getting care at our institution for 15 years. The surgeon said that he would waive his fee, but we would need to get the hospital to cooperate as well. The associate director of the hospital told me that it was a considerable expense to the hospital do a transplant. Even if they waived all charges, the patient would be unable to pay for his transplant medications in the long run.

I implored him to pursue it and see if MediCal (California's Medicaid) would be willing to provide Luis with coverage, given his long time living in the country. The administrator claimed that they tried but MediCal refused. We were incensed, but the hospital's decision was final. Our only hope was to get him to another hospital that might try harder to get MediCal approval. Fortunately, a fellow who was training in liver disease was as frustrated as my residents and I were. He contacted the other liver transplant programs in the region. One of them agreed to take Luis. We learned that they were able to get MediCal to authorize the procedure, and he was placed on the transplant waiting list.

On the face of it, this episode had a good outcome. The reality, though, was that the system had failed Luis. If the medical team had not figured out that he would be able to take his medicines consistently, that his parents were extraordinarily supportive, and that his time in the country was a mitigating circumstance that might get him a new liver, Luis would have been sent home to die. In American health care, some lives are cheap. When they are extinguished, few take note. In cases like this one, the problem isn't the tunnel vision of the doctors but the misplaced priorities of a health system that stand in the way of patients getting the care they need.

The Patient: Do Everything!

Frances, a 73-year-old social worker, served critically ill individuals. Despite a past diagnosis of aggressive breast cancer, Frances survived and kept working. One day, she was admitted to the hospital with a serious infection, which led to extreme elevation of her blood glucose level and a loss of consciousness. She was treated for the infection, but her mental status did not return to normal. She was transferred to our hospital, where she did poorly. Her white blood cell count became extremely elevated, indicating that the infection was getting much worse despite treatment. There was further deterioration in her mental function. Strenuous efforts to save her were unsuccessful. She lapsed into coma, and several of her organs failed as she slid relentlessly toward death.

Frances had not completed an advance directive that would have specified her preferences for treatment when there was little or no chance of meaningful recovery. Frances's daughter, who worked with patients in intensive care, understood the hopelessness of the situation and did know her mother's preferences. But then two of Frances's brothers, who lived overseas, came into town. They were intensely religious and presented the medical team with nonnegotiable demands that she be kept on life support.

Their niece clearly did not agree, but she deferred to the authority of her uncles. We tried to reason with them that several of her organs had failed, no treatments were helping, and intubating her so that a ventilator could breathe for her was going to cause additional suffering in a hopeless situation. They insisted that it was contrary to their religion not to "do everything." Frances endured several more weeks of intensive care treatment on a ventilator until her family relented and allowed her to die.

Unlike the previous case, the issue here had nothing to do with insurance. It was instead about ethical decision-making. Some patients or their families make it difficult to do what is humane and most appropriate for an individual or to use health care resources in socially responsible ways, with the goal of ensuring that *everyone* has access to care with the meaningful potential of increasing their quantity or quality of life.

Such issues are common and a central concern of ethics consultation services in the United States. "Patient autonomy" (discussed in chap. 2) can become a mandate to allow a family member to make decisions, supposedly on behalf of the patient, but often for reasons of their own that in the end extinguish the patient's voice, rather than represent it.

The Medical Student: It Would Be a Waste

David was a medical student doing his third-year clerkship in internal medicine. This is a crucial learning experience in which students are exposed, often for the first time, to a large array of diseases and situations, typically while caring for patients who require input from other specialty groups, like surgery, radiology, and psychiatry. David was smart and highly motivated. I was the supervising faculty member on his team, which also included a resident and two interns. David's knowledge of diseases and their treatment was at a high level for someone in the third year. He interacted extremely well with the members of his ward team and with the nursing staff. He also was terrific with the patients: sensitive and open, caring and committed. He obviously loved what he was doing.

I shared my impressions with David, telling him that I believed he would be an outstanding resident in internal medicine. He acknowledged that he loved the rotation and could imagine himself in internal medicine. However, he added, other students had advised him not to do that. "Your test scores and grades are too good. It would be a waste." They were not saying that knowing a lot and doing well would be unhelpful in internal medicine. They were telling him that his level of medical school performance would qualify him for one of the high-paying medical specialties. Nonetheless, he promised to think about what I had said.

The way in which the health system pays for services shapes the choices that physicians and physicians-to-be make about their careers and about how they practice medicine. In fields like radiology, orthopedic surgery, dermatology, and anesthesiology, practitioners make a lot more money by doing procedures. Internists, family physicians, and pediatricians, who earn much less, spend more time talking to patients, examining them, and getting to know them. They do this in order to diagnose and treat their patients' problems, educate and comfort them, and provide support without performing high-priced medical procedures. Several months after our conversation, David came by my office and asked if I would write a letter of recommendation for him for residency. I was happy to provide one, but I was disappointed to learn that he had chosen to go into anesthesiology.

It is likely that David will be a terrific anesthesiologist. That discipline, like my own, needs fine physicians like him. It is unfortunate that money drives such decision-making. While every specialty is a legitimate choice, awareness of what it means financially is, in a sense, a corrupting influence upon the career decisions of medical students.

At first glance, some of these stories may appear to be to be tangential or even irrelevant to the main problems facing the health care system. In the ensuing chapters, I show that they are not. In considering these issues, I devote chapters to the people who receive medical care (the patients and their families), the physicians who provide medical care, the system of medical education, the corporations that organize and deliver much of medical care, the scientists and scientific organizations and their priorities, the producers of treatments and medical machines, and the roles of government and the insurance industry.

I draw on my personal experiences and observations, and on relevant literature in developing the themes in each chapter. In so doing, I explore three sets of factors that shape expectations about health and how we think about it, as well as about the organization, provision, and experience of health care today.

The first factor is the conception, organization, and effectuation of health care, and the treatment of health and of life itself not as inherent rights of all members of society, but rather as commodities (things that are valued and exchanged within a market). All parties—corporations in the health sector, providers, recipients of care, and scientists—want to maximize their shares of the goods.

The second factor is health care as a venue in which participants (medical practitioners, scientists, educators, scientific and professional organizations, government officials, and the people who seek medical care) pursue their nonmaterial needs, mediated by their personalities, values, and priorities. I characterize these attributes as "consciousness."

The distortion of communication regarding health and health care that occurs among the actors in the health care system and throughout society is the third factor. This intensifies and reinforces attitudes, beliefs, expectations, perceived needs, behaviors, and policies that are already in evidence, thereby impeding corrective action.

We need to identify effective "treatments" for the problems of health care and its afflictions. In order to do this, we need to gain insight into all three of these factors and their interactions. Therefore the final four chapters of the book bring together the issues discussed above. They also provide a framework for thinking about how we got into this mess, what it may take to escape our current predicament, and what the prospects are for creating a health care system that is more equitable, effective, efficient, compassionate, and just.

I include in the book a prologue, an epilogue, and a series of dialogues that appear between chapters. These are imagined conversations between a professor and her student on the issues raised. They are modeled after the often adversarial, apparently fictional discussions about justice between Socrates and his interlocutor, Thrasymachus, in Book I of Plato's *Republic*. Here, the conversations represent two things: my own search for answers in developing this book and the kind of discourse that I believe needs to occur if we are to make meaningful progress.

This book focuses upon the United States. A health care system like that in the US can become somewhat more humane without broader transformation. Things are now so bad that some bandages may at least staunch the bleeding. But all industrialized societies will have to have a reckoning. Health care eventually could consume entire domestic budgets or lead to the inability, even in generous public programs, to cover costs of some treatments that are essential to health. Such developments would be particularly harmful to individuals who do not have access to other resources to pay for such services. A broad conversation on this topic is needed urgently, as these problems have the potential to disrupt all such societies.

Note
1. Psalm 34:5; 1 Samuel 21:8–15.

| Dialogue #1 |

Professor: Well, what have you learned so far?

Student: This really is complicated. There are so many things going on.

Professor: That is true.

Student: I don't see why it has to be this complicated. Maybe expanding Medicare will be enough.

Professor: Wouldn't it be better to have some clarity about what all of the problems are? That would allow us to anticipate the likely impact of an intervention.

Student: I suppose so, but I really want to start addressing the problems.

Professor: You can do that, but we still need a diagnosis if we want to figure out what treatment will be needed to cure this "condition." It will feel less overwhelming if we take on the problems of health care one at a time.

Student: Where should we start? How about with the insurance companies?

Professor: Oh, we should get to them, eventually. If we start there, with a problem that is undoubtedly enormous in the United States, we might lose sight of other elements that also may be important.

Student: Well, you said that patients were one of the groups you want to look at. Why don't we start with them? I think that we will find that patients aren't the problem. They are the innocent victims of the health care system.

Professor: I like your idea of starting with the patients. Since we want to develop a comprehensive understanding of what is going on, it may be useful to start somewhere other than with the usual suspects. As for whether they contribute to the problem, how sure are you that they don't? Isn't it possible that their demands for care drive some of the use and rising costs?

Student: I see your point. But shouldn't we emphasize how the system fails to meet their needs?

Professor: We'll get to that. For now, you might want to look at this less from the perspectives of micro- and macroeconomics than from those of psychology and sociology. It would be terrific to get at patients' motivations through a deeper dive into some of their stories.

Student: Professor, the main problems of health care are econometric: access, quality, and outcomes. Quantitative data measure them. Anecdotes will tell us nothing.

Professor: You might be correct. But just as in medical care, the story that patients (or others) tell—"the history of the present illness"—is perhaps the most important part of the process of getting to a diagnosis. I have a bunch of examples of this, but we need to identify themes across these cases.

Student: I see what you are saying. I remain skeptical about this approach, but let's get started.

2

A Heart in a Heartless World

What Patients Want and Need

To cure sometimes, to treat often, to comfort always.
—Folk saying with various attributions

A Life without Connections

Ruth was in her fifties and a tough nut to crack. I inherited her from a wonderful, committed, empathic physician who had been at her wit's end trying to take care of Ruth. She had lots of minor health problems and was creative in finding ways not to follow the doctor's recommendations. At the same time, she was needy, came in frequently, and phoned often. She lived with her young adult son, Billy, who was as disorganized as she was. Their financial situation, like much of her life, was chaotic. On one occasion Ruth called me to say she could not take it anymore. She and Billy were going to be evicted shortly for failure to pay rent for the motel room where they had been living. Billy was off playing basketball with his friends.

"Oh, Dr. Shapiro," she said, "I just can't go on. I'm going to kill myself."

I told her that she needed to go to the emergency room of our hospital (which was a little more than one mile away) immediately.

"I don't have money for a taxi."

"Take the bus."

"I don't have money for a bus. Dr. Shapiro, could you please come here and help me?"

I had no choice. I headed over to Ruth's place. She brightened up when she saw me. I gave her $4 to pay for a cab. (It was a short ride.) She talked for a while, saying I made her feel better by coming over and that she didn't feel like killing herself anymore.

"Dr. Shapiro, would you mind if I spend this money on cigarettes?"

I sighed in resignation, and undoubtedly some despair and frustration. I did not deny her the cigarettes, but I determined not to respond with a visit the next time she called in desperation. I advised her a bit on things she might do to induce compliance from Billy when there were urgent tasks at home. We settled into a relationship in which I could not do much to affect her behavior. And I certainly stopped asking her to quit smoking!

The journey through the many influences upon contemporary health care and its afflictions begins, perhaps paradoxically, with its intended beneficiary. The word "patient" is derived from the Sanskrit word *pati*, meaning suffer. The Latin word *patiens* has a similar meaning: one who suffers. Today, the term is applied more broadly to all people encountering the health care system as recipients of service. These individuals are not always suffering from a disease, at least not in the sense that most doctors would consider to be one. Nor are they merely consumers seeking a commodity (although that is a nontrivial part of their relationship to health care, as we shall see). Arguably, many patients do have some kind of suffering from which they seek relief or repair.

These individuals are generally interested in optimizing their well-being, but they also bring to encounters the context of their lives, their values, their fears, their aspirations, their disappointments, and their challenges. All of these can have a decisive impact on their encounters and on the system as a whole. In so doing, they may act in ways that are rational, irrational, or both, directed toward goals that range from easy to discern to opaque and that confront their providers with needs and expectations that can be straightforward to evaluate, complex and difficult to address, or a mix of the two.

As a general internist, I take care of inpatient and outpatient adults with a broad range of problems and needs, ranging from primary care to managing problems at the end of life. In my career, I have encountered many patients whose interactions with me were heavily influenced by their life experiences and were much more complicated as a result.

Some came wrapped in entitlement, others inundated by despair. Some were burdened by anxieties or panicked about the waning of life. Many came with entourages of relatives or friends with attitudes or agendas. Many of their problems did not originate in anatomical, biochemical, or physiological aberrations, but all were expressed in the context of seeking medical care.

The examples in this chapter are illustrative of common problems that precipitate the pursuit of medical care or affect the care sought and received. In some cases, I was able to respond to the situation more or less effectively. In others, I was frustrated because there was so little that I could do. Together, they paint a picture of the roles played by consciousness and social existence—and their interplay—in the seeking of medical care in contemporary society.

Ruth stands out in my mind because in some ways she was an affliction for me, at least until I realized that it was beyond my ability to intervene successfully. I continued to see her in my office and tried to allay her anxieties and distress, but eventually I realized that her existential problem was something that I could not fix, given her lack of motivation or belief in her ability to proceed in life in a different way. She declined psychotherapy, and social workers made little headway with her. She did not seem to have any friends. Her son was not a source of strength. She sought solace and companionship through the pursuit of medical care.

Was Ruth an anomaly? In one American study, the combination of psychological distress and social isolation increased the use of medical care as much as fourfold.[1] According to an analysis of data from the US Health and Retirement Study, among persons over the age of 60, between 37% and 56% were lonely in 2012, depending on the definition used. Those who were lonely were more likely to be unmarried, nonwhite, with less education and income, with more depressive symptoms and disabilities, and more likely to rate their health as fair or poor. They also visited the doctor and were hospitalized more often.[2] Increased use of medical care among the lonely also was observed in a British study.[3] Dutch general practitioners taking care of patients who were chronically lonely reported feelings of frustration and powerlessness, given the lack of available therapeutic options to address the underlying problem.[4]

As I learned in Ruth's case, loneliness cannot be treated medically because it reflects the disintegration of communities in which people barely know their neighbors. Without another adult in the household, people often have little contact with others yet may decline referrals to community resources. The patient, in despair, may seek solutions, or at least companionship, through receipt of medical care. Doctors oblige with medical visits but are ill-equipped to solve the underlying problems. Other societal resources may not meet those needs.

Desperate to Stay Healthy

Ann lived with her mother until she was in her early fifties. She never married. She cared for her aged mother and then for her older sister, who developed cancer. After her mother and sister died, Ann had the resources to support herself but had become quite fixated on her health, particularly after her sister died in her mid-sixties. She went to doctors frequently. She had many scans and x-rays. The doctors she saw attempted to allay her anxiety about her health with medical tests. It was never enough. Late in life, a physically disabled man became Ann's companion, in some ways reproducing her role as caregiver for her mother. He was demanding, and taking care of him became an additional source of stress for her. Medical care and her doctors provided some solace.

The pursuit of medical care as the front line in addressing psychosocial challenges is not limited to individuals who are in as much disarray as Ruth was. They can be reasonably functional. They may not chase cosmetic or chemical solutions for what ails them, but they often pour their anxieties into the pursuit of answers or reassurance from their doctors. Ann was not frustrating to her providers. She was charming and had good interpersonal skills. As a relatively high utilizer of care, she had identified a group of physicians who were happy to oblige her with visits and procedures on a regular basis. Win-win.

"Some Strong Bond Which Is to Be"

Alfred, Lord Tennyson, "In Memoriam A.H.H.: Is It, Then, Regret for Buried Time"

Helena was a lovely lady in her mid-forties when I first saw her. She was married to a man who was about 15 years older. A Jewish Holocaust survivor, her husband was a nice man but with dark experiences that he rarely would discuss. Helena was not Jewish and came from a Mediterranean country. She worried a lot about her mother's health and even brought her to Los Angeles to see me. Helena had no children. She always came to clinic with gifts for my kids, generally really nice stuffed animals. She worried constantly about her health but was very healthy, with only mild hypothyroidism. She wanted regular laboratory tests. When I did obtain some, it would calm her. She often called repeatedly when there had been a minor abnormality of any test, even though I would reassure her as best I could that it was of no consequence and posed no danger.

Patients like Helena sometimes are not even aware of their anxieties but manifest the dis-ease through visits to the doctor, during which they press for more tests. I must admit, I did order more tests than she needed at times, but I tried to limit my profligacy.

Helena's life was good in many ways, but the relationship with her doctor was essential to maintaining her equilibrium. Around the time that I moved away from Los Angeles, her husband (by then in his mid-eighties) died. His death was hard on her. Even though she had a new physician, she continued to call me from time to time to talk about how much she missed him.

"'Twas Like Midnight"

Emily Dickinson, "It Was Not Death I Stood Up For"

I cared for Dalileh for many years. She became my patient in her late fifties, an immigrant from Iran after the Iranian Revolution. She came in often and had many complaints: headaches, backaches, bellyaches, chest pain, knee pain, hip pain. At each visit she complained something different. Objective evaluations never found a source for these problems. She always seemed depressed. I also cared for her husband, who was much happier, and I spoke regularly with their son. Her family recognized that she was depressed, reporting that it had been a long-standing issue.

I rarely gave Dalileh satisfaction because I would not prescribe anything stronger than a nonsteroidal inflammatory drug like ibuprofen or naproxen for her pain. She would not talk about the problems she had; she remained focused on the physical pain. Dalileh's affect (mood) was depressed. Her face looked grim. She did not want to talk to a counselor or therapist. I prescribed her antidepressants, but she stopped them after a few days, saying that she could not tolerate them and that her problem was the pain.

Up to 30% of visits to a primary care physician are triggered by emotional problems.[5] Yet for many patients, somatic complaints are amplified and poorly tolerated; overcoming them is inconceivable. The symptoms are closely related to depression, anxiety, and other mood disorders.[6] Such cases are the most challenging for a primary care physician. Often, these patients will not seek psychologic care or see a social worker, only wanting treatment for the perceived source of their dis-ease. Many psychiatrists do not take insurance, and it can be hard to find mental health providers whom patients can afford. Yet the reflex antidepressant prescription can only take the patient so far, even when they are willing to take the pills. Some other treatment modalities are needed. Cognitive behavioral therapy is a popular one right now, but it is not an answer for everyone.

Compounding the challenge in Dalileh was the cultural distance between her and me. The "idioms of distress" and suffering can vary widely across cultures. Drawing on the expertise of someone familiar with these expressions in a particular culture is needed to be able to address the problem.[7]

Much of medical care is consumed by the investigation of somatic complaints for which an "organic" cause cannot be found. I think that I might have had more success with Dalileh had I been more familiar with her culture or able to speak her first language. Even translators can only help so much. They are not trained in psychology or in interpretation of nonverbal communication. In Los Angeles, many Iranians were reluctant to see a psychotherapist, social worker, or psychiatrist who spoke Farsi, for fear that word about their stigmatized condition would get around the community. When caring for a depressed patient, one feels the sadness. Visits with Dalileh were not a happy time, since I never could give her what she wanted.

Existential Panic: "Shrill Peals That Waver and Crack and Break"
Aldous Huxley, "Panic"

Olivia, in her early thirties, came to my office for a new patient visit. Her opening statement was remarkable. She was a handsome woman, well-dressed, clearly attentive to her appearance. She spoke with urgency and a certain edginess.

"Doctor, you've got to help me," she pleaded. "I have been to over 200 doctors and none of them have been able to figure out what is wrong. You are my last hope."

An actress whose career had not gone well, Olivia was not earning a living from her profession. She was not isolated, like Ruth, but she was "out of joint." She could not look at the reality of her life and figure out another path. Her symptoms were vague (tightness in her throat and chest). In the absence of positive findings from numerous investigations, they strongly suggested a psychological basis. When it came to my entreaties to consider seeing a therapist, Olivia would have none of it, convinced there was a physical basis for her symptoms.

Some patients are tireless in pursuit of a medical explanation for what ails them. This was a frustrating case. Olivia had had numerous tests and countless doctors' visits but never received an answer that she considered satisfactory. She wanted the doctors to identify a disease that was responsible for what made her feel bad and was unwilling to accept the idea that it might be psychological. Her life was a perpetual search that consumed medical care and would never give her the answer that she desired. She wanted no stone left unturned, no body part left unscanned, no laboratory test left unordered, perhaps multiple times.

"The Judgment"

Franz Kafka, "The Judgment"

Georg was in his late twenties when came to see me, complaining of headaches and neck pain. He had had scans that revealed no deformity. A neurologist who evaluated him excluded the possibility of atypical migraine and suggested that he had muscle tension headaches. Georg had a PhD, and he was not impressed with this diagnosis, insisting that something else was going on. He was a postdoctoral scholar but was unable to work effectively because of his symptoms. He made sure that everyone knew that his father was a distinguished researcher at another institution when he asked for additional studies to explain his symptoms. Finally, a study revealed a possible trapped nerve near Georg's armpit. He was offered surgery but also was warned that it might not help. He went ahead with the surgery, but it did not improve his symptoms. He continued to look for a cure.

Sometimes it is evident what the underlying problem is, but it still is not easy to promote insight into the "lesion." Despair may reflect fear of not living up to family's expectations. Although I couldn't be sure, since he was not accessible to psychological discussions, I thought that Georg had an underlying fear of failing to live up to what he perceived as the expectations of his famous father. The pursuit of an elusive medical diagnosis offered a way to rationalize his sense of failure. This was both sad and frustrating: he was doing well professionally, but it was not going to be enough in his own eyes.

Unrequited: "Come to Dust"

William Shakespeare, "Fear No More the Heat o' the Sun," *Cymbeline*, Act 4, Scene 2

Andrew was 65 the first time that I saw him. He came in for a physical examination, but his agenda was that he wanted a refill of his testosterone prescription. He claimed to have a low testosterone level, but when I checked it, it was only slightly below the middle of the normal range. I informed him of the result and encouraged him not to continue to use testosterone, but he was insistent. Andrew was professionally successful, but none of his relationships had lasted more than a few months. He continued to look for love in what I thought were all of the wrong places, seeking partners who were at least 40 years younger. He felt that he needed chemicals to perform at the level to which he aspired. His latest flame was half a continent away, but that fire did not endure.

Sometimes, doctors try to mollify such perceived needs by ordering unnecessary tests, procedures, and medications, and even provide labels for the complaints that imply a physiological basis for what ails the patient. Chemicals were not going to solve Andrew's problems. I declined to prescribe testosterone. He also asked me about growth hormone, but I would not give him that, either. Accordingly, he went to the antiaging "specialist" whom he had seen previously, whose practice apparently was almost entirely devoted to the provision of such "therapies," and obtained his refill. As in other areas of life, enterprising individuals may take advantage of those who want to feel better and think that medical treatments are the answer. Thanks to heavy promotion and direct-to-consumer advertising, many men are seeking this particular fix.[8]

Nondisease for What Ails You

When I was a resident physician, I undertook a community research project: we screened people in shopping centers for hypertension and kept track of the results. It was an interesting project in which we identified many people with uncontrolled hypertension. One puzzling finding was that when we asked participants if they had ever been told that they had high blood pressure, some reported that they had been informed that they had low blood pressure and had been treated for it with vitamin B_{12}, veal liver extract, and other such concoctions, none of which are recognized treatments for blood pressure problems. We then did a systematic study in which we found that quite a few people in that community had had such treatments.

When we looked further into the matter, we found that low blood pressure emerged as a popular diagnosis as early as the 1920s, when J. F. Hallis Dally gave it a medical-sounding name: hypopiesia. The clinical description suggested that the symptoms were more likely due to depression: "they are difficult to awaken in the morning and start the day badly. For many hours during the day, however, they are capable of rousing themselves in response to necessary activities."[9] The diagnosis was widely acknowledged even in medical textbooks in the 1930s.[10] A contrary view was expressed in a 1940 article, asserting that hypotension was not a disease but rather "an ideal blood pressure level."[11]

Textbooks in 1947 and 1950 acknowledged the doubts but still offered the possibility of treatment. Comments in *Cecil's Textbook of Medicine* seemed to recognize the association with depressive type symptoms: "psychoneurotic states, including neurocirculatory asthenia have been ascribed to hypotension."[12] Another textbook in 1950 acknowledged that it "cannot be called a definite clinical entity" but still described potential therapies such as open-air activity and an interesting occupation.[13] By 1956, the diagnosis of primary hypotension as a distinct clinical entity had disappeared from the textbooks.[14]

The temptation may be strong to give the patient a "treatment" for their symptoms, no matter how improbable the benefit therefrom. I learned upon further reading that this was far from the only such "nondisease" to be described in the literature. In 1965, Meador wrote in a leading medical journal about "the art and science of nondisease," cataloging several, including "non-Cushing's disease" (Cushing's is a disorder in which to much cortisol is produced by the adrenal glands due to a pituitary tumor), "nonhypothyroidism," and "nonanemia." He said they were conditions that bore vague resemblances to known diseases but did not meet diagnostic criteria.[15]

Since then, other nondiseases have gained fashion: "nonhypoglycemia," "candidiasis hypersensitivity syndrome," "chronic fatigue syndrome" due to Epstein Barr virus infection, and others.[16] Occasionally, a clinical trial produces evidence that diminishes the popularity of such a diagnosis, but like whack-a-mole, new ones pop up to replace them.[17]

Why do these diagnoses continue to appear? I believe that it is because patients perceive a need, and many practitioners are looking for an "explanation" that can get the patient out of the office. Providing support for someone whose symptoms probably lack a physical basis is a complex challenge. The longitudinal relationship between a patient and a medical provider can be complicated. While some patients have few, if any, chronic complaints, and other have physical or emotional ailments that are easy to diagnose, still other have vague or obscure symptoms that evade diagnosis.

Explaining to a patient that their symptoms may have no physical basis is not easy, and many patients are reluctant to accept such explanations. Discussion of such matters requires delicacy, empathy, patience, and some psychological sophistication. As will be clear in chapter 5, these are not the attributes that form the basis of selection of students for medical school. Medical schools do little, if anything, to nurture these skills in their students. It is far easier for clinicians to put a label on the symptoms. Medical "science" has obliged by offering some labels for the symptoms to fulfil this need.

Many patients do not care to have their problems characterized as psychologically—or socially—mediated. On one occasion, I was at an event celebrating an accomplishment by a family friend. One of the guests, who was known to find some such occasions challenging, lay down on the floor during dinner, announcing that it was an attack of hypoglycemia, thereby becoming the center of attention for a period. He did not have diabetes and was not manifesting any of the classic signs of hypoglycemia. The reality is that blood values of glucose can be well out of the normal range without causing any symptoms. Yet this entity (dubbed as non-hypoglycemia) was liberally diagnosed for a time in the 1970s.[18]

In addition to the nondiseases mentioned above, there are many more described in the medical literature, such as fibrocystic breast disease and dermatological "conditions" of the face, scalp, and genital areas.[19] Classifying these conditions as diseases may be largely a response to the patient's need for a diagnosis, but the doctor who affixes the label is an enabler, either lacking the patience or capacity to talk empathically to the patient about the true source of their problems, benefitting financially by being able to order a test or do a procedure, or being disinclined to spend time with the patient to explain why there is no diagnosis that can be affixed to their situation.

There are other conditions or situations that may well have physiological correlates but raise questions about whether it is most beneficial to treat them medically. One article reported the results of a survey of the readers of the *British Medical Journal* and identified 20 such conditions, including unhappiness, cellulite, and loneliness,[20] to which we might add alcoholism (now characterized medically as "alcohol use disorder," but for which Alcoholics Anonymous does at least as well as any medical program) and chronic back pain (for which physicians do extensive studies and frequent medical procedures that are rarely beneficial and often harmful).

Ivan Illich refers to medicalization of many aspects of life as a kind of "medical imperialism" and "the appropriation of health." Symptoms that may be attributable to life dissatisfaction (such as anxiety and hopelessness) receive medical labels and medical treatments that may be wildly inappropriate. Illich blames the medical establishment, which he asserts "has become a major threat to health."[21] It is the practitioners, more than the establishment, that do the enabling, but none of this would matter if there were not a "receptor site" in the patient, searching for some form of relief from the whips and scorns of life.

In addition to these manifold diagnoses, we now are inundated by the promotion of lifestyle treatments that rage against the progress of life. The medical marketplace offers goods for every taste: botulism toxin injections and surgery for wrinkles, fillers in the lips and elsewhere to enhance self-image and appearance, breast augmentation or reduction, liposuction to remove fat from the abdomen and elsewhere, minoxidil to treat baldness, phosphodiesterase inhibitors to enhance erections, testosterone for virility, amphetamine derivatives to improve academic performance in people who do not have evidence of attention deficit disorder, growth hormone to increase the height of children or to enhance performance of athletes, and other treatments to hide your veins, lose weight, fall asleep, and so on. The producers of these treatments are not shy about touting their wares, and many patients desperately want them. One study estimated that care for medicalized conditions in the US cost about $77 billion in 2005.[22]

"King of Kings": The Aggressive Demand
Shelley, "Ozymandias"

Kevin came to my office for an urgent appointment. A man in his early forties, he was attired in a suit and tie. Clearly, he had taken some time off work to attend this appointment. He told me that he had a cold. Generally, there is nothing to do for a cold except treat the symptoms with such medicines as antihistamines, decongestants, and cough medicines. In this instance, as often is the case, he insisted on antibiotics. Antibiotics attack the cell wall of a bacteria. Cold viruses do not have cell walls, so antibiotics don't help.

Kevin had heard that explanation before, but he insisted, "every time I have a cold, it turns into sinusitis [which sometimes is treated with antibiotics]. I am going out of town tomorrow for my work as a medical malpractice attorney. I absolutely have to have an antibiotic to take with me, or I will have a serious problem."

Individuals who have ample resources often will use their persuasive skills to extract what they want from medical encounters. Kevin did that with the skill of a prize fighter: with an impressive uppercut, combined with a decisive left hook! (I had not asked him about his profession, much less his area of legal practice, but he wanted me to know.) He clearly believed that antibiotics would help him and was not prepared to wait and see how he did. Many patients insist on antibiotics, and doctors often give them what they want. They prefer not to spend a lot of time arguing with a patient who may give the doctor a low satisfaction rating either online or in an institutional survey if not satisfied with the "service." The overprescribing of antibiotics in this way contributes to the development of resistance, making them less effective for the people who really need them.[23]

Autonomy: The Relatives Show Up (It Is Written)

In other instances, it is members of the family who make demands for medical care. Sometimes, near the end of life, they stand in the way of withdrawing futile care as a way of showing love to the patient. Not infrequently, it is relatives who are distant or even estranged from a dying patient who present the most difficulty in this regard.

That was the situation in the case of Frances, whom I discussed in chapter 1, whose uncles had come from overseas and would not allow us to withdraw care. It was a sad experience for me. I had cared for her for years, and I enjoyed a good relationship with her. I regret that I never had gotten her to complete an advance directive. Consequently, we did not have that available to help her negotiate her final days in the way that she and her daughter would have chosen. Religious dogma can get in the way of humane care. Nothing in the New Testament, the Torah, or the Koran dictates use of modern life-supporting technologies. Yet patients and families often defer to religious authorities, some of whom are reasonable while others (for reasons probably more psychological than theological) not infrequently prolong the dying process.

Autonomy: Regrets "When the Blasts Denote I Am Nearing the Place"
Robert Browning, "Prospice"

I began to care for Shapur in his late sixties. When he entered his mid-eighties, he began to speak less and less. It turned out that he had a form of progressive dementia in which expressive aphasia (the inability to produce spoken or written language, even when comprehension is intact) is a primary characteristic. He was physically able to get around. He seemed to understand what was happening around him. He just had very few words in him. Eventually, other manifestations of dementia became apparent. I discussed all of this with his family, who understood the situation. We all recognized that there was little to do as Shapur's condition progressed. One day, he came to the emergency department with his family. I was not notified that he was there and did not learn about his admission until some weeks later, when I received a request from the decedent affairs office to sign his death certificate. I let them know that I had not been aware that he was in the hospital.

I contacted the team that had been involved and asked what had happened. It turned out that Shapur had presented with advanced dementia and aspiration pneumonia (a common complication with dementia, and a situation that is often the terminal event) and had not responded to treatment for the pneumonia. The team had suggested to the family that they limit care, since he was not going to recover. They refused. They insisted on extensive treatment that prolonged his dying. Since Shapur could not express himself, the family's decision was the final word. I felt bad not to have been there. Perhaps I could have encouraged them to do less when there was no hope of meaningful recovery. Even an advance directive regarding his preferences for care near the end of life might have made a difference, but we did not have one in place before Shapur was no longer able to convey that information.

While no one would suggest that patients and their families should not have a say in their care, there has to be a reasonable limit. When families insist on life-extending treatment in futile situations, the people being subjected to that care occupy beds in intensive care units and draw on resources such as ventilators, hospital beds, medications, specialty consultations, and nursing care. This increases the direct and indirect costs of medical care and may deprive others of care that they need and that has a much better chance of being beneficial.[24] The patient and their family may not think about the consequences of their request. The providers of medical care (some of whom also contribute not infrequently to perpetuating futile care) have a responsibility to be attuned to those implications, but it is challenging to convince family members to take such issues into consideration. If Shapur's family had been able to get past the panic that they were about to say goodbye to their loved one, they might have considered how their decisions affected the care of others.

Sometimes the physician is a reluctant participant. Other times, the physician is a willing accomplice in the overuse of medical care. In the case of the elderly, many treatments can help prolong life. Families are desperate to "save" their beloved relative from further decline and death. Yet, even when there is no evidence that it prolongs life or appreciably affects its quality, and even geriatric guidelines recommend against it, many patients with advanced dementia receive feeding tubes that are inserted into the stomach through the wall of their abdomen because they lack swallow reflexes and cannot eat.[25]

Scenarios such as the one that arose with Shapur occur frequently. Physicians and nurses find it demoralizing to provide such "futile care."[26] This problem arises in hospitals caring for the well-insured and in municipal hospitals taking care of the poor. The issues involved in responding to such situations often are framed in relation to one of the basic precepts of modern medical ethics: *autonomy*. This concept holds that the patient (or their surrogate) should be able to make decisions regarding care.

This is far removed from the situation several decades ago, when Eliot Freidson, a medical sociologist, wrote that professional autonomy—the doctor as the sole decision maker—is illegitimate. He regarded the medical profession as "a rather special source of advice" on "what treatment is necessary and therefore what technical limits are imposed on the alternatives for management." In this context, "lay choice is quite legitimate and professional autonomy illegitimate."[27] Yet allowing patients or their families to make decisions with few constraints other than their out-of-pocket costs (which affect lower-income individuals preferentially) can drive up utilization of procedures, days in hospital, and occupancy of intensive care unit beds.

Autonomy: Consequences for Others[28]

Laurent, a French citizen in his late thirties, was living in Los Angeles. He had acute myelogenous leukemia that was unresponsive to treatment, and he had been hospitalized for several weeks, during which he'd had repeated episodes of pneumonia and urinary tract infections. Laurent also had severe thrombocytopenia (a low platelet count in the blood-stream, making him prone to serious hemorrhage) and urinated blood constantly. Needing daily red cell and platelet transfusions as well as supplemental oxygen, he knew that he had little time left.

"I want to go home to Paris," he told me.

The resident physicians were able to arrange with Air France to transport Laurent and his wife to Paris, so long as they were accompanied by a physician and a nurse. The residents were not given leave to ac-company him, so I did, since I was going off service anyway.

The airline arranged to have oxygen available, and we brought an array of medications and blood products intended to get him safely to Paris. We were concerned about the effects of changes in cabin pressure during takeoff, given Laurent's thrombocytopenia and the risk of intracranial bleeding. Takeoff was mostly uneventful, but he began to breathe rapidly. Because of the noise of the aircraft's engines, it was difficult to hear through a stethoscope what was going on in his heart and lungs, so we gave him an injection of a strong diuretic medicine. He seemed com-fortable but continued to breathe rapidly.

About 30 minutes into the flight, the copilot approached us. "We made a mistake," he reported. "We did not board enough oxygen to get to Paris. Would you like us to land in Chicago to pick up some more?"

I was unsure about what to do. The thrombocytopenia had not led to catastrophe on takeoff, but how would an additional landing and takeoff affect him? I asked for time to consider the situation.

As it happened, there was another patient being transported on a stretcher to Paris on the same flight, a woman in her early twenties en route from Tahiti, where she had sustained a subarachnoid hemorrhage (bleeding from a ruptured blood vessel in the brain). She was comatose. She was accompanied by a French physician. I approached him about my dilemma regarding landing in Chicago.

He looked me squarely in the eye. "My patient's blood pressure was unstable when we landed and took off at Los Angeles," he told me.

"Landing in Chicago would be a big risk for her. Your patient is dying. My patient has a small but real chance of long-term survival. My patient's needs should take precedence."

I was taken aback. Should I place Laurent at greater risk of dying on this flight in the interest of the well-being of another patient? The nurse shared my misgivings, but we concurred that our patient was certain to die very soon. I informed the copilot that we would take our chances with the available oxygen.

Laurent made it to Paris and survived five days after a meaningful reunion with his family. I recall vividly the joy tempered by sorrow on the faces of his two brothers as we emerged from Customs and Immigration in the airport. Notwithstanding that, I feel that we made the right decision in this instance. We were in a situation where one patient's needs conflicted directly with those of another. Yet they were essentially in the same boat. In the end, we all are, so the episode was clarifying.

There are two problems with unrestricted patient autonomy. When patients address their anxieties, disappointments, family conflicts, or impulses by insisting upon more medical care, it can lead to considerable waste. At the same time, there is unlikely to be much, or even any, consideration of the consequences for others when these decisions are made. Were the resource recognized as part of what is owed to everyone in society, then everyone would be in the same boat when it comes to receiving that care. Ideally, patients, providers, and the larger society would look upon health care expenditures as societal costs and would think about the availability, appropriate use, and allocation of health care resources as decisively affecting health outcomes. What benefits one patient might harm another.

Sometimes, in seeking to fulfill patients' wishes, clinicians are unwitting accomplices in such misallocation. In the most unusual circumstance described above, the allocation decision, which is usually made without any other affected patients in mind, was an explicit choice between the interests of two very ill people who were literally in the same "boat." I came to realize that I had been complicit in being prepared to allocate a substantial resource to a man who was about to die, and potentially in a way that could have harmed another individual.

Trust (and the Lack Thereof): "All the World Is Made of Faith, and Trust, and Pixie Dust"

J. M. Barrie, "Peter Pan"

Harold, a middle-aged African American man, came to my clinic for the first time. He was pleasant and soft-spoken. He wore a baseball style cap that commemorated his visit to the old city in Jerusalem. He was generally healthy but had a few common problems: hypertension, prostate disease, and occasional back pain. There were a few tests that were indicated, and he needed an adjustment in his blood pressure medication. I prescribed that and asked him to return several weeks later to recheck his blood pressure and to review his laboratory results. When Harold returned to clinic, his wife came with him. In contrast to her husband's easygoing manner, she was formal and unsmiling. She interrogated me and treated me as a hostile witness! Most of her questions had to do with why I was not ordering a whole series of other tests.

I patiently explained my thinking. She remained skeptical. At his next visit, she again questioned and challenged me at several points, although the interaction was not as tense. Over the years, she often came with Harold to the appointments. When he developed hoarseness that had not gone away after several weeks, I sent him for laryngoscopy, and we discovered a malignant tumor, which was treated successfully. That seemed to be a turning point in the relationship. She had come to believe that I was acting consistently in her husband's interest.

Physicians often differ from the populations they serve. About 90% of physicians come from families above the median income. Relatively few are members of racial/ethnic minorities. When there is a socioeconomic or cultural chasm between patients and providers, there can be other problems. For one, the relationship is unequal, and providers tend to assume a more authoritarian role in care.[29] When doctors do not speak the language or understand the culture or experience of the patient, they may make assumptions. They may not share decision-making to the same degree as they do with someone who is socioculturally similar to them. For another, as a corollary, patients who come from backgrounds that differ from those of their doctors are less trusting. Hence, when decisions need to be made, for example, about limiting care at the end of life, such patients are less likely to accede to suggestions about futility of care.[30] It takes a lot of work to reach across such a divide and build a trusting relationship.

In this case, there was a lack of trust initially because of the sociocultural distance between Harold and his wife and myself. There was a presumption, I think, that I might do less for a Black patient than a white patient. I had to earn their trust. That required patience, persistence, and demonstration of commitment to his well-being. It also called for empathic recognition that the concerns were grounded in the reality that many African Americans are less likely to receive critical tests and treatments than are white patients.[31]

Entitlement: "Some Animals Are More Equal Than Others"

George Orwell, *Animal Farm*

When my son Matthew was 11 years old, he went in for repair of a hernia in his groin. He was a little apprehensive. His parents (both physicians) worked hard not to manifest our own concerns about complications. On the appointed day, we trooped into the ambulatory surgery center of our health system. There were three or four people in line in front of us registering for their procedures. When we got to the front of the line, we presented the insurance card and had begun to answer the questions of the person at the desk, when she received a brief phone call. After she hung up, she told us to step aside. Someone else would be processed before us. A couple of minutes later, a man walked over from the elevator, accompanied by a member of the medical center staff. He was a famous actor. He was whisked in for his procedure. After that, we were allowed to return to the desk and continue registration.

Health care systems treat patients differently all the time. There may be an assumption that some people should receive special treatment, but it means that others get treatment that is less special. Sometimes, the consequences are trivial, other times, less so.

This was a little thing, but it was a disruption when we wanted to have things go smoothly for Matthew. Yet in American health care, some people expect preferential treatment, and they get it. In most medical centers, very important people get very special treatment. A patient of mine whose father was a donor to the medical center was admitted for a serious health problem. The hospital director checked in on him regularly. Even in routine situations, many of the affluent expect and receive better service than is reasonable for others to expect. The obverse is that someone else is getting deprioritized, and no one notices or cares. When Ronald Reagan was diagnosed as having colon cancer, he had surgery to remove the tumor the next day.[32] It would have been scandalous if he had had to wait weeks or months. Is it less so when that is the case for a poor person with the same disease?

The Help

We visited the home of Judy and Mark, who lived in an exclusive, gated community. My wife was about seven months pregnant with our first child. As it happens, Judy also was well along in what was her third pregnancy. My wife mentioned some minor symptoms that she had been having. Judy asked, "What did your OB say?"

"I haven't spoken to her about it. I don't have an appointment until next week."

"Don't you ever call her?"

"No, I haven't done that."

"Well, I have called my OB about 50 times during this pregnancy." (The pregnancy was uncomplicated.)

Clearly, Judy expected people to service her needs and felt no responsibility to limit her calls to her doctor to occasions when she could not work it out herself. Does any of this matter? I think that it does. For one thing, many people lack any ability to reach their doctor when they need to. Until recently, the Los Angeles County Health Services Department's clinics did not assign faculty physicians to be responsible for ongoing care of patients, even the ones with chronic diseases, and did not give them set appointment times. Instead, there were "cattle calls." Patients often would have to wait for hours to be seen, while missing work or paying someone else to care for a family member. As for being able to call the doctor when they had a truly urgent problem, forget it. Go to the emergency department, where patients, even those with serious problems, sometimes leave without being seen, after waiting a very long time.[33]

Entitlement is so ingrained in many affluent individuals that not a few now sign up for so-called concierge care. This system ensures enrollees immediate access to their physician for an annual fee, ranging from several hundred dollars to $10,000 or more a year. The physician, in turn, makes sure that the patients get what they want done expeditiously. This model is increasingly popular with wealthy patients and the physicians who cater to them. The extravagant use of medical resources in this way can affect what is available to others. The poor die quietly.

In some cases, those who possess resources will go even further. One physician I knew, who was a nice man, had an elderly parent who was admitted to the intensive care unit in late December. The situation was hopeless, but the family wanted to keep the parent alive until after midnight on December 31, because the tax laws were changing and it would be financially advantageous for them for the parent to die after the law changed. This is autonomy truly run amok!

The Scream: "People Living Deeply Have No Fear of Death"

Anaïs Nin, "People Living Deeply Have No Fear of Death"

Christine was in her late twenties when she came to see me. Her older sister had been diagnosed with breast cancer, and Christine wanted magnetic resonance imaging (an MRI) to determine whether she did as well. I suggested that we could do that if there were any ambiguity in a mammogram and ultrasound, but she would have none of that. Even though she did not have a genetic type associated with breast cancer (such as BRCA1), Christine was certain that someone with early breast cancer in the family should be eligible for an MRI. There was (at the time) no guideline suggesting that this was the appropriate diagnostic approach, but Christine browbeat me into doing it.[34]

Sometimes, it is not one's socioeconomic class that drives care as much as one's "informed" decision-making, mediated by intense, personal experiences. There are scads of tests that are often done without scientific evidence of their utility in particular situations. When a physician finds a rationale for ordering a test in a way that will be covered by insurance in order to mollify their patient, or perhaps to earn a fee for a procedure, it drives up the cost of medical care for everyone. It is harder to say no, especially in an era when it is easy for patients to share their dissatisfaction widely.

Passing Time

Irene first came to see me when she was in her mid-eighties. She lived with her daughter, Jane. Irene wasn't too worried about her health (which was generally pretty good), but Jane was totally preoccupied with her mother's well-being. She called me a lot about little things. She brought her mom in more often than was necessarily, seeking tests for this or that. At their visits, Irene was relaxed and smiling; Jane was all business with her list of issues that needed to be addressed. Jane did not have a job and did not seem to have any kind of a relationship, other than with her mother. Her mother was her whole world, and she used medical care for her mother as a tool for expressing her love and devotion. Now, that is not always a bad thing, but Irene did not need a lot of medical care. Exploratory conversations about Jane's life never revealed much. She always directed them back toward issues regarding her mother.

I am not sure what to make of this case. It felt to me as though Jane was not well connected to the rest of the world. For some, the doctor visit is a way of marking time and making contact in a situation in which the individual is unable to acknowledge that there aren't many other markers or contacts in their lives. If our society were one in which everyone was looking out for everyone else, someone might have engaged with her to broaden and enrich her range of life experiences.

None of this is to say that doctors shouldn't respond to social distress, health crises, psychological challenges, and even routine encounters with empathy and support. Far from it. At the same time, some of the need is driven not by biology but by circumstances.

How can we synthesize these clinical experiences? I think that they break down into a few categories:

1. First are the patients who are deeply dissatisfied with life, who look to the doctor for companionship that is not available elsewhere. This reflects a society rife with loneliness. In an earlier time, religion provided the solace for such individuals, a "heart of a heartless world,"[35] but it seems to be far less able to do so now.

2. There are some individuals who are mildly anxious and others who are panicked about existential problems (career failures, perceived disappointment of others, etc.), who come looking for medical diagnoses to explain their dis-ease or medical tests to calm them down. In these cases, the lack of an empathic community to whom they are connected, and who can soothe, reassure, or redirect them to other dimensions of life, seems to be part of the problem.

3. Some people have difficulty coping with serious health issues. Their maladies are not reflections of societal issues, but these individuals need connections with a doctor to help them come to terms with their situations. Some doctors are attuned to these issues and are pretty good at helping their patients, but others are not. We will consider this issue in chapter 4.

4. Next are the patients or families that want more treatment, even when it is futile, sometimes reflecting reluctance to understand the inevitable, sometimes because of bad advice from religious authorities, sometimes because of conflicts within families, but always oblivious to the impact this has on others: the frustration of the medical caregivers, the effect on the availability or cost of care for others, and even needless suffering of those who are dying.

5. There are the demanders: people who feel entitled or are convinced that more care is better—whether it is antibiotics, a feeding tube, an MRI, a cosmetic procedure, or the constant availability of a doctor to address every whim.

6. Some patients make requests without realizing their implications, and their doctors may go along without telling them about the trade-offs and consequences to other patients in the same boat.

7. Some patients demand more care because they have experienced discrimination in the past, and their sociocultural distance from the provider does not give them any confidence that it won't happen again.

8. A context affecting most of the instances that I have described, and many others that I have not, is the way in which health care is organized and delivered. Health care is treated as a commodity—a thing that is bought and sold—by many of the participants in the system, as discussed in the next several chapters. It is natural for patients (for whom care is not guaranteed) to regard it in that way: to see health care as a good of which they want their share, and even to see life as a commodity as well.

What would it take to better address these problems? In some cases, doctors can and should offer advice, perform tests, and suggest potential approaches when the presenting complaints appear to be connected to physical or mental illness. When such connections are less clear, they have an obligation at the very least to empathize with their patients, offer potential insights about the problems, and identify appropriate resources that might help. In many instances, however, a more cohesive society in which "every man is a part of the main"[36] and in which individuals recognize each other's anguish, and try to help address it, is what would make a big difference.

Notes

1. A. C. Kouzis and W. W. Eaton, "Absence of Social Networks, Social Support, and Health Services Utilization," Psychological Medicine 28, no. 6 (November 1998): 1301–10, https://doi.org/10.1017/s0033291798007454.

2. Kerstin Gerst-Emerson and Jayani Jayawardhana, "Loneliness as a Public Health Issue: The Impact of Loneliness on Health Care Utilization among Older Adults," *American Journal of Public Health* 105, no. 5 (May 2015): 1013–19, https://doi .org/10.2105/AJPH.2014.3024.27.

3. Hanyuying Wang et al., "Is Loneliness Associated with Increased Health and Social Care Utilisation in the Oldest Old? Findings from a Population-Based Longitudinal Study," *BMJ Open* 9, no. 6 (June 2019): e024645, https://doi.org/10.1136 /bmjopen-2018-024645.

4. Jonne van der Zwet, Marije S. Koelewijn-van Loon, and Marjan van den Akker, "Lonely Patients in General Practice: A Call for Revealing GP's Emotions? A Qualitative Study," *Family Practice* 26, no. 6 (December 2009): 501–9, https://doi.org /10.1093/fampra/cmp059.

5. "Percentage of Mental Health-Related Primary Care Office Visits, by Age Group—National Ambulatory Medical Care Survey, United States, 2010," *Morbidity and Mortality Weekly Report* 63, no. 47 (November 28, 2014): 1118, https://www.cdc .gov/mmwr/preview/mmwrhtml/mm6347a6.htm.

6. Arthur J. Barsky et al., "The Amplification of Somatic Symptoms," *Psychosomatic Medicine* 50, no. 5 (September–October 1988): 510–19, https://doi.org/10.1097 /00006842-198809000-00007.

7. Mark Nichter, "Idioms of Distress Revisited," *Culture, Medicine and Psychiatry* 34, no. 2 (June 2010): 401–16, https://doi.org/10.1007/s11013-010-9179-6; Roberto Lewis-Fernandez and Laurence J. Kirmayer, "Cultural Concepts of Distress and Psychiatric Disorders: Understanding Symptom Experience and Expression in Context," *Transcultural Psychiatry* 56, no. 4 (August 2019): 786–803, https://doi.org /10.1177/1363461519861795.

8. Mohit Khera, "Controversies in Testosterone Supplementation Therapy in Older Men," *Asian Journal of Andrology* 17, no. 2 (March–April 2015): 175–76, https://doi.org/10.4103/1008-682X.148728; Carol Cardona Attard and Stephen Fava, "Benefits and Risks of Testosterone Therapy," *Minerva Urologica e Nefrologica* 71, no. 3 (June 2019): 217–29, https://doi.org/10.23736/S0393-2249 .19.03301-0.

9. J. F. Hallis Dally, *Low Blood Pressure: Its Causes and Significance* (New York: William Wood, 1928), 66.

10. E. V. Allen, "Vasodilating Disturbances (Hypotension; Low Blood Pressure)," in *Internal Medicine: Its Theory and Practice*, 3rd ed., ed. John H. Musser (Philadelphia: Lea & Febiger, 1938), 519–21.

11. Samuel C. Robinson, "Hypotension: The Ideal Normal Blood Pressure," *New England Journal of Medicine* 233 (September 12, 1940): 407–16, https://doi.org/10.1056 /NEJM194009122231103.

12. Russel L. Cecil, ed., *A Textbook of Medicine*, 7th ed. (Philadelphia: Saunders, 1950), 458.

13. Jonathan C. Meakins, *The Practice of Medicine*, 5th ed. (St. Louis: Mosby, 1950), 458; Henry A. Christian, *The Principles and Practice of Medicine*, 16th ed. (New York: Appleton-Century, 1947), 1133.

14. Jonathan C. Meakins, *The Practice of Medicine*, 6th ed. (St. Louis: Mosby, 1956), 1017–18.

15. Clifton K. Meador, "The Art and Science of Nondisease," *New England Journal of Medicine* 272 (January 14, 1965): 92–95, https://doi.org/10.1056/NEJM196501142720208.

16. Joel Yager and Roy T. Young, "Non-Hypoglycemia Is an Epidemic Condition," *New England Journal of Medicine* 291, no. 17 (October 1974): 907–8, https://doi.org/10.1056/NEJM197410242911713; Donna E. Stewart, "Emotional Disorders Misdiagnosed as Physical Illness: Environmental Hypersensitivity, Candidiasis Hypersensitivity, and Chronic Fatigue Syndrome," *International Journal of Mental Health* 19, no. 3 (1990): 56–68, https://doi.org/10.1080/00207411.1990.11449173.

17. William E. Dismukes et al., "A Randomized Double-Blind Trial of Nystatin Therapy for the Candidiasis Hypersensitivity Syndrome," *New England Journal of Medicine* 323 (December 20, 1990): 1717–23, https://doi.org/10.1056/NEJM199012203232501.

18. Yager and Young, "Non-Hypoglycemia."

19. John A. Cotterill, "Dermatologic Non-Disease," *Dermatologic Clinics* 14, no. 3 (July 1996): 439–46, https://doi.org/10.1016/s0733-8635(05)70371-5; Susan M. Love, Rebecca S. Gelman, and William Silen, "Fibrocystic Disease of the Breast—A Nondisease?," *New England Journal of Medicine* 307 (October 14, 1982): 1010–14, https://doi.org/10.1056/NEJM198210143071611.

20. Richard Smith, "In Search of 'Non-Disease,'" *BMJ* 324, no. 7342 (April 13, 2002): 883–85, https://doi.org/10.1136/bmj.324.7342.883.

21. Ivan Illich, *Limits to Medicine: Medical Nemesis—The Expropriation of Health* (London: Marion Boyar, 1975), 3.

22. Peter Conrad, Thomas Mackie, and Ateev Mehrotra, "Estimating the Costs of Medicalization," *Social Science and Medicine* 70, no. 12 (June 2010): 1943–47, https://doi.org/10.1016/j.socscimed.2010.02.019.

23. Carl Llor and Lars Bjerrum, "Antimicrobial Resistance: Risk Associated with Antibiotic Overuse and Initiatives to Reduce the Problem," *Therapeutic Advances in Drug Safety* 5, no. 6 (December 2014): 229–41, https://doi.org/10.1177/2042098614554919.

24. Than N Huynh et al., "The Frequency and Cost of Treatment Perceived to Be Futile in Critical Care," *JAMA Internal Medicine* 173, no. 20 (November 11, 2013): 1887–94, https://doi.org/10.1001/jamainternmed.2013.10261.

25. Daniel Fischberg et al., "Five Things Physicians and Patients Should Question in Hospice and Palliative Medicine," *Journal of Pain and Symptom Management* 45, no. 3 (March 2013): 595–605, https://doi.org/10.1016/j.jpainsymman.2012.12.002.

26. Somaye Rostami et al., "Perception of Futile Care and Caring Behaviors of Nurses in Intensive Care Units," *Nursing Ethics* 26, no. 1 (February 2019): 248–55, https://doi.org/10.1177/0969733017703694.

27. Eliot L. Freidson, *Profession of Medicine: A Study of the Sociology of Applied Knowledge* (New York: Dodd Mead, 1973), 345. For more recent perspectives on the

evolving relationship of physician and patient in the area of autonomy of decision-making, see, e.g., Ezekiel J. Emanuel and Linda L. Emanuel, "Four Models of the Physician-Patient Relationship," JAMA 267, no. 16 (April 22/29, 1992): 2221–26.

28. Adapted from Martin F. Shapiro, "Considering the Common Good: The View from Seven Miles Up," New England Journal of Medicine 374, no. 21 (May 26, 2016): 2006–7, https://doi.org/10.1056/NEJMp1601144. Copyright © 2016 Massachusetts Medical Society. Reprinted with permission.

29. Thomas S. Szasz and Marc N. Hollander, "A Contribution to the Philosophy of Medicine: The Basic Models of the Doctor-Patient Relationship," Archives of Internal Medicine 97, no. 5 (May 1956): 585–92, https://doi.org/10.1001/archinte.1956 .00250230079008.

30. L. Ebony Boulware et al., "Race and Trust in the Health Care System," Public Health Reports 118, no. 4 (July–August 2003): 358–65, https://doi.org/10.1093/phr/118 .4.358; Laura B. Shepardson et al., "Racial Variation in the Use of Do-Not-Resuscitate Orders," Journal of General Internal Medicine 14, no. 1 (January 1999): 15–20, https:// doi.org/10.1046/j.1525-1497.1999.00275.x; Carole A. Winston et al., "Overcoming Barriers to Access and Utilization of Hospice and Palliative Care Services in African-American Communities," Omega—Journal of Death and Dying 50, no. 2 (March 1, 2005): 151–63, https://doi.org/10.2190/QQKG-EPFA-A2FN-GHVL.

31. "Executive Summary," in Institute of Medicine Committee on Understanding and Eliminating Racial and Ethnic Disparities in Health Care, Unequal Treatment: Confronting Racial and Ethnic Disparities in Health Care, ed. Brian D. Smedley, Adrienne Y. Stith, and Alan R. Nelson (Washington, DC: National Academies Press, 2003), https://www.ncbi.nlm.nih.gov/books/NBK220355/.

32. Robert H. Sorensen et al., "President Reagan's Lifesaving Colectomy and Subsequent Historical Implications," Military Medicine 179, no. 7 (July 2014): 704–7, https://doi.org/10.7205/MILMED-D-14-00034.

33. David W. Baker, Carl D. Stevens, and Robert H. Brook, "Patients Who Leave a Public Hospital Emergency Department without Being Seen by a Physician: Causes and Consequences," JAMA 266, no. 8 (August 28, 1991): 1085–90, https://doi.org/10 .1001/jama.1991.03470080055029.

34. Debra L. Monticciolo et al., "Breast Cancer Screening in Women at Higher-Than-Average Risk: Recommendations from the ACR," Journal of the American College of Radiology 15, no. 3 (March 2018): 408–14, https://doi.org/10.1016/j.jacr.2017 .11.034; Albert L. Siu and US Preventive Services Task Force, "Screening for Breast Cancer: U.S. Preventive Services Task Force Recommendation Statement," Annals of Internal Medicine 164, no. 4 (February 16, 2016): 279–96, https://doi.org/10.7326/M15 -2886.

35. Karl Marx, "Toward the Critique of Hegel's Philosophy of Law: Introduction," in Writings of the Young Marx on Philosophy and Society, ed. and trans. Lloyd D. Easton and Kurt H. Guddat (Garden City, NY: Anchor Books, 1967), 250.

36. John Donne, "No Man Is an Island."

| Dialogue #2 |

The professor is reading a copy of report that was given to her by the student.

Student: What do you think?

Professor: We have some good material here. Clearly, some utilization is driven by the patients for a variety of reasons. We need to make sure that we don't paint a picture that blames the patients for all the problems.

Student: Before we started, I said that I was worried about that. I do agree now that some patients make demands that contribute to overuse and costs, but there are many other factors. Also, it looks like there are lots of things going on in their lives that motivate their behavior. I am having trouble seeing how we fix these kinds of problems. And we really need to make sure that we don't convey the impression that all the problems with the system are attributable to an insatiable appetite for medical care. If we don't make it clear what the real problems are, the patients will get the blame.

Professor: I agree. We have shown that patient-driven overuse is a contributing factor. What would you suggest that we examine next?

Student: I know that you don't want to jump to the insurance industry. How about physicians and their role? It sure seems that many of them are complicit in increasing costs and demand.

Professor: Good. Think about how paying for each medical act, and how much gets charged for each act, affects both what doctors do and the overall costs of the system.

Student: I'm no economist, but wouldn't a universal health insurance program be able to address that by regulating doctors' fees and cutting costs?

Professor: Perhaps, but we should see what we can learn about physicians and how the payment system affects their behavior. We also should try to understand how we got to this point, why it isn't changing, and whether things are different in other countries.

Student: Is this going to be a takedown of doctors? The problem is the system!

Professor: We'll get to "the system," as you call it. Let's see what we can learn about physicians.

Student: All right, but I'm concerned that this will end up being an exercise in blaming the doctors and more of a distraction than a useful insight. The problem is the system!

3

Doctors and Dollars

Antecedents, Actions, and Consequences

No physician, insofar as he is a physician, considers his own good in what he prescribes, but the good of his patient.
—Plato, *The Republic*, Book I

My friend Henry was a busy internist who practiced in an affluent area. He was extremely bright and seemed to have good values. We got together from time to time over dinner to talk about life, love, and politics. On one such occasion, he commented that he sometimes felt bad about ordering pulmonary function (breathing) tests on asymptomatic nonsmokers (people without breathing difficulties), "but I have to pay the rent." I was shocked to hear that, not that I didn't know that such things went on, but rather because I thought that Henry would be immune to such crass and unethical use of his position as a doctor to extract as much money as he could from an encounter.

In exploring the implications of such decisions, let's consider the following questions: How much should doctors be paid? How should their remuneration be calculated? To this end, how should different kinds of clinical activity be valued? How does pay compare across specialties in the United States? How does physician pay, and pay across specialties, compare to that in other countries? What effect does this have on the health care system as a whole and on the relationships between doctors and patients?

Praecipuus Pecuniam: The Centrality of Money

A brief survey of the history of physician compensation puts in perspective the trends over the last several decades and the behavior that we see today. For thousands of years, physicians have received income from their professional work. The Code of Hammurabi (which dates to about 1754 BC) specified that a physician in ancient Babylon should be paid more for the care of someone of higher social status. The ancient Greeks disagreed as to whether medicine was a liberal art (the perspective of Aristotle and Socrates) or a craft (the view of Sophocles). If the latter, they should be paid. If the former, it was more in the category of philosophy and poetry, and fees should not be collected. Some of the physicians who took the side of the art, such as Hippocrates and Galen, came from wealthy families, so there was less of a pressing need to ask for money. Galen's nuanced position on this matter was that he would never ask for payment but would accept it if offered.[1]

Over the ensuing millennia, doctors generally have been well compensated. Today, few physicians look upon their work as a liberal art to be done for the love of humanity alone, but more as a craft for which they expect to be well paid. Perhaps that is why so many (including me) lament the inattention to the art of medicine in favor of the technological interventions and compensation. Literature is rife with discussions of this matter.

As early as the thirteenth century, Chaucer describes the physician in the preface to the *Canterbury Tales* as having "a special love for gold."[2] In medieval Europe, some cities, such as Venice, hired physicians to care for the poor who could not afford the fees that other doctors charged. In Boston, a "fee bill" was developed by the local medical society in 1780, setting minimum fees that could not be undercut; the prices on this list subsequently inflated more rapidly than the cost of living. Prices charged by physicians often varied, according to what the members of a community could afford. Distinguished physicians like William Osler (who helped create the foundation for the specialty of internal medicine and introduced it to North America; who practiced at McGill University in

Montreal, University of Pennsylvania in Philadelphia, Johns Hopkins University in Baltimore, then at Oxford University in England; and after whom my elementary school in Winnipeg was named) charged fees to those who could afford them but provided free care to the poor.[3]

The Social Standing and Income of the Physician

Early in the twentieth century, the American physician was firmly in the upper middle class. Physicians did not become extremely rich, but neither were they likely to fall into poverty. Prior to the Great Depression, even graduates of elite medical schools did not typically belong to the economic elite. A 1937 survey of Harvard Medical School graduates from 1907, 1917, and 1927 found that doctors 10 to 30 years after graduation (presumably well-established by then) were earning on average $5,000 to $10,000 (somewhat more than the average US physician at that time, but not remarkably so).[4] Several graduates from 1927 were earning less than $2,500 per year, and only five from all years were earning more than $20,000. As one participant in the Harvard survey commented, "I am satisfied with medicine as a life's work. However, I should recommend it only for the man who has plenty of money back of him. Many men never make much in medicine." In commenting on this in the 1970s, Lewis Thomas noted that the evolution of the specialties led to more scatter of incomes in medicine.[5]

After 1929, physicians' position relative to other groups began to change. The net income after office costs and other expenses in the United States increased by about 125% from 1929 to 1949, compared to 46% for lawyers and 67% for dentists, whose incomes had been comparable to those of physicians in 1929. That trend continued. Physician incomes increased by an average of 8.3% per year from 1939 to 1975, compared to 5.9% for other professional fields. Specialist physicians in non-salaried practices always had earned more than generalists, but the differences up to 1949 were not that great. As late as 1949, when the mean income of non-salaried physicians in the US was $11,744 (equivalent to $127,422 in 2020), only 12.6% were earning $20,000 or more ($215,453 in 2020). Accordingly, income in a specialty such as cardiology (mean income $15,589) was only about 23% higher than that of internists ($12,637) in non-salaried practice.[6]

The lack of scatter of physician incomes in the first half of the twentieth century, compared to the situation today, is eye-opening, as discussed later in this chapter. True enough, some chose to work among the poor, others among the rich, and there were consequences of those choices, but the differences in earnings were not generally extreme. Today, that salary differential in the United States is substantial and is greater than in other countries.[7]

The differential between physicians and other full-time workers in the United States also began to increase. That ratio was 4.03 in 1951, 4.98 in 1965, and 5.39 in 1975.[8]

Physician incomes are higher in the United States than in Canada, France, Germany, and the United Kingdom. According to a 2009 report by the Organisation for Economic Co-operation and Development (OECD) on physician incomes in member countries, specialists earn more than generalists in almost all of those. The ratio of physician incomes to per capita gross domestic product in the US (5.7 for specialists and 4.1 for generalists) was among the very highest.[9]

In the context of exciting developments in care, there has been substantial augmentation not only of the incomes of physicians relative to the rest of society, but also of the incomes of physicians in particular specialty areas relative to other medical fields. Physicians who engage in "cognitive" services (talking to patients, examining them, and writing prescriptions) earn less than those who do procedures (surgeons, gastroenterologists, cardiologists, anesthesiologists, radiologists, and dermatologists). Why has this occurred? There was nothing in the writing of the ancients that hinted at distinctions in compensation between generalists and doctors who did procedures. In those days, almost all physicians were generalists. Nor, until recently, did anyone talk about "cognitive services." The primary work of almost all doctors was to examine, diagnose, and prescribe treatments for patients whom they knew over time.

The Growth of Specialization

In the 1860s, American medicine began to become more specialized, particularly in cities, although an ophthalmologist who advertised his area of specialization was censured by his state medical association in 1865 for this transgression. As late as 1925, an ophthalmologist was initially excluded from the American Ophthalmological Society for allowing the term "oculist" to be used after his name.[10] With the introduction of antisepsis and anesthesia, as well as accelerating developments in diagnostic technologies and therapeutics, many more specialties began to emerge in the first half of the twentieth century, and even further subspecialization developed after that.

An indicator of the growth of specialization in medicine was the founding of the American Board of Medical Specialties in 1933. Its mission is to set "professional standards for medical specialty practice and certification" in partnership with the certifying member boards in the specialties. Four specialties joined in 1933 (dermatology, obstetrics and gynecology, ophthalmology, and otolaryngology). By 1937, eight more had become part of the organization (orthopedic surgery, pediatrics, psychiatry and neurology, radiology, urology, internal medicine, pathology, and surgery). Since then, another twelve specialties have joined: four surgical fields (neurosurgery, colon and rectal, plastics, and thoracic), anesthesiology, allergy and immunology, physical medicine and rehabilitation, medical genetics and genomics, nuclear medicine, emergency medicine, preventive medicine, and family medicine.[11]

The specialty examination in internal medicine was instituted in 1936. Five years later, the American Board of Internal Medicine introduced subspecialty certifications in three fields: cardiovascular disease, gastroenterology, and pulmonary disease. There was then a long gap before they added five more subspecialty certifications in 1972 (endocrinology, diabetes and metabolism, hematology, infectious disease, nephrology, and rheumatology). Twelve more have been added since then.[12]

While there were some differences in what physicians earned in the different specialty fields, the differences were not as substantial as they later became. In the United States, a key development was the enactment of Medicare in 1965 and the implementation of its fee schedule. The health care system offers mighty temptations. We have come a great distance from the era when a physician could sit, hold the patient's hand, and offer occasional remedies but mostly comfort. Now the treatments are more effective, and there are lots of procedures that can be done.

What is salient here is that the physician has conflicts of interest. *The system of paying for medical care rewards the physician for doing procedures* much more than for talking to patients and their families, comforting them, or even making difficult diagnoses or judgments about therapy. Beyond that, physicians can derive additional income by marketing drugs or devices to their patients at a profit, or with financial incentives from manufacturers.[13]

Medicare Fees and Their Consequences

Starting in the late 1960s, Medicare based payment on "usual, customary and reasonable" charges for medical procedures, which varied by region and community. In 1991, as I discuss below, a fee schedule was established for every procedure, subject to periodic updates. Even before the fee schedule was implemented, disparities in pay across the specialties began to grow. Part of the problem was that there were limited changes in fees over time for existing clinical acts. For cognitive doctors, there was only one set of procedure codes relevant to their work: those for evaluation and management (taking a history, doing a physical examination, and prescribing medications).

In contrast, almost every technical procedure evolved or changed dramatically over time. When a new technology (like magnetic resonance imaging, MRI) or a new technique (like transesophageal echocardiography) was introduced, a new fee had to be negotiated, and it was often substantially greater than the fee for the procedure that it replaced (such as chest x-ray or transthoracic echocardiography). Specialties have been able to make the case that the new procedures are difficult or time-consuming and should be paid for at higher rates than the older procedures. Thus the fee for performing and reading a computed tomography (CT) scan of the chest was about $325 in 2020, while that for a chest x-ray was about $70.[14] This has led to mother lodes of revenue in some specialties, with several consequences.

First, the physicians in those fields have an enormous incentive to spend their time doing procedures, not examining, counseling, and managing patients. One commonly sees the physician who does a procedure only at the time of the procedure.

Second, the pressure to do procedures generates other costs, including paying staff for the procedures, maintaining the equipment, processing specimens (such as biopsies during a colonoscopy, which then lead to pathologists' fees and lab fees), and so on. When procedures need to be performed in hospitals, that increases costs substantially.

Third, specialties often push the envelope of indications for procedures, of doing more procedures or more complex versions of procedures, and of doing them more often. This also drives up costs. (Thus Medicare reimbursement for a series of plain abdominal x-rays is about $93, whereas reimbursement for CT of the abdomen without injection of contrast material is about $130, with contrast material $256, both with and without contrast $288, and CT with and without with angiography $401.) Reimbursement for these procedures is far higher from commercial insurance.[15] It is hard for a clinician who will be paid for the test to be indifferent to the choice of one of these procedures.

The fundamental issue with physician pay is not the amount, but rather the structure of the incentive and its consequences. Physician incomes are only about 20% of the cost of health care. The problem is that they make more money when they do more procedures, and the procedures generate substantial additional expenses other than the actual income accruing to the physician. Thus one could imagine that if physicians' only incentive was to work more hours and get paid by the hour, they would cease to feel compelled to generate additional expenses, well beyond their salaries, for the health care system. Arguably, paying specialists as much for consultations that do not lead to additional procedures (and their attendant costs) as we do for performing the procedures could save money overall.

Meanwhile, health care costs have risen relentlessly to crisis levels, from about $146 per person in the United States in 1960 to $11,582 in 2019.[16] Where is this money spent? According to the Center for Medicare and Medicaid Services, 31% of expenditures go to hospitals. Of the remainder, physician and clinical services accounted for 20%, retail prescription drugs 10%, dental care 4%, home care 3%, nursing homes 5%, durable equipment 2%, other medical products 2%, other professionals 3%, and other health, residential, personal health services 5%.[17]

Arguably, the 20% or so of medical expenditures that go to physicians could be diminished by a quarter and they still would be able to live comfortably, but that would only amount to 5% of all expenses. Much more consequential is the effect of having so many doctors with an incentive to do more and more procedures that are associated with costs other than physician fees. There often are facility fees as well. If the procedure is an operation, then other physicians and treatments come into play, including anesthesiology and the medication used, the cost of an operating room, the charge for processing laboratory tests and pathology specimens, and the other things that may get done to the patient on the basis of the results of the procedures (such as more tests and procedures, management of complications, and so on). In many instances, the physician fee is as little as one-tenth of the total cost of the procedure. Interventions that lower those fees might cause clinicians to compensate by increasing the numbers of procedures they do. The result would be an increase in the cost of care.[18]

Colonoscopies and Their Periodicity

Guidelines exist for use of procedures, but specialty societies (and the specialists themselves) tend to push in a direction consistent with their economic interests. As one example, colon cancer screening is now widely accepted as having some utility. If you find a lesion early, there is a better chance of cure. A randomized trial did show improved outcomes with a combination of testing the stool for blood and performing a sigmoidoscopy. There have been no randomized trials of colonoscopy, the most expensive procedure, but that is what is generally done now because of indirect evidence from case-control studies and observational studies (neither of which is the gold standard for evidence). The guidelines of the US Preventive Services Task Force and the American Cancer Society advocate some form of periodic testing after the age of 45 in persons of average risk. The Affordable Care Act specified that patients should be offered a choice between stool testing or structural (visual) examination with sigmoidoscopy, colonoscopy, or CT colonography. (If any other test is positive, a colonoscopy should be done.)[19]

Notwithstanding the lack of definitive answers and the availability of other effective forms of testing that can be substantially less expensive, colonoscopy has become the norm. A typical recommendation is colonoscopy every 10 years after the age of 45, stopping at age 85. When the procedure is performed, gastroenterologists often do biopsies, however benign any lesions appear to be. That is a source of additional revenue. The patient is told to come back sooner if there are certain kinds of polyps seen.

A brief digression into my own colonoscopy history is illuminating. I have had this procedure done at regular intervals. In my family, two of my father's sisters and the son of one of them had colon cancer. Notably, two of them had histories of inflammatory bowel disease, which greatly increases the risk of cancer. When I had a colonoscopy done in Los Angeles after I turned 50 (the recommended age to start screening at that time), guidelines suggested that if a first-degree relative (parent, sibling, or child) has had cancer, one might benefit from more frequent procedures or starting at an earlier age (for example, 10 years before the age at which your parent or sibling was diagnosed). My doctor said that with two second-degree relatives, I might want to have a repeat procedure in 7 years. When I moved to New York, the doctor there who elicited my family history asked if I was having colonoscopies every 3 years, given that history! (I was not.)

Was my doctor's question a reflection of her economic interest? No, she was a primary care physician who refers for the procedure. What it speaks to is that in the pervasive culture in medicine, it is considered acceptable to have a low threshold for performing billable tests, and in effect to "run the till." In contradistinction to the notion of evidence-based medicine, many decisions get made on the basis of what is often referred to as the "standard of care" (what "everybody" does). This approach to decision-making is evident in the patterns of care of many practitioners, including those who do not necessarily benefit financially.

The distortion of pay for procedures acts as an enormous incentive to do more of them. Specialists, whose work schedules differ by no more than a few hours per week, if at all, from those of generalists, can earn two or three times as much. Still, it is not just the highly paid specialists who are focused upon cash collections. Even in the cognitive fields, doctors often do what they can to maximize billing. For example, there are five levels of charges possible for an initial evaluation and management visit and five for a follow-up visit. There are guidelines as to what needs to be done and documented for each such charge level. "Upcoding" (charging more for a service by billing at a higher level than is justified) is becoming more commonplace. In cases where doctors need to spend a lot of time—for example, managing multiple health and social problems, or carefully assessing a patient with subtle neurological abnormalities, or arranging for appropriate support services—these higher codes are entirely justifiable. In other situations, such as when a specialist spends five minutes examining an ear or a rash, they are not. From 2001 to 2010, the proportion of evaluation and management follow-up visits coded at levels 4 and 5 (the highest levels) increased from about 24% to 41% and the percentage of level 5 follow-up hospital visits increased from 32% to 48%, while those of lower complexity and reimbursement declined. Similarly, for emergency department visits, the proportion of visits coded at level 5 increased from 27% to 48%.[20]

Running the Till

There are other ways that physicians, whose work is mostly evaluation and management, can maximize revenue. One is to add certain procedures to routine visits, whether they are indicated or not. My friend Henry, who ordered the unnecessary breathing tests "to pay the rent," was an example of someone who did this with some regularity. As I said above, I was shocked at his revelation but should not have been. In the fee-for-service system, this temptation is there for everyone, and there is no reprobation for such inappropriate and unethical behavior.

He was doing in a small way what proceduralist physicians do all day, every day. Doctors can earn more money doing a procedure that might take 30 minutes than they would providing monthly care for an individual for a year or even more. The fee schedule is structured to reward procedures. Thus the threshold for doing them is lower for many—but by no means all—physicians than it should be, to the point that, for many specialists, consulting them means getting the procedure done.

Get On with the Test

When I was in training, there was a joke among the residents about some of the cardiologists, that they only had two indications for getting a heart catheterization: "lub" and "dub." Traditionally, these are the two heart sounds that we can always hear when we listen to the chest! The incentive structure may cause some physicians, who make most of their money doing procedures, to evaluate a patient far less carefully than they should.

Art Schwabe, a wonderful doctor, was chief of the division of gastroenterology at the University of California, Los Angeles (UCLA). A relative of mine came to town with a complicated problem in his area and needed a consultation. After they met, my relative commented on how thorough he was, how carefully Dr. Schwabe had reviewed his history, and how much time he had taken to carefully explain his interpretation of the symptoms and options for treatment. Afterward, I let Art know how exemplary we felt that his consultation had been. He lamented to me about the relative rarity of that kind of clinical care in gastroenterology.

"Years ago," he said, "it was normal for the gastroenterologist to spend an hour or more with a new patient, then a lot of additional time reviewing the [x-ray] films. Nowadays, many of the docs just spend a few minutes with the patient, then order the procedure."

Repeat Testing

Medical care costs can escalate surreptitiously. Sometimes, a doctor orders an x-ray and the radiologist reads it carefully, suggesting that the patient have another test to confirm or rule out a condition. For example, a patient in the hospital with pneumonia may get a CT scan or an MRI even though the diagnosis was clear from the much less expensive x-ray. The test may be repeated even though the patient is improving, and the abnormalities seen on the initial test are unlikely to resolve in less than five to six weeks. The initiative for additional tests may come from the treating physician or the radiologist, but both should know better. In most patients, those additional studies are extremely unlikely to affect management. Inpatient doctors often order standing "daily labs" and repeated imaging studies that do not affect management but do add greatly to the cost of care.

Residents and students may order such unneeded or redundant studies to avoid any possible criticism by their superiors for failing to do so (sometimes referred to as CYA, for cover your assets, so to speak). When I was in training in Montreal, the professors often would challenge us as to why we had ordered a particular test. When I moved to Los Angeles and became a faculty member at UCLA, I emulated that practice. I learned that doing so was not at all part of the culture there.

Archie Cochrane, a visionary clinical epidemiologist, wrote, "before ordering a test decide what you will do if it is (a) positive, or (b) negative, and if both answers are the same don't do the test."[21] It would help if there were systems in place to encourage more practitioners to pay attention to that wise rule.

Add-Ons

Even when a procedure is indicated, the physician may add bells and whistles that increase the cost and complexity of care. One of these add-ons is the participation of an anesthesiologist in a colonoscopy to administer conscious sedation—basically being put under anesthesia but not to the level at which the patient would need a tube down their throat so that a machine could breathe for them. It has become the norm in the United States for colonoscopy to be performed with conscious sedation. Afterward, people are drowsy, and they need to have someone available to make sure they get home safely. In many other countries, conscious sedation is rarely done for colonoscopy. My most recent experience with the procedure is instructive as to how entrenched the use of a discretionary add-on procedure can become.

"Perchance to Dream": My Colonoscopy, Again

Several years before I moved to New York, when I had a colonoscopy, I was given a form consenting to the use of conscious sedation. I asked Dennis, the gastroenterologist who was to perform the procedure, if I could receive no medicine and stay awake throughout. He agreed. He told me that when he had his own colonoscopy, he had it without sedation and had done fine. He said that he was supposed to chair a meeting after the procedure, so he wanted to be awake, alert, and able to do that. He noted that one problem with his being awake during colonoscopy was that, given his expertise, he could not help but guide the device with his hand through his own abdominal wall during the procedure! When I had mine, I kept my hands at my sides. I endured it with minimal discomfort and went back to work.

When it was time to schedule my next colonoscopy in New York, I told them that I did not want anesthesia. On the day of the procedure, I reminded the staff of my preference. They put me in a room, and the doctor came in. He asked if I really did not want anesthesia, and I affirmed. A few minutes later, the anesthesiologist came around. I told her that I would not be having anesthesia. She asked if I was sure. I said that I was. She asked me if I wanted her to be in the room for the procedure, just in case I changed my mind. I said that I did not.

I tolerated the procedure well. Afterward, I asked the nurse how often they had done the procedure without an anesthesiologist. She told me that in the several months that this particular large and busy practice location had been open, only one patient had declined anesthesia. I told two physician colleagues about these experiences, and when they asked to have their colonoscopies done without anesthesia, they were not given that option. One was told by the gastroenterologist (without evidence) that he might be more likely to miss a lesion in those circumstances.

Colonoscopy can detect colon cancer before it spreads. The cost of the procedure and the inconvenience and disruption to the patient are substantially greater when conscious sedation is administered and when an anesthesiologist is involved. I am not an individual who is renowned for remarkable pain tolerance. If the default was no anesthesia unless necessary, it would be used less. At the very least, patients should be offered the option to proceed without anesthesia. It may be even more difficult for women, who tend to express preferences to decline such care less forcefully. Both men and women without medical backgrounds ought to be informed that proceeding without sedation is an acceptable option.

Some doctors and clinics are open to performing colonoscopies without anesthesia. Of note, Jaime Zighelboim of the Mayo Clinic, Eau Claire, Wisconsin, reports that although most patients prefer anesthesia, "almost everyone who requests to do this without sedation is very pleased and will do it again without the sedation the next time they need to do it."[22] Indeed, in many countries, it is the normal approach to do colonoscopy without sedation.[23] In the United States, it is not, and it is the kind of thing that contributes to the high cost of medical care.

Likewise, patients should know how much the procedure costs before they get the bill. As I discussed previously, the cost of specialty care extends well beyond the professional fee of the specialist who is doing the procedure. For example, Medicare (which pays less than private insurance) paid for almost 2 million colonoscopies in fee-for-service Medicare patients in 2015. The physicians performing them received about $417 million for the procedures, approximately $212 for each one on average. Some colonoscopies cost more because additional things were done at the time of the procedure, such as removing a lesion. But the total cost was $1.874 billion, or about $950 per colonoscopy, or four and a half times the colonoscopist's fee. The other costs included anesthesiology and sedation (which averaged $84), pathology ($75), and "facility charges" (the fee charged by the place where the procedure was done, $470). These numbers do not include the fee for an anesthesiologist, if one was involved, as is now usually the case, which can add several hundred dollars to the total cost.[24]

The facility costs are clearly a substantial item. The nonprofessional fee costs often differ dramatically, depending on whether the procedure is done in a hospital outpatient department or in an ambulatory surgery center. In 2018, Medicare paid $380 to an ambulatory surgery center as a facility fee for colonoscopy, compared to $749 to a hospital outpatient department. For arthroscopy of the knee with repair of a meniscus, the respective facility fees were $1,024 and $2,116. Clinical groups and organizations have a clear incentive to do procedures in the facilities that generate the higher fees.[25] Health systems have a substantial incentive to move their procedures into hospital clinics to accrue that additional revenue.

The issue of unneeded anesthesia/sedation is not limited to colonoscopy. Getting clinicians not to do things that you don't want done can be more difficult than pulling teeth.

When my son Daniel was having his wisdom teeth removed, I discussed with him the option of not having sedation/anesthesia. I told him that the area would be frozen. He seemed satisfied with that, and we informed the dentist's office ahead of time. When we showed up for the procedure, the staff presented me with the bill, which included the cost of anesthesia and the services of an anesthesiologist. I told them that my son did not need those components. We proceeded to the waiting room, where an anesthesiologist was sitting. I told him that my son would not be needing his care. The dentist came out and queried me again about it.

I reiterated our plan. A few minutes after my son went to the procedure room, the dentist came out and said, "your son really wants to be asleep for the procedure."

I had no choice but to accede to this. I had no doubt that he talked my son into it, and that he and the anesthesiologist benefited financially from this approach. This might seem like a minor issue, but the crazy cost of medical care in the United States is built upon a latticework of components that are not essential to health.

Guidelines to Reduce Waste?

There now is considerable literature to suggest that much of medical care does not improve health, regardless of the cost. One national study of several medical procedures found substantial variation in the use of such procedures as upper gastrointestinal endoscopy, and review of medical records of patients who had had these procedures showed that a nontrivial minority (17% for endoscopy, 32% for carotid endarterectomy) were inappropriate, according to the judgments of expert consensus panels.[26]

As the recognition has grown that we do too much of everything in medicine, one strategy that has emerged for addressing this issue is the promulgation of guidelines. By their nature, guidelines are suggestions. It was presumed that physicians would want to incorporate this information into their practices. While guidelines for selected conditions had been around for a while, initially there was considerable new momentum for them in the 1970s and 1980s in the United States. Many of these were produced by "experts" in a consensus development program of the National Institutes of Health (NIH). Various specialty societies began to produce their own guidelines. The American College of Physicians (mostly an organization of general internists) developed a Clinical Efficacy Assessment Project in the 1980s. Since then, it has blossomed into an ongoing program of production of clinical practice guidelines and "guidance statements."[27]

The federal Agency for Healthcare Research and Quality (AHRQ) and its predecessors participated in creating a National Guidelines Clearinghouse in 1990.[28] The US Preventive Services Task Force, created in 1984, focused upon recommendations that weighed the evidence for various preventive services.[29] The movement for guidelines was driven in part by the rising cost of care and by recognition that there were issues of quality of care that were not addressed sufficiently by assessment of the credentials of practitioners. It was influenced by emerging efforts to make medical practice more "evidence-based" through "the conscientious, explicit, and judicious use of current best evidence in making decisions about the care of individual patients."[30]

Inevitably, there has been pushback against guidelines development, and it has not always been genteel. Gynecologists, who were in the habit of performing Pap smears on women's cervixes annually, or even more often, to screen for cancer, were unhappy about guidelines that suggested not doing the test more than once every three years, if there had been two consecutive normal tests. A firestorm erupted when a guideline from the US Preventive Services Task Force recommended not doing mammograms in normal-risk women under the age of 50, and to stop doing the test in old women.[31]

Guidelines can be helpful in standardizing practice. The committees that produce many guidelines are not without conflicts of interest, however. For example, the American Society for Gastrointestinal Endoscopy produces guidelines for use of the procedures that represent the major source of income for many of the members of the organization.[32] Their guidelines disclose committee members' conflicts of interest associated with ownership participation in corporations relevant to the guidelines, but not conflicts of interest relevant to their own practice revenue. Other specialties' guidelines are enmeshed in similar conflicts of interest.[33]

Conflicts of interest pertaining to ownership participation in or other financial relationships with corporations that produce drugs or medical devices often do involve clinicians. There is additional concern about practice guidelines from specialty societies regarding drug therapies. A Danish study found that among 45 such guidelines that they studied, 43 committees had one or more members who were paid by drug manufacturers either as a consultant, researcher, equity holder, or speaker—a clear conflict of interest. In only two of the cases was the conflict disclosed.[34]

Choosing Wisely or Calculatedly?

In an attempt to calm the rhetoric, in 2012 the American Board of Internal Medicine Foundation launched the Choosing Wisely Campaign, which "seeks to advance a national dialogue on avoiding unnecessary medical tests, treatments and procedures."[35] As of February 2020, 77 specialty societies in the United States were participating in this initiative. All told, the program has generated recommendations in their fields (more than 550 to date) about clinical acts that should be avoid because they are not evidence based, are duplicative, are not free from harm, or are not truly necessary. This is a well-intentioned campaign, and some good comes of it. What is interesting, but not surprising, is that many of the specialty societies' recommendations do not threaten their revenue flow. When specialty societies were asked to identify procedures that were unnecessary or of "low value," they rarely recommended changes in patterns of use of their procedures.

In the case of the American Academy of Orthopedic Surgeons, none of their five recommendations call for avoiding surgery in situations in which it may not be beneficial. Instead, they talk about avoiding the use of splints of the wrist after carpal tunnel surgery; avoiding lateral wedge insoles to treat patients with symptomatic medial compartment osteoarthritis of the knee; avoiding glucosamine, chondroitin, and needle lavage of the knee in osteoarthritis; and avoiding postoperative screening (that would be performed by another specialty) for deep vein thrombosis after knee or hip surgery.[36]

The American Association of Neurological Surgeons and Congress of Neurological Surgeons similarly participates with five guidelines, two recommending avoidance of medications in certain situations and three avoiding imaging studies for low-risk situations, but none discouraging use of neurosurgical procedures (although, arguably, the avoidance of some imaging studies might lead to fewer surgeries, on occasion).[37]

In contrast, some specialties direct some of their recommendations toward more evidence-based care that can have revenue implications for them. The American Society for Radiation Oncology recommends not to initiate "non-curative radiation therapy without defining the goals of treatment with the patient and considering palliative care referral."[38] The American Society for Echocardiography also includes recommendations that would avoid tests in low-risk situations, and another not to repeat tests that detected minimal abnormalities.[39] Three of the guidelines from the American Gastroenterological Association deal with the frequency of their procedures, but two others address certain kinds of medicines and the need for x-rays (that are performed and billed for by radiologists).[40]

Thus some specialties are acting in the spirit of the initiative, but others (including among the highest-earning specialties, as discussed below) are not. One analysis of the overall program found that almost two-thirds targeted services that were revenue-neutral to the specialty societies recommending them.[41] Whether any of these efforts have much effect on what practitioners are motivated to do, and are rewarded for doing, is another question entirely.[42]

Skinflints

There are distinct benefits to some fields not to "choose wisely." One of the highest-paying fields in medicine is dermatology. Dermatologists do not have long hours and rarely have night call. In fact, on average, they work about 12% fewer hours than general internists, pediatricians, and family physicians.[43] They run patients through their offices with extreme efficiency and can log a lot of visits in a week.

As financially rewarding as that is, dermatologists can make even more money if they perform procedures. These include treatments that clearly are indicated, such as removal of basal cell carcinomas and actinic keratoses (which can progress to cancer), as well as removal of more serious forms of cancer such as melanoma. They also include procedures that are more cosmetic, such as botulinum toxin injections for wrinkles, laser removal of aging spots, and other similar procedures. Cosmetic procedures are not covered by insurance, so doctors can charge whatever they like. Granted, their clients presumably can afford the service, but it is a far cry from spending time taking care of people with serious problems that could benefit from their care.

The Choosing Wisely contributions of the American Academy of Dermatology do little to challenge their revenue stream. Of their ten recommendations, five relate to avoidance or more appropriate use of antibiotics or antifungal medicines in certain situations, two to avoiding certain tests (probably performed in labs or by allergists), one to not using steroids (which might be injected for a fee or taken by mouth), and only two to avoiding procedures that generate significant revenue and that dermatologists might do: more extensive (Mohs) surgery in low-risk skin cancers and lymph node biopsies in early-stage melanomas (which do not improve survival in that circumstance).[44]

Where the Money Is

When I was in my final year of medical school, I had a vague notion of differences in specialty incomes, but it never occurred to me that such differences would affect specialty choice. When Peter, a classmate of mine, mentioned that he was going to specialize in radiology, I was shocked. He seemed like a nice man with good interpersonal skills. Why was he opting for a field in which he would have little or no contact with patients?

I later came to realize that some specialties generate a lot of income partly because they don't involve much time interacting with each patient. These include radiology and its subspecialties, pathology, and anesthesiology. Specialists in fields such as those earn two or three times as much as doctors who provide ongoing care in nonprocedural specialties. In so doing, they rarely work nights, hardly ever get calls from patients, and the hours are terrific. A radiologist friend of my wife took 10 weeks of vacation per year.

The choice of a medical specialty has enormous consequences for the livelihood of the physician. According to a survey by Doximity, the average neurosurgeon earned about $610,000 in 2015, orthopedic surgeons made $536,000, thoracic surgeons $471,000, cardiologists $437,000, vascular surgeons $429,000, plastic surgeons $408,000, radiologists $404,000, hematologists $377,000, otolaryngologists $370,000, general surgeons $360,000, anesthesiologists $357,000, ophthalmologists $343,000, emergency medicine doctors $320,000, and obstetrician-gynecologists $320,000. In contrast, family physicians and internists earned $228,000 and $223,000, respectively, while nonprocedural medical subspecialists earned $218,000 (endocrinology), $206,000 (infectious diseases), and $245,000 (rheumatology). Psychiatrists averaged $227,000, general pediatricians $207,000, and neurologists (some of whom do procedures) $243,000.[45]

Whatever the motivations for all the procedures that certain specialties do, it is clear that the income differences across specialties are substantial and a far cry from the slight disparity in incomes evident in 1949, as discussed above. Now, the incomes of physicians in the cognitive/nonprocedural fields certainly are not bad. They are generally four or five times the wage of the average worker, but the differences between their incomes and those of the specialists are perceptible. The disparities in income have increased even more since the 1970s, when I was oblivious to them.[46] Today, the differences are so large that they can't be missed and have a profound effect upon specialty choice of graduating medical students.

Analyses of data from two studies, a national probability sample of physicians who participated in the National Physicians' Practice Costs and Income Survey in 1983–84 (which had a response rate of 67.7%) and a survey in 2018–19, using different methods but including over 30,000 physicians, found that the net income of all specialties increased substantially (in the case of internists, from an average of $85,371 to $243,000. But the disparity in incomes between procedural and nonprocedural fields increased. General surgeons earned 30% more than internists in 1983–84 and 49% more in 2018, urologists jumped from 34% to 68% greater, ophthalmologists from 46% to 51% higher, cardiologists from 57% to 77% more, and orthopedic surgeons from 67% to 98% higher.

Psychiatrists, pediatricians, and family physicians earned less than internists.[47]

Other specialties have been able to identify their own sweet spots to augment revenue flow. As Art Schwabe lamented to me, gastroenterology has become a procedural business for most practitioners: upper and lower endoscopies; procedures involving the pancreatic duct, esophagus, and stomach; biopsies of the bowel and the liver. They averaged $417,000 in the 2018–19 survey. Dermatologists, who have very little night call, averaged $419,000.

In addition to their procedure fees, doctors in some specialties have other ways to embellish income from what they do. Medical oncology has become one of the highest paying of the medical specialties, averaging $359,000 in 2018–19. Oncologists can make a lot of money, in part because the chemotherapy drugs that they administer are sold by their practices to the patients at a profit. Since many of these drugs are increasingly expensive, incomes have risen. Thus oncologists have an incentive not only to do procedures (administer chemotherapy), but also to sell drugs.[48] Some oncologists in academic practices can generate incomes of $1 million or more in this way, and many more are close to that level of income.

Cancer is scary. Shouldn't these doctors get paid whatever it takes to save some lives? When the incentives are misaligned, this can have consequences for the patient. There is ample evidence that many patients continue to receive treatments that can be toxic until shortly before they die, for cancers for which successful treatment is uncommon after failed treatment.[49]

Shortly after I moved to Los Angeles, I attended a Grand Rounds at which a physician from St. Christopher's, the pioneering London hospice founded in 1967 by the visionary Cicely Saunders, spoke about their approach to care. As he described the effort to limit treatment and suffering for a particular patient, the chief of hematology and oncology at UCLA raised his hand and interrupted the presentation. It was a dramatic moment. I cannot recall another occasion when I witnessed a faculty member interrupting a speaker during Grand Rounds, which typically is a rather formal performance with a question-and-comment period at the end. "Clearly, your patients are different from ours," said the UCLA professor. "Our patients want us to do everything possible to prolong their lives."

"Well," the speaker responded, "it depends what you say to them. If you say that you have a treatment that may prolong their life, of course they will want it. If, on the other hand, you say that you have a treatment that will give you nausea, vomiting and diarrhea, that it may well suppress your bone marrow and lead to an infection that will result in spending time in the hospital, and that there is no evidence that it will prolong your life, they might give you a different answer."

Well said.

Patients Choosing Wisely?

Financial conflicts of interest may propel clinicians to misrepresent the need for diagnostic procedures such as echocardiography, endoscopy, or heart catheterization, from which they earn income, or for inserting a device such as a pacemaker, which generates a procedure fee and perhaps a profit from its sale. They may also overstate the likely benefit from ongoing cancer treatment or a more expensive form of chemotherapy, or of need for a surgical procedure such as a hysterectomy or gall bladder resection.

One could imagine a way of mitigating this: carefully structured, precise, data-driven explanations of the prospects for survival of someone with cancer, where the likely impact of a particular treatment on survival is articulated clearly. Likewise, for someone with cardiac symptoms, one could lay out explicitly the actual level of risk of not getting a pacemaker in a particular situation. Physicians often speak in generalities. Many patients are capable of understanding information if the physician is willing to take the time to explain it in a way that they can understand. Doing so would put patients in a position to choose, and to be able to opt out when they judge that the potential health benefit is outweighed by financial costs, inconvenience to the family, or other hardships.

Some groups try to empower patients to be true partners in "shared decision-making" by providing them with the information, tools, and opportunities to decide whether to have a particular procedure, including things like interactive videos. Establishing such methods in routine clinical practice has proved evasive, particularly when doing so might well have implications for practice revenue.[50]

The Relative Value Scale

In an effort to restrain accelerating health care expenditures, the US government has pursued fixes to the fee schedule that were intended to curtail procedural fees. One notable effort was the resource-based relative value scale (RBRVS), developed by Hsiao and his colleagues at Harvard and implemented as a Medicare fee schedule in the 1990s.[51] It assigned a value to each medical act based upon an estimate of the work involved and the practitioner's associated costs. It reduced procedural fees a bit and gave a little more to evaluation and management.

There was considerable unhappiness at first in the procedural fields, but the sky did not fall. The system attempted to account for practice expenses and how hard the work was for each kind of task. In establishing the RBRVS fee schedule, it was presumed that time spent doing a procedure was intense and should be rewarded somewhat better, but that the differences in pay were larger than could be justified by the data. The RBRVS still overestimated time and cost for the proceduralists, but it should have closed the gap somewhat. As the income data cited previously suggest, the changes did not interrupt a long-term trend toward even more disparity in income across the specialties.[52]

Adding vinegar to that wound, the inspector general of the Department of Health and Human Services has tracked patterns of coding for intensity of service for evaluation and management, and reviews physician billing at higher levels of intensity. This is easy to do by running Medicare data. In contrast, figuring out which procedures should not have been done is more complicated. It is analogous to an investigative television series going after the small-time cheater and letting the big one get away with far more.[53]

A new Physician Payment Review Commission[54] and successor organizations attempted to address these stubborn trends. One identified concern was that practice expense allowances for doctors performing procedures were inflated because they were based on practice volume rather than on actual expense (since procedure doctors efficiently covered what little office expense that they had through high-priced procedures, often spending much of their time in procedure or operating rooms).[55] Some other factors appeared to have had greater impact.

The Relative Value Scale Update Committee: A Monument to Self-Interest

With the procedure-performing societies up in arms about the RBRVS, the American Medical Association convened a Relative Value Scale Update Committee (the RUC) to advise the government on changes in the Medicare fee schedule. All the specialties care a great deal about this committee and its deliberations. The procedural fields have a singular vision: protect the revenue for their disciplines and increase it if possible. The cognitive disciplines would like to see some redistribution of income away from procedures and to "evaluation and management," the things that they do. Since the agenda has to do with *relative* payment of the specialties, it is a zero-sum game, and the RUC's composition is crucial to their deliberations. As of 2017, there were 31 members, of whom 23 were clinicians who were entirely or largely proceduralists, and 8 were clinicians (including a dietician) whose work was primarily diagnosis and management.[56]

As we would expect, committee members advocate for their own specialties, and the proceduralists carry the day. Not surprisingly, the committee has not opposed higher reimbursement for diagnostic and management services, *but not at the expense of procedures*.[57] In one analysis, occupying a rotating seat on the committee was positively correlated with increased payment to a subspecialty.[58] This would be analogous to allowing real estate tycoons to establish the rules for how much taxes major players in their line of work should pay.

That is not to say that there are no altruistic or more broad-minded specialists, but their representatives are on the RUC to serve the interests of their constituencies, and the overwhelming priority of those constituencies is not to scale back what they get paid for their services. The federal agency that establishes rates of payment for services through Medicare lacks the personnel to independently evaluate the cost of services, so it almost always goes along with the committee's recommendations. Even though the federal administrator responsible for Medicare and Medicaid from 2001 to 2004 warned that "the existing structure makes objective assessment and reallocation almost impossible," nothing has changed since then.[59]

The nonprocedural fields are extremely frustrated by this situation. Since the government is not about to inject more funds into the system, it is entirely predictable that the current structure supports the status quo. It even has managed to heighten the imbalance between primary and cognitive care and the procedural fields in some respects, as new procedures enter the equation. As a result, and contrary to the promise of the RBRVS, the disparities have increased.

Bodenheimer identifies four reasons for this. One is the composition of the RUC and the ability of the procedural specialties that control it to shape the fee recommendations to the government. Another is the increase in the volume of diagnostic and imaging procedures that are performed by the procedural fields. A third is that Medicare's formula for controlling physician payments penalizes primary care physicians. Finally, private insurers tend to pay higher rates than Medicare for procedures, but not for primary care.[60]

Medical students are savvy. They understand how to position themselves in order to get into medical school. They also are aware of what doctors in the various specialties earn. Some websites keep them fully informed in this regard.[61] Students are also exposed to physician faculty and can see how their lifestyles and incomes affect their job satisfaction. At many medical schools, numerous faculty members in procedural fields earn incomes exceeded only by those of the senior administrators of their hospitals and the football and basketball coaches. It's good work if you can get it.

The disparities in pay by specialty have grown so large over the decades that they now dominate medical student specialty choice. A large proportion seeks fields that pay a great deal (like orthopedics or neurosurgery) or that provide high incomes with less demanding work schedules (like dermatology or anesthesiology). Out of about 100 entering medical students at Cornell's medical school in a recent year, 15 expressed a preference for orthopedics. When I was seeking a residency in internal medicine, I was nervous about my prospects because most of the strongest medical students seemed to be going into that field.

Now, it is the high-paying fields that attract the students. Often, students wait to see if their test scores are good enough for a procedural field, then, if needed, settle for a cognitive field if they are not. The chair of a department of internal medicine at an East Coast medical school resignedly mentioned to me that when the dean touted the proportion of their students applying to highly competitive specialties, internal medicine was not mentioned as being one of them. As one would expect, within fields like internal medicine and neurology, many physicians go on to subspecialize in the more procedural (and higher-paying) components of those disciplines, such as gastroenterology, cardiology, epilepsy, and critical care neurology. Each of these subspecialties does involve some evaluation and management, but the procedures come to define them and the nature of much of their clinical activity.

To be sure, many of the procedural fields involve examining patients. Surgeons are supposed to provide the postoperative care for their patients, and they are paid a "global fee" for all of the services related to the surgery. That fee is calculated on the basis of the expected amount of such care. Over the decades, they have provided less and less of such care. In the hospital, they tend to hand everything other than wound care to the internist. I used to be puzzled as to why someone was admitted to the hospital with a broken hip was sent to the internal medicine ward until the surgeons were ready to operate, then came back to us after the operation. Now I understand that it has become the norm. After hospitalization, follow-up with the surgeon is less extensive than the amount that went into the "relative value" calculation of global rates for the procedures. The result, according to a recent analysis, is that surgeons are overpaid.[62] The drift away from postoperative care in and outside of the hospital gives the surgeon more time to maximize income. It also turns many of them into something more like technologists. The human dimension of the relationship is diminished by the economic realities.

The Medical Act as a Commodity

In fee-for-service medicine, practice is piecework, and doctors are selling pieces of medical care. As in any retail business dealing in any commodity, it is good to sell more pieces, and it is even better to sell pieces that bring in more revenue (generally the ones that cost more). Certainly, in the specialties, the payments that physicians receive for what they do provide plenty of motivation to gin up procedure rates. Hospitals love surgeries, which are efficient generators of revenue. They particularly like elective surgeries because they mostly allow hospitals to avoid people with poor insurance. Filling surgical beds allows these institutions to generate substantial physicians' fees while they garner considerable additional revenue from operating room charges and other aspects of care. Inevitably, many clinicians share this passion for doing more revenue-generating procedures and target patients with generous insurance or other resources. When I was advocating in a meeting of my department at UCLA for placing some of our clinics in areas where disadvantaged patients reside, a professor of dermatology piped up that his group were establishing a Botox injection program in Beverly Hills!

As we have seen, doing procedures generates income more efficiently than spending that time with patients. Thus "invasive" cardiologists earn about $150,000 more per year than their well-paid "noninvasive" colleagues. In one study of doctors' wages, investigators examined what physicians earn per hour. They found some variation in the length of the work week (42 to 68 hours), but much more in hourly income ($50 to $132), with the pay rate being higher in the surgical fields and the technical medical specialties than in primary care.[63]

In the pursuit of more revenue, there is an incentive to spend less time talking to the patient. That is also true of the doctor who provides cognitive services, but the opportunity cost of spending more time with the patient is less if you aren't foregoing procedures. Move the patients through quickly, and you will amass more "relative value units" of billable care. Bring the patient back sooner for a repeat colonoscopy on some pretext. Perform a Pap smear more often than the guideline suggests. Order another expensive imaging study on a patient recovering from pneumonia, just to be sure that the image is consistent with the clinical improvement. The clinical rationale may be tenuous, but the payment is not.

Is There a Psychiatrist in the House?

Mental health care is hard to come by in the United States. More than 40 million Americans have a behavioral health issue each year. Psychiatrists are not the front line in treating most of them. Fully 51% of counties in the US do not have a psychiatrist, and 37% lack a psychologist.[64] Among physicians, psychiatry is not a particularly popular specialty. There are few procedures to do. The level of reimbursement for mental health services is comparable to that for primary care, and it is not sufficient to meet the needs of many psychiatrists (whose visits often take longer than those of general physicians). Accordingly, psychiatrists tend to congregate in metropolitan areas where it is possible to attract a clientele that can afford their services even if health insurance doesn't cover them. Psychologists and psychiatric social workers are variably available, but not nearly enough for those most in need of care.

Yet even in major cities, much of the mental health care is provided by primary care physicians or by nonphysicians, since few patients can afford to pay out-of-pocket prices for treatment. Consequently, many of the people most in need of mental health services are unlikely to get them from mental health professionals. When I worked at UCLA, few faculty psychiatrists accepted insurance payment for ongoing outpatient care. The only way for a patient to be seen through their insurance was by a trainee. Otherwise, a single visit could cost $300 or more. If patients are sick enough to be hospitalized, they do get care. That is a bit of a respite from the inflated pricing of outpatient psychiatric care. Even those who are insured report cost as a barrier to mental health care. Like much of the health care system in America, mental health services are crazily expensive and out of touch with the reality of many people's ability to pay for the treatment they need.[65]

At Your Service

As mentioned in chapter 2, concierge medicine is flourishing among doctors who specialize in diseases of the affluent. The term "concierge" originated in France and designated the warden of a house castle, prison, or palace. It likely was derived from the Latin *conservus*, meaning fellow slave. Some practices charge as much as $40,000 to $80,000 to be constantly available to an individual or family, respectively, although others' fees are much more modest.[66] By practicing in this model of care, physicians can make a great deal of money. A concierge doctor who charges 200 patients $5,000 or $10,000 each per year generates revenue of $1 or $2 million per year. For primary care doctors and others who provide ongoing principal or chronic care, there has been some movement to pay them for coordinating the care of their Medicare patients, but these fees are miniscule by comparison.[67]

Concierge medicine reinforces the current reality in the United States of different levels of care/service for different socioeconomic classes of patients. The clientele of these practitioners is limited to an even thinner slice of society socioeconomically than the people who can see doctors who decline to take Medicaid patients.

Open a Business

Some doctors get rich by doing lots of procedures, like a transplant surgeon I knew. This surgeon worked hard but also supposedly had 15 fancy sports cars. Others get rich because they start a clinic business, owning many office locations, hiring lots of physicians, and making far more than they could on their own in even the most efficiently extractive medical practice. The doctor from my medical class who most succeeded in this regard was a poor student, perhaps the weakest in the class, but he clearly was a clever businessman.

Deceit

A doctor who admitted patients to a Southern California hospital specialized in the treatment of pancreatic cancer. She was aggressive in treatment, giving intense chemotherapy every two or three weeks. The medical residents hated taking care of her patients because she always painted an optimistic picture of prognosis. Even though about 95% of patients with that disease will die and virtually the only survivors are those diagnosed very early with small tumors that can be removed, she would tell patients whose cancer was inoperable (because the disease had spread) that she was giving drugs to shrink the tumor so that they could then have surgery and hopefully be cured. She was dishonest about prognosis, but it was not appropriate for the residents to contradict her to the patients. Sometimes, when disease was advanced, a physician would confront her about needlessly torturing a patient. She would say, "OK, you take care of him" and walk away from the case. She made a lot of money administering those drugs.

The dash for cash can have untoward effects on vulnerable patients if a physician is so committed to procedural interventions to generate revenue that the patient is put in harm's way. Compassionate end-of-life care does not pay nearly as well. It may well be that this physician had limited interpersonal skills and could not comfortably handle difficult conversations about prognosis, but it was clear that such incapacity was in her financial interest.

The Junk Medical Visit

When I received my first medical license in Quebec, I was sworn in by an executive of the province's College of Physicians. In so doing, he said to me, "there are some doctors in this province who see 70 patients a day. Don't be one of those doctors."

A Portuguese physician whom I visited in Lisbon came up with an apt characterization of medical encounters that weren't long enough to assess patients' needs adequately. In their hospital clinic, many patients were seen for only two or three minutes because of overwhelming demand and lack of resources. He characterized this situation as "the junk medical visit."

Unlike professions such as law, in which attorneys are paid by the hour, most doctors are paid fee-for-service. The more acts, the more money. In our system, the issue is not resources or overwhelming demand; it is the lust for revenue. As explained above, there can be different levels of fees charged within a particular kind of service. For a follow-up office visit, even the charge for the highest level of complexity does not pay nearly as much as a charge for an initial consultation or for a minor procedure. If a patient needs to talk, needs reassurance, needs things explained several times, that can consume the visit. The meticulous, conscientious doctor will give a patient as much time as he or she needs. Another doctor moves patients through at a rapid pace. The meticulous doctor sees fewer patients than the doctor who has mastered the junk medical visit.

So-Called Productivity

Multispecialty medical groups expect their members to be clinically busy, as measured by numbers of visits of a certain value. These relative value units (RVUs) are the score of "productivity" and can be a major contributor to stress and burnout.[68] Many groups set explicit expectations in relation to national or regional data on RVUs for a particular centile of that score. Standards for academic medical groups are a little different, since they need to account for time for teaching and the like. Nonetheless, it is medicine on the assembly line. The executives promoting more productivity really want less time per patient per RVU.

One is reminded of Charlie Chaplain's character in the film *Modern Times*, who worked on an assembly line. The boss increased the speed of the assembly line in order to increase profits. Charlie couldn't keep up, moved down the assembly line to compete his task, and eventually got caught up in the machinery. One of my professors talked about Dr. John Lawrence, a mentor of his whom he sought to emulate. "He never compromised on a physical examination," he said. That would not be looked upon favorably in today's era of RVUs. Lawrence, who became the founding chair of the Department of Internal Medicine at UCLA after career stops at Vanderbilt, Harvard, and the University of Rochester, might not have survived the early phases of his career had such productivity metrics been in place during his day.

In the context of the additional work inflicted by electronic medical records and the pressure to produce RVUs, it is not surprising that generalists are unhappy and that fewer of them than in other specialties indicate that they would make that choice again (64% for general internal medicine and 67% for family medicine, compared to 90% to 96% for dermatology, orthopedics, oncology, plastic surgery, ophthalmology, cardiology, otolaryngology, radiology, and gastroenterology).[69]

Caring for the Disadvantaged

For the physicians whose idealism has not been entirely extinguished by their medical education, the consolidation and corporatization of medical practice present additional problems that we shall consider in chapter 7. At one time, many doctors would accept a certain amount of "charity care" for people who had no insurance and could not afford their fees. Practicing in a large health system or medical group deprives the clinician of autonomy in deciding for whom he or she will provide care.

Eugene, a patient of mine who was a community activist, devoted his life to making the world a better place. He wanted to heal the world but was never in a situation to be able to get health insurance. I used to sneak Eugene into clinic for a physical examination and to write the prescriptions that he needed. I could not sneak him into the laboratory, so getting any tests was an insurmountable problem. The organization charged more to those without insurance than to anyone with insurance. That is how fees get set. It was possible to ask for a discount, but even if granted, it was never down to the level that my own health insurance would pay.

Individual physicians in these practices do not have the option to contravene corporate policy and provide service gratis. Whereas a physician practicing alone would have the discretion to treat a patient in need for no charge, that is nearly impossible in a large clinical organization, where every patient must be registered and present an insurance or credit card for every service. To be sure, some such organizations do take on some care for the disadvantaged, but it is far from a major emphasis.

When I asked a leader of one academic health system, which was placing clinics in neighborhoods where the patients were all middle class or above, what their view was of who would care for people in predominantly poor, minority neighborhoods, he responded, "our affiliates will provide that care." (The affiliates were public hospitals and their clinics.) How can individual doctors respond to that approach? They may feel that they are let off the hook, because it was not their choice to exclude patients with Medicaid or no insurance. I find that to be a flimsy rationalization. They are accepting the values of the place where they chose to work. Clinicians who work in academic institutions, for the most part, are no more virtuous than nonacademic ones.

Doctors in Public Hospitals and Clinics

There are some wonderful, idealistic physicians working in public clinics and hospitals, but many others do not always view their mission as being to provide care comparable to that available through the private sector. When Mitch Katz, a friend of mine, became the director of the Los Angeles County Department of Health Services, he was determined to ensure continuity of care for at least the sickest patients in the system (of whom there were hundreds of thousands). Up until then, patients who came to county clinics were seen by whoever was on that day, not by a regular doctor, and often had to wait several hours to be seen by someone who would never see them again. If they had a problem between appointments, there was no doctor whom they could call. When he issued his directive, many doctors were initially resistant. They didn't think it was their job to be responsible for particular patients on an ongoing basis and available to take their calls.

The World Health Organization (WHO) defines continuity of care as care that "reflects the extent to which a series of discrete health care events is experienced by people as coherent and interconnected over time and consistent with their health needs and preferences." WHO observes that those receiving private sector care expect their care to look like that. The absence of such care puts people at risk.

> Without good continuity or coordination of care and support, many patients, carers and families experience fragmented, poorly integrated care from multiple providers, often with suboptimal outcomes and risk of harm due to failures of communication, inadequate sharing of clinical information, poor reconciliation of medicines, duplication of investigations and avoidable hospital admissions or readmissions. This is a particular problem for people with chronic or complex conditions that require care and support, many of whom have multiple conditions associated with low income or complex circumstance, who are often underserved.[70]

Given that doctors working in public institutions are the subset of the profession most committed to the care of the poor, the bifurcated health care system in the United States has established deep and strong roots, and many practitioners are numbed to its consequences. In theory at least, the country has judged that separate cannot be equal in education. That point of view has not yet prevailed in health care.[71]

The Virtuous Citizens

I have perseverated here about the shortfall in values, the cynicism, and even the corruption of many medical practitioners, although it is essential to understand that they behave this way in a system that gives them permission to do that. Nonetheless, I would be remiss not to talk about some of the people who are different. There are physicians who break the mold and devote their lives to the disadvantaged, sometimes at considerable cost in both income and convenience. There are many doctors who are wonderful people who work to make the world a better place and are relatively indifferent to how much they get paid.

Davida

When I volunteered at a free clinic in the Venice area of Los Angeles, one of the people who worked there was a pediatrician named Davida. She had a faculty position at UCLA, but she spent about half of the year working in refugee camps in the most dangerous places in the world, including Biafra, Honduras, and the Middle East, and working to improve health systems in Africa, Haiti, India, and Nicaragua. She also established a program for substance users in the United States and was a political activist who worked alongside Cesar Chavez, Pete Seeger, Martin Sheen, and others.

I was in awe of her. She thought nothing of the sacrifices that she made to serve people who were truly the wretched of the earth, ignored by so many. She died recently, after a lifetime of such work. As I ponder my career and ask if I have done enough to make the world a better place, she is one metric of what is possible, and of what a medical profession that is committed to its potential to heal humanity can accomplish.[72]

Steve

Steve is a general pediatrician in Los Angeles. I first met him when he was an intern at Los Angeles County Hospital. He was a firebrand. He proudly wore a button that read, "health care for people not profits." He had grown up in Chicago and attended college and medical school there. As an undergraduate, he had been active in the anti–Vietnam War movement, as well in anti-apartheid activities. He worked at a free clinic in uptown Chicago, where members of the Black Panther party used to bring in patients. While a pediatric resident in Los Angeles, he was consistently involved in health reform efforts, in a Los Angeles Health Organizing Committee, then with Physicians for a National Health Program, and later as president of the board of the California Physicians' Alliance. Through that organization, among other things, he was part of a successful effort to get undocumented children in California health insurance coverage.

As a clinician, he spent two years in Mozambique to provide care in a medium-sized city there. When he returned from Africa, he went to work for Kaiser Permanente in the Los Angeles area, eventually becoming head of their pediatrics group. At Kaiser in Inglewood and West Los Angeles, the vast majority of his patients were African American or Hispanic. They were working-class individuals, often in government jobs that did not pay much. Many parents were single mothers. When they had kids with chronic illnesses like asthma and diabetes, they faced many challenges filling prescriptions, getting transportation to the hospital, and ensuring that the child took their medications. Often there were many social problems to address, including parents separated by immigration authorities, violence in the neighborhood, and the like, which traumatized the children. Steve had to work closely with social workers to address these problems.

He says that his sociopolitical values were a valuable asset. He needed to gain the patient's and parent's trust, particularly when there were immigration issues involved. "Progressive values give you persistence. When there is a problem, you dig a little deeper and push the system to make sure that your patient gets the help they need," he told me. He loved providing patient care but never stopped trying to make the world more just. Now, mostly retired from Kaiser, he keeps a hand in clinical practice and all four limbs firmly in efforts to transform the US health care system.

Susana

Susana is a general internist at Cornell's medical college in New York. Her grandparents moved to New York from Puerto Rico, and she grew up in the Bronx. In college, she was a "campus trouble-maker," being active in Latino and Puerto Rican student organizations and a South Africa solidarity committee during the apartheid era. She attended medical school at Columbia, where she also did her residency. She took a position there as a clinician and educator for several years before moving to Cornell. At both institutions, she has been heavily involved in efforts to increase the racial and ethnic diversity of the training programs by "attracting more black and brown people into medical careers," and training young physicians-to-be "to provide culturally-competent and compassionate care to all patients." She hopes that the physicians she trains will in turn become activists who "fight to provide excellent care" for all patients.

She tells me that her commitment to health equity has led her to care largely for underserved patients throughout her career. "Patient care informs my advocacy," she says. "Learning about the barriers my patients face keeps me grounded about what to prioritize." That has included working with AIDS organizations at the peak of the HIV epidemic, speaking engagements, and lending a prominent voice in New York to publicizing the need to address inequities faced by disadvantaged populations in the context of the COVID-19 pandemic. She has been able to pursue her agenda of equity, diversity, and advocacy through her federally funded Diversity Center of Excellence and as vice chair for diversity in Cornell's Department of Internal Medicine.

Susana notes that she has not always been wise in taking on institutional responsibilities related to diversity and justice, often finding that they were uncompensated and left her scrambling to cover her salary. She now mentors many other faculty members with similar interests, so that they can be successful and not exploited in their roles as champions of diversity. Her efforts have contributed to the medical school identifying diversity as one of their core principles and goals, and helping Cornell achieve no less than 25% African American and Latino representation in the internal medicine residency program each year.

Tom

Tom was my colleague for many years at UCLA. He is strongly committed to social justice. In medical school, he spent time in a teaching general practice in England and was drawn to the fact that they collected and analyzed research data and were well connected to their community. Another formative experience in medical school was that he organized students from his class to travel to Holmes County, Mississippi, to work in a free clinic in the spring and summer of 1971. That program was funded by the Robert F. Kennedy Foundation. Going there and seeing the great need for decent health care, along with the other challenges that the people faced, is seared in his memory.

After graduating from medical school at Georgetown, he completed his residency and chief residency in internal medicine at Harlem Hospital in New York and Cook County Hospital in Chicago. He says that Quentin Young, who was chair of medicine at Cook County, was a progressive and inspirational leader. The greatest influence on Tom during that time was a progressive study group of young doctors in the training program, all of whom carried their values forward in their careers.

Tom then returned to Harlem Hospital, where he worked for a decade as a general internist. After that, he came to UCLA, where he worked in the university hospital and spent time at a public hospital and in an affiliated free clinic. Tom often ended up caring for multiple generations in a family. He was one of the rare doctors who did house calls, seeing patients in their environments and gaining insight into their social problems.

At UCLA, he was one of the most beloved teachers and very best clinicians. He was extraordinarily conscientious and consistently took more time with each patient than the schedule allowed. He was no friend to RVUs! His notes were exhaustive. In the era before electronic records were instituted, he was known for his small handwriting, which allowed him to capture every detail.

He is a quiet man but is held in the deepest respect by all. His clinical judgment is superb. Tom was my physician. He was always an ally in efforts to nudge our health system toward social responsibility. Many students who saw his devotion to his patients and his love of what he did followed him into primary care. He recently retired from UCLA and is working in an academic program in Washington, where he is developing a curriculum on the social determinants of health. He is the least materialistic doctor with whom I ever have worked. He is great at all of the important things.

There are many more idealistic, giving physicians like Tom, but they are more exceptions than the rule. The business of medical practice is a commercial activity that affects what many physicians choose to do and what gets done to the people who seek medical care. This reality is an important obstacle to creating a better health care system. Can this be fixed with policy interventions to transform the financing of care? That could help, perhaps considerably, but many other problems with the ways in which physicians view themselves and their work, as well as the competencies (and lack thereof) that they bring to bear and the organizations that represent their interests, would remain substantial obstacles. We will discuss these in chapter 4.

Notes

1. Tom Warren, "A Brief History of Physician Remuneration," *University of Western Ontario Medical Journal* 78, no. 2 (2008): 38–40, https://citeseerx.ist.psu.edu /viewdoc/download?doi=10.1.1.1084.5240&rep=rep1&type=pdf.

2. Geoffrey Chaucer, "The Prologue," in *The Canterbury Tales*, l. 454, accessed July 27, 2021, https://www.dvusd.org/cms/lib011/AZ01901092/Centricity/Domain /2891/Canterbury%20Tales%20prologue.pdf.

3. Warren, "Brief History."

4. An income in this range in 1937 was the equivalent of about $90,000 to $180,000 in 2021. "CPI Inflation Calculator," US Bureau of Labor Statistics, accessed September 18, 2021, https://www.bls.gov/data/inflation_calculator.htm.

5. Lewis Thomas, "A Brief Historical Note on Medical Economics," in *The Medusa and the Snail: More Notes of a Biology Watcher* (New York: Penguin, 1995), 118–20.

6. William Weinfeld, "Income of Physicians, 1929–49," *Survey of Current Business* (July 1951): 9–26, https://fraser.stlouisfed.org/files/docs/publications/SCB/pages /1950-1954/4374_1950-1954.pdf; "US Inflation Calculator," accessed April 10, 2020, https://www.usinflationcalculator.com.

7. Leslie Kane et al., "International Physician Compensation Report 2019: Do US Physicians Have It Best?," Medscape, accessed June 13, 2020, https://www.medscape .com/slideshow/2019-international-compensation-report-6011814#1; Leslie Kane, "Medscape Physician Compensation Report 2019," Medscape, accessed June 13, 2020, https://www.medscape.com/slideshow/2019-compensation-overview-6011286#1.

8. Zachary Dykman, Executive Office of the President, Council on Wage and Price Stability, "Income of Physicians, Dentists, and All Professional and Kindred Workers, 1939–1976," in *A Study of Physicians' Fees: Staff Report* (Washington, DC: US Government Printing Office, 1978), 73–93, table IV-1, https://babel.hathitrust.org /cgi/pt?id=umn.31951d00827889m&view=1up&seq=93; see also Daniel H. Weinberg, "Evidence from Census 2000 about Earnings by Detailed Occupation for Men and Women, May, 2004," accessed April 10, 2020, https://www.census.gov/library /publications/2004/dec/censr-15.pdf, which reported a median income for all workers of $33,000; John C. Langenbrunner, Deborah K. Williams, and Sherry A. Terrell, "Physician Incomes and Work Patterns across Specialties: 1975 and 1983–84," *Health Care Financing Review* 10, no. 2 (Winter 1988): 17–24; Organisation for Economic Co-operation and Development, "Remuneration of Doctors, Ratio to Average Wage, 2015 (or Nearest Year)," in *Health at a Glance* (OECD: Paris, 2017), https://doi.org/10.1787/88933604704.

The following table summarizes data on physician income since 1929 from the sources cited in this section:

Physician income in the United States by year, adjusted for inflation

Year	Income	Inflation Adjusted to 2020
1929	$5,224	$79,132
1949	$11,744	$127,422
1955	$16,107	$155,110
1965	$28,960	$237,182
1995	$180,930	$305,771
2003	$202,982	$284,175

9. "Average Compensation in U.S. Dollar Purchasing Power Comparing Specialists' and General Practitioners' Incomes Across Countries," Organisation for Economic Co-operation and Development, accessed July 6, 2021, https://journal.practicelink.com /vital-stats/physician-compensation-worldwide/.

10. Rosemary Stevens, *American Medicine and the Public Interest* (Berkeley: University of California Press, 1998), 43–47, 101.

11. "About ABMS," American Board of Medical Specialties, accessed June 17, 2020, https://www.abms.org/about-abms/faqs/.

12. "Exam Administration History," American Board of Internal Medicine, accessed June 17, 2020, https://www.abim.org/about/exam-information/exam-administration-history.aspx.

13. "More Security for Doctors Profiting from Medical Devices They Use," ProPublica, accessed June 17, 2020, https://www.propublica.org/article/more-scrutiny-for-doctors-profiting-from-medical-devices-they-use.

14. Prices vary, depending on where the test is done. "Physician Fee Schedule Search," Centers for Medicare and Medicaid Services, accessed May 19, 2020, https://www.cms.gov/apps/physician-fee-schedule/search/search-criteria.aspx; "Standard Charges," Sparrow.org, accessed May 19, 2020, https://www.sparrow.org/patient-resources/financial-resources/standard-charges.

15. Commercial insurers pay about $202, $750, $1,164, $1,164, and $1,939, respectively, for those abdominal imaging tests. See "Standard Charges."

16. "Historical," and "NHE Summary, Including Share of GDP, CY 1960–2019 (ZIP)," Centers for Medicare and Medicaid Services, accessed October 9, 2021, https://www.cms.gov/Research-Statistics-Data-and-Systems/Statistics-Trends-and-Reports/NationalHealthExpendData/NationalHealthAccountsHistorical; "Infographic—US Health Care Spending: Who Pays?," California Health Care Foundation, June 28, 2021, https://www.chcf.org/publication/us-health-care-spending-who-pays/.

17. "National Health Expenditure Data," Centers for Medicare and Medicaid Services, accessed March 5, 2022, https://www.cms.gov/Research-Statistics-Data-and-Systems/Statistics-Trends-and-Reports/NationalHealthExpendData.

18. Joseph Bernstein, "The Policy Implications of Physician Income Homeostasis," *Journal of Health Care Finance* 24, no. 4 (Summer 1998): 80–86, PMID 9612740.

19. Andrew M. D. Wolf et al., "Colorectal Cancer Screening for Average-Risk Adults: 2018 Guideline Update from the American Cancer Society," CA: *A Cancer Journal for Clinicians* 68, no. 4 (July 2018): 250–81, https://doi.org/10.3322/caac.21457. The USPSTF is nondirective about the choice of a procedure but favors some form of testing. "Final Recommendation Statement Colon Cancer: Screening," US Preventive Services Task Force, accessed June 7, 2021, https://www.uspreventiveservicestaskforce.org/uspstf/recommendation/colorectal-cancer-screening.

20. Daniel R. Levinson, *Coding Trends of Medicare Evaluation and Management Services* (Washington, DC: Office of Inspector General, Department of Health and Human Services, May 2012), OEI-04-10-00180, https://oig.hhs.gov/oei/reports/oei-04-10-00180.pdf.

21. Archie L. Cochrane, *Effectiveness and Efficiency: Random Reflections on Health Services* (London: Nuffield Provincial Hospitals Trust, 1972), 43.

22. "Skipping Sedation: A Quicker Colonoscopy," Mayo Clinic Health System, last modified February 21, 2017, https://www.mayoclinichealthsystem.org/hometown-health/patient-stories/skipping-sedation-a-quicker-colonoscopy.

23. Yuuichi Takahashi et al., "Sedation-Free Colonoscopy," *Diseases of the Colon and Rectum* 48, no. 4 (April 2005): 855–59, https://doi.org/10.1007/s10350-004-0860-0.

24. "Colonoscopy-Related Costs, Medicare Fee-for-Service Beneficiaries Who Received a Screening or Diagnostic Colonoscopy, 2015," Office of the Assistant Secretary for Planning and Evaluation, Department of Health and Human Services, accessed October 22, 2021, https://aspe.hhs.gov/system/files/pdf/255906/DHNAdditionalInfor.pdf. Anesthesiologists submit a separate bill for their participation in the procedure. One analysis of colonoscopies insured by Medicare or private insurance found that participation of an anesthesiologist increased the average procedure cost by $358 in 2007 and about $200 in 2015. Whereas only about 13% of procedures involved anesthesiologists in 2003, that proportion was 58% in 2015. John M. Inadomi et al., "Projected Increased Growth Rate of Anesthesia Professional-Delivered Sedation for Colonoscopy and EGD in the United States: 2009 to 2015," *Gastrointestinal Endoscopy* 72, no. 3 (September 2010): 580–86, https://doi.org/10.1016/j.gie.2010.04.040; Anna Krigel et al., "Substantial Increase in Anesthesia Assistance for Outpatient Colonoscopy and Associated Cost Nationwide," *Clinical Gastroenterology and Hepatology* 17, no. 12 (November 1, 2019): 2489–96, https://doi.org/10.1016/j.cgh.2018.12.037.

25. Laura Dyrda, "CMS Posts Payment for ASCs and HOPDs: Medicare Pays $359 Less for Colonoscopy, $1,092 Less for Knee Arthroscopy," Becker's ASC Review, last modified November 28, 2018, https://www.beckersasc.com/asc-coding-billing-and-collections/cms-posts-payments-for-ascs-vs-hopds-medicare-pays-ascs-359-less-for-colonoscopy-1-092-less-for-knee-arthroscopy.html.

26. Mark R. Chassin et al., "Variation in the Use of Medical and Surgical Services by the Medicare Population," *New England Journal of Medicine* 314, no. 5 (January 30, 1986): 285–90, https://doi.org/10.1056/nejm198601303140505; Mark R. Chassin et al., "Does Inappropriate Use Explain Geographic Variation in the Use of Health Services? A Study of Three Procedures," *JAMA* 258, no. 18 (November 13, 1987): 2533–37, https://doi.org/10.1001/jama.1987.03400180067028.

27. "Clinical Guidelines and Recommendations," American College of Physicians, accessed February 10, 2020, https://www.acponline.org/clinical-information/guidelines.

28. "Guidelines and Measures," Agency for Healthcare Research and Quality, accessed February 10, 2020, https://www.ahrq.gov/gam/index.html.

29. "About the USPSTF," US Preventive Services Task Force, accessed February 10, 2020, https://www.uspreventiveservicestaskforce.org/Page/Name/about-the-uspstf.

30. David L. Sackett et al., "Evidence-Based Medicine: What It Is and What It Isn't," *BMJ* 312, no. 7023 (January 13, 1996): 71–72, https://doi.org/10.1136/bmj.312.7023.71.

31. "Major Cancer Agencies Respond to USPSTF's New Mammography Guidelines," Cancer Network, last modified December 15, 2009, https://www.cancernetwork.com/view/major-cancer-agencies-respond-uspstfs-new-mammography-guidelines.

32. "ASGE Guidelines," American Society for Gastrointestinal Endoscopy, accessed May 19, 2020, https://www.asge.org/home/resources/key-resources/guidelines.

33. David C. Classen and Leonard A. Mermel, "Specialty Society Clinical Practice Guidelines: Time for Evolution or Revolution?," JAMA 314, no. 9 (September 1, 2015): 871–72, https://doi.org/10.1001/jama.2015.7462; Institute of Medicine (US) Committee on Standards for Developing Trustworthy Clinical Practice Guidelines, *Clinical Practice Guidelines We Can Trust*, ed. Robin Graham et al. (Washington, DC: National Academies Press; 2011), https://doi.org/10.17226/13058; "Conflicts of Interest and Development of Clinical Practice Guidelines," in *Conflict of Interest in Medical Research, Education, and Practice*, ed. Bernard Lo and Marilyn J. Field (Washington, DC: National Academies Press, 2009), chap. 7, https://www.ncbi.nlm.nih.gov/books/NBK22928/; Julie Bolette Brix Bindslev et al., "Underreporting of Conflicts of Interest in Clinical Practice Guidelines: Cross Sectional Study," *BMC Medical Ethics* 14, no. 19 (2013): https://doi.org/10.1186/1472-6939-14-19.

34. Bindslev et al., "Underreporting."

35. "Choosing Wisely," website of the ABIM Foundation, accessed February 10, 2020, https://www.choosingwisely.org.

36. "Clinician Lists: American Association of Orthopaedic Surgeons," Choosing Wisely, accessed February 10, 2020, https://www.choosingwisely.org/clinician-lists/#parentSociety=American_Academy_of_Orthopaedic_Surgeons.

37. "Clinician Lists: American Association of Neurological Surgeons and Congress of Neurological Surgeons," Choosing Wisely, accessed February 10, 2020, https://www.choosingwisely.org/clinician-lists/#parentSociety=American_Association_of_Neurological_Surgeons_and_Congress_of_Neurological_Surgeons.

38. "Clinician Lists: American Society for Radiation Oncology," Choosing Wisely, accessed February 10, 2020, https://www.choosingwisely.org/clinician-lists/#parentSociety=American_Society_for_Radiation_Oncology.

39. "Clinician Lists: American Society of Echocardiography," Choosing Wisely, accessed February 10, 2020, https://www.choosingwisely.org/clinician-lists/#parentSociety=American_Society_of_Echocardiography.

40. "Clinician Lists: American Gastroenterological Association," Choosing Wisely, accessed October 9, 2021, https://www.choosingwisely.org/clinician-lists/#parentSociety=American_Gastroenterological_Association.

41. Ishani Ganguli et al., "Longitudinal Content Analysis of the Characteristics and Expected Impact of Low-Value Services Identified in US Choosing Wisely Recommendations," JAMA *Internal Medicine* 182, no. 2 (February 1, 2022): 127–33, https://doi.org/10.1001/jamainternmed.2021.6911.

42. Elizabeth J Rourke, "Ten Years of Choosing Wisely to Reduce Low-Value Care," *New England Journal of Medicine* 386, no. 14 (April 7, 2022): 1293–95, https://doi.org/10.1056/NEJMp2200422.

43. J. Paul Leigh et al., "Physician Wages across Specialties: Informing the Physician Reimbursement Debate," *Archives of Internal Medicine* 170, no. 19 (October 25, 2010): 1728–34, https://doi.org/10.1001/archinternmed.2010.350.

44. "Clinician Lists: American Academy of Dermatology," Choosing Wisely, accessed February 10, 2020, https://www.choosingwisely.org/clinician-lists/#parentSociety=American_Academy_of_Dermatology.

45. James Hamblin, "What Doctors Make: Variations in Salary Are Drastic and Opaque," *The Atlantic*, January 27, 2015, https://www.theatlantic.com/health/archive/2015/01/physician-salaries/384846/.

46. In 1975, general surgeons earned about 12% more than internists in the United States. Langenbrunner et al., "Physician Incomes"; Hamblin, "What Doctors Make"; "Physician Starting Salaries by Specialty: 2018 vs. 2017," Merritt Hawkins, accessed June 29, 2019, https://www.merritthawkins.com/news-and-insights/blog/job-search-advice/physician-starting-salaries-by-specialty-2018-vs-2017/.

47. Langenbrunner et al., "Physician Incomes"; John Elflein, "Annual Compensation Earned by U.S. Physicians As of 2020, by Specialty," Statista, accessed July 12, 2020, https://www.statista.com/statistics/250160/median-compensation-earned-by-us-physicians-by-specialty/.

48. Reed Abelson, "Drug Sales Bring Huge Profits, and Scrutiny, to Cancer Doctors," *New York Times*, January 26, 2003, https://www.nytimes.com/2003/01/26/us/drug-sales-bring-huge-profits-and-scrutiny-to-cancer-doctors.html; Roxanne Nelson, "Oncologist Getting 6% of Drug Price Is 'Financial Conflict,'" Medscape, March 7, 2018, https://www.medscape.com/viewarticle/893547.

49. Jonas B. Green et al., "Physician Variation in Lung Cancer Care at the End of Life," *American Journal of Managed Care* 23, no. 4 (April 2017): 216–23, PMID 28554208.

50. Anne M. Stiggelbout et al., "Shared Decision Making: Really Putting Patients at the Centre of Health Care," *BMJ* 344 (January 27, 2012): e256, https://doi.org/10.1136/bmj.e256; Tammy C. Hoffman, Victor M. Montori, and Chris Del Mar, "The Connection between Evidence-Based Medicine and Shared Decision Making," *JAMA* 312, no. 13 (October 1, 2014): 1295–96, https://doi.org/10.1001/jama.2014.10186; Michael J. Barry and Susan Edgman-Levitan, "Shared Decision Making—Pinnacle of Patient-Centered Care," *New England Journal of Medicine* 366, no. 9 (March 1, 2012): 780–81, https://doi.org/10.1056/NEJMp1109283; Glyn Elwyn et al., "Shared Decision Making: A Model for Clinical Practice," *Journal of General Internal Medicine* 27, no. 10 (October 2012): 1361–67, https://doi.org/10.1007/s11606-012-2077-6.

51. William C. Hsiao et al., "Estimating Physicians' Work for a Resource-Based Relative Value Scale," *New England Journal of Medicine* 319 (September 29, 1988): 835–41, https://doi.org/10.1056/nejm198809293191305.

52. David C. Colby, "Impact of the Medicare Fee Schedule," *Health Affairs* 11, no. 3 (Fall 1992): 216–26, https://www.healthaffairs.org/doi/pdf/10.1377/hlthaff.11.3.216. This 1992 paper suggested that much larger shifts, such as 30% drop in procedural payments and 30% increase in evaluation and management payments, would be forthcoming. For example, when fully implemented in 1996, the Centers for Medicare and Medicaid Services anticipated that payment would decline for hip replacement by 30%, cataract removal by 40%, pacemaker insertion and coronary artery bypass surgery by 47%, coloscopy by 38%, and transurethral prostate resection by 30%. For cognitive services, the fee for a new patient evaluation was supposed to rise by 49% and for a follow-up visit by 32%. Such changes, in theory, would have decreased specialty income differences substantially. It did not happen that way.

53. Levinson, *Coding Trends*.

54. Philip R. Lee and Paul B. Ginsburg, "Building a Consensus for Physician Payment Reform in Medicare: The Physician Payment Review Commission," *Western Journal of Medicine* 149, no. 3 (September 1988): 352–58, PMID 3051680.

55. Eric A. Latimer and Edmund R. Becker, "Incorporating Practice Costs into the Resource-Based Relative Value Scale," *Medical Care* 30, 11 suppl. (November 1992): NS50-60, https://doi.org/10.1097/00005650-199211001-00005.

56. Six members were on the RUC for reasons other than representing their specialty, of whom four were proceduralists: the chair (cardiovascular surgeon), the vice chair (emergency medicine physician), an endovascular radiologist, and a pulmonary/critical care physician. The other two were generalists: an osteopath and a dietician. The other twenty-five slots were filled from specialty societies. Nine permanent seats belong to surgeons (general surgery, neurosurgery, obstetrics and gynecology, ophthalmology, orthopedics, otolaryngology, plastic surgery, thoracic surgery, and urology), and six others are held by other procedural fields (cardiology, dermatology, emergency medicine, pathology, anesthesiology, and radiology). Six more permanent seats belong to fields that could be cognitive or procedural: family medicine, geriatrics, and psychiatry are all cognitive, but internal medicine, pediatrics, and neurology could be either. In 2017, two of these were occupied by proceduralists, a cardiologist and a sleep medicine neurologist. Of the four remaining seats, two were rotating subspecialties of internal medicine—at the time, allergy (largely procedural) and rheumatology (mostly cognitive, but with some minor procedures)—one was a rotating primary care seat, and one a rotating seat in a specialty (at the time, vascular surgery). "Composition of the RVS Update Committee (RUC)," American Medical Association, accessed June 28, 2017, https://www.ama-assn.org/about-us/composition-rvs-update-committee-ruc.

57. Uwe E. Reinhardt, "The Little-Known Decision-Makers for Medicare Physician Fees," *New York Times*, December 10, 2010, https://economix.blogs.nytimes.com/2010/12/10/the-little-known-decision-makers-for-medicare-physicans-fees/.

58. Y. Nina Gao, "Committee Representation and Medicare Reimbursements—An Examination of the Resource-Based Relative Value Scale," *Health Services Research* 53, no. 6 (2018): 4353–70, https://doi.org/10.1111/1475-6773.12857.

59. Thomas A. Scully, "Testimony before the Senate Finance Committee," Senate Finance Committee, accessed July 4, 2020, https://www.finance.senate.gov/imo/media/doc/Scully%20Statement.pdf.

60. Miriam J. Laugesen, Roy Wada, and Eric M. Chen, "In Setting Doctors' Medicare Fees, CMC Almost Always Accepts the Relative Value Update Panel's Advice on Work Values," *Health Affairs* 31, no. 5 (May 2012): 965–72, https://doi.org/10.1377/hlthaff.2011.0557; Thomas Bodenheimer and Hoangmai H. Pham, "Primary Care: Current Problems and Proposed Solutions," *Health Affairs* 29, no. 5 (May 2010): 799–805, https://doi.org/10.1377/hlthaff.2010.0026.

61. See, e.g., "Physician Starting Salaries."

62. Andrew W. Mulcahy, Katie Merrell, and Ateev Mehrota, "Payment for Services Rendered—Updating Medicare's Valuation of Procedures," *New England Journal of Medicine* 382, no. 4 (January 23, 2020): 303–6, https://doi.org/10.1056/NEJMp1908706.

63. Leigh et al., "Physician Wages across Specialties."

64. C. Holly A. Andrilla et al., "Geographic Variation in the Supply of Selected Behavioral Health Providers," *American Journal of Preventive Medicine* 54, no. 6, suppl. 3 (June 2018): S199–S207, https://doi.org/10.1016/j.amepre.2018.01.004.

65. Kathleen Rowan, Donna D. McAlpine, and Lynn A. Blewett, "Access and Cost Barriers to Mental Health Care, by Insurance Status, 1999–2010," *Health Affairs* 32, no. 10 (October 2013): 1723–30, https://doi.org/10.1377/healthaff.2013.0133; "America's Mental Health 2018: Attitudes and Access to Care," Cohen Veterans Network, National Council for Behavioral Health, accessed May 20, 2020, https://www .cohenveteransnetwork.org/AmericasMentalHealth/.

66. Nelson D. Schwartz, "The Doctor Is In. Co-Pay? $40,000," *New York Times*, June 3, 2017, https://www.nytimes.com/2017/06/03/business/economy/high-end -medical-care.html.

67. Catherine S. Hwang et al., "Bridging to Value with Codes That Promote Care Management," *American Journal of Managed Care* 26, no. 11 (November 2020): e344–e346, https://www.doi.org/10.37765/ajmc.2020.88528; "What Is Medicare Chronic Care Management (CCM)?," American Academy of Family Physicians, accessed October 22, 2021, https://www.aafp.org/family-physician/practice-and -career/getting-paid/coding/chronic-care-management.html; Disha Patel, "New Reimbursement Codes You Can Use Now," ACP Internist, April 2020, https:// acpinternist.org/archives/2020/04/new-reimbursement-codes-you-can-use-now .htm; "How to Code for Chronic Care Management of Patients with One Disease," AAP News, August 1, 2020, https://www.aappublications.org/news/2020/08/01 /coding080120.

68. Mark Linzer et al., "Worklife and Wellness in Academic General Internal Medicine: Results from a National Survey," *Journal of General Internal Medicine* 31, no. 9 (September 2016): 1004–10, https://doi.org/10.1007/s11606-016-3720-4.

69. Sarah Grisham, "Medscape Physician Compensation Report 2017," April 5, 2017, https://www.medscape.com/slideshow/compensation-2017-overview -6008547#39.

70. World Health Organization, *Continuity and Coordination of Care: A Practice Brief to Support Implementation of the WHO Framework on Integrated People-Centered Health Services* (Geneva: WHO, 2018), 9.

71. Emily Friedman, "Public Hospitals Often Face Unmet Capital Needs, Underfunding, Uncompensated Patient-Care Costs," *JAMA* 257, no. 13 (April 3, 1987): 1698–701, https://doi.org/10.1001/jama.1987.03390130016003.

72. Richard Sandomir, "Dr. Davida Coady, Medical Missionary, Is Dead at 80," *New York Times*, May 11, 2018, https://www.nytimes.com/2018/05/11/obituaries/dr -davida-coady-public-health-activist-is-dead-at-80.html.

Dialogue #3

Student: It looks to me like a big part of the problem is doctors chasing the money. The system is set up to reward the ones who do that most efficiently. Your doctor friends who aren't that way are exceptions to the rule.

Professor: There are lots of doctors who are more interested in doing good than in making more money. I'll grant you that the opportunity to earn high incomes colors the choices many doctors make about their specialties. It also affects what they do for individual patients. We've documented that, but I feel like something is still missing here. What do you think?

Student: Maybe it isn't just about the money. Perhaps docs in specialties that mostly do procedures just like what they do. But we need to be careful. We don't want to let them off the hook, using career satisfaction as a rationalization. The lust for money sure looks like it's the root of much of the overuse in medicine.

Professor: No doubt, but don't jump to that conclusion too quickly. Your idea is a good one. Of course, money is a factor but surely not the only one. *Why* do they like what they do? We should figure out if anything else is going on. Perhaps some procedural doctors are more comfortable doing clearly defined tasks like passing a tube or cutting out a tumor than with the ambiguities and open-endedness of talking to patients about problems in the context of their lives.

Student: I guess that's possible, but how important could it be?

Professor: We won't know unless we explore that. Also, we haven't said anything about other aspects of practicing medicine that could be as satisfying as doing procedures. How could so-called cognitive care be a meaningful focus for a career?

Student: OK, I will look into that. I do see the relevance of those issues, but I'll be surprised if we find that they're as important as the economic rewards.

4

Procedural Proficiency or Human Connection?

Attitudes, Aptitudes, and Opportunities

Who is that on the other side of you?
—T. S. Eliot, "The Waste Land"

When I was a fourth-year medical student on a gynecology rotation, I was instructed to examine one of the patients, then report back to the resident physician. When I returned, I began with a brief history of the patient that included a description of her social circumstances. The resident interrupted me. "Below the waist and above the knees," he said.

The prospect of earning a lot of money decisively affects the choices that many physicians make and the ways in which they practice. At the same time, while many medical schools identify altruism, empathy, and genuine connectedness with patients as core values, these considerations seem to have less influence than the financial ones do upon the actions of their graduates. Achieving proficiency in technical tasks, such as procedures, can be challenging, but for many trainees, that may seem more achievable than the prospect of building meaningful relationships with patients. To understand fully the problems in health care today, we must look beyond financial motivations to other influences upon the practitioners. In reality, while some physicians are loving, empathic, and devoted to their patients, many others appear to lack the intrinsic characteristics, training, and inclination to be good at interacting with patients, much beyond obtaining their consent for, and cooperation during, a procedure. Why is that?

Ideology: "Words Fly Up, but Thoughts Remain Below"

Shakespeare, *Hamlet*, Act III, Scene 3

One influence upon clinicians is what might be called the implicit ideology of the profession. An ideology is a set of ideas or doctrines. Many groups form around a clearly delineated set of ideas. In others, like the medical profession, there may be less consensus about the core beliefs, and some of the ideology may be less explicit. When we consider some core values that the medical profession as a whole professes publicly, attentiveness to the patient's needs would seem to be one of the most important. Modern variants of the Hippocratic Oath, traditionally recited upon graduation from medical school, and more recently in so-called white coat ceremonies upon entrance (discussed in chapter 5), speak to idealistic commitment to patients and humankind as a whole.

In part, the classical version reads: "Whatever houses I may visit, I will come for the benefit of the sick, remaining free of all intentional injustice."[1] An updated version, adopted by the World Medical Association at its general assembly in Geneva in 1948, includes the following text: "I solemnly pledge myself to dedicate my life to the service of humanity . . . The health of my patients will be my first consideration."[2]

Although not explicit, there is an implication that the physician will provide what the patient needs and will not be primarily concerned with her or his own well-being. As we saw in chapter 3, physicians often fail to do this. The groups in which they practice regularly turn their backs on patients with the wrong insurance, incentivize their members to generate more revenue, and frown upon clinicians who take more time with each patient. This implicit *entrepreneurial ideology* overwhelms any residual commitment of many physicians to the flowery words of their oaths. In one survey of practicing physicians, only 26% indicated that their oaths had "a lot" of influence upon their medical practices (compared to 92% citing their personal sense of right and wrong).[3] To understand why this happens, we need to consider the innate and learned personality traits of the practitioners, their moral and ethical perspectives, their psychological challenges and needs, their awareness of the broader world, their sense of their own capabilities, and the influence of those with whom they associate.

Failure to Communicate

Many encounters with patients are complicated: patients can be difficult people. One needs to talk to them about sensitive issues in their lifestyles and aspects of their behaviors that are difficult to change, often because of the circumstances of their lives. Anyone can develop a serious health problem, and they are entitled to be informed about their prognosis and their options. Most people would want in such circumstances to talk to someone who is sensitive, empathic, and nonjudgmental.

Beyond those serious and unavoidable episodes, many people want and need little from their doctors. Others have needs but have difficulty communicating them. Still others are unaware of problems they are facing that pertain to their health, either because they are in denial or because they are oblivious. Yet others do not feel entitled to take the time of a physician to address their problems and concerns. When the physician does provide answers or advice, it is common for people not to understand what the doctor tells them, as they may be nervous or distracted, or they may not comprehend the words that are said.

To sort all of this out requires that a clinician show patience, be attuned to nonverbal cues, and be prepared to ask difficult, exploratory questions. Instead of doing that, many doctors barely listen to patients, and when they communicate with them, they may not make sure that they are well understood. In a pioneering study of doctor-patient communication, Barbara Korsch and her colleagues recorded 800 pediatric patient visits and analyzed the communication as well as the parents' perspectives on the interviews. They found that 24% of parents were not satisfied. In more than half of the cases, the pediatricians used difficult technical language. In the words of one participant, they "talked medical." Another asked someone to explain "in English" what the doctor had said.[4]

In another study, Beckman and Frankel reported in 1984 that patients had an opportunity to complete an opening statement about why they were there in only 23% of cases recorded.[5] A follow-up study 15 years later found little improvement: only 28% of patients were able to complete their opening statement. When they did interrupt, the doctors redirected the conversations after an average of 23.1 seconds.[6] It is not as though there has been no attention in medical training and in the medical literature to the importance of improving doctor-patient communication. Why have things not changed very much?

From what I have observed, while some physicians are interested and effective in engaging their patients in conversations about their experiences of illness, or about the context in which they deal with their illness, many others are not. There could be a number of reasons for this.

First, intellectually, much of the medical profession is closely allied with a kind of biological reductionism, where disease is biology. This stands in contradistinction to much social and psychological research on the interaction between biology, psychology, and social forces in producing disease. Like my resident supervisor in the gynecology clinic, many physicians and other providers do not consider social circumstances to be areas in which they need be expert. They only focus upon them when they are disruptive. Even then, the reaction may be to discard or avoid patients with such problems as dominating concerns.[7]

Medical training is directed at promoting certain kinds of curiosity. The focus upon the biological does not obliterate curiosity, but it can contribute to its misdirection. Instead of being curious about the patient's totality, many physicians tend to be searching for the interesting case, the rare diagnosis, or the unusual manifestation of a more common disorder. Up to a point, that is fine, but the pursuit of clinical "zebras" can be inefficient, and much else can be lost. By definition, this does not represent the reality of most patients, who are not "interesting cases" but nonetheless deserve the attention of the physician. It may also lead to physicians performing procedures or administering other treatments that prove to be harmful as "bodily cures" for problems that often are psychological, social, or environmental, even when evidence of any benefit is lacking.[8]

Biological reductionism also promotes intellectual narrowness of the specialties and subspecialties of medicine, which leads to emphasis on less than the whole (even of the biological system). The patient ceases to be a whole person, merely a focused clinical problem. This in turn reinforces a culture in which social context is ignored and care is dehumanized. While the gynecology resident who was supervising me was explicit and rather crass in this respect, much of the practice of specialty medicine has a gaze no broader than that.

The intellectual narrowness of super-specialized medicine is reflected in the extent to which clinicians attend medical conferences across specialty boundaries. In an academic medical center, there are regular conferences for each specialty: cardiology, gastroenterology, infectious diseases, nephrology, and so on. There also are conferences for the broader fields like internal medicine (so-called Grand Rounds). Some specialist physicians have wide-ranging interests, but most rarely attend talks on more diverse topics at Grand Rounds when they are outside of their specialty areas, and they almost never go to subspecialty conferences of other fields. Likewise, the national meetings that they attend are in their own specialized fields. All of this reflects what they think about and are interested in. Paul Beeson, a famous, beloved professor of medicine, told me that even after he had retired, he maintained his custom of always attending Grand Rounds, no matter the topic. That perspective is not widely shared. When the gaze of the specialist is limited to their particular discipline, it often falls far short of embracing the patient's humanity in its entirety.

A specialty or subspecialty often has a proprietary interest in a component of care, manifested through creation of rules about who can perform certain procedures or even take care of certain categories of patients in specialized hospital units. Along with procedural skills, the specialty may put little effort into sharing their specialized knowledge with other providers.[9] Even though experience is more important than certification for providing high quality of care,[10] depriving practitioners outside of the subspecialty of the opportunity for meaningful involvement in care of patients in certain clinical situations leads to atrophy or extinction of skills in that area, thereby solidifying the subspecialty's exclusive franchise.

Second, while many medical school admission committees attempt to account for the strength of applicants' interpersonal skills, including their ability to communicate and to empathize, these characteristics are far from determinative in the selection process, as discussed in chapter 5.[11] Many physicians have a narrow and limited appreciation for the world of their patients. They have little understanding of the relevance of history, culture, emotions, social forces, disadvantage, race and ethnicity, gender identity, and many other factors to the experience of their patients. The occasional course on medical anthropology or history may affect some students meaningfully, but it has little impact on most.[12] Numerous disciplines possess tools that have the potential to improve communication and empathy, and increase clinicians' comfort in clinical encounters, but they are rarely used.[13]

Third, providers may not connect with the emotional or social problems of their patients, precisely because they have unresolved personal issues that are aggravated by engaging patients with certain kinds of needs or problems. Some of these issues may be related to the stress of their jobs. Lack of resources to support the practitioner (as often is the case for physicians in the cognitive domains) may lead to burnout.[14] Another intrinsic stress of the jobs of physicians is "compassion fatigue," which can affect physicians who spend a great deal of time talking to patients who are in difficult situations or who have bleak futures. The caring physician may bear the brunt of that stress but may not always get the help that they need.[15]

Sandra was a good friend and colleague of mine who was in her late thirties. She was a wonderful clinical oncologist, ethical, industrious, smart, and devoted to her patients. One day she told me that she was depressed. I helped her identify a psychiatrist, who treated her with psychodynamic psychotherapy. It became clear that the trigger for Sandra's depression was having recently taken care of a series of women about her age with advanced breast cancer. It was difficult to set emotional limits when she identified closely with these women.[16] Through her therapy, Sandra came to understand the need to establish limits. She was able to accomplish that goal, and she recovered.

Some of what Sandra encountered might have been avoidable if there had been a mechanism in place to address stressors encountered in practice by the clinician. Figuring out how to give patients what they need without being sucked into a whirlpool of grieving can be a delicate balance. In Sandra's case, her ability to empathize was a great attribute, but it was also a threat to her well-being. In similarly fraught clinical situations, many doctors close themselves off from their patients' emotional needs.

One mechanism that can mitigate the impact of psychologically draining patients is "Balint groups." These were originally developed by psychoanalysts to help clinicians improve their relationships with patients, increase satisfaction, and diminish burnout. In these groups, one clinician presents a case and then listens to a discussion among the other clinicians about how to proceed. Such groups have had salutary effects but are not used widely in American medical practice outside of family medicine training programs.[17]

Jeffrey was an intern who was genteel but emotionally distant. Once a week, a psychiatrist named Herb Weiner joined our hospital rounds. Herb liked to explore psychological dimensions of care. The case on one occasion was a man seriously ill with three different kinds of cancer. The psychiatrist asked the patient how he was doing, and eventually engaged him in a discussion of his dreams. The patient reported that he dreamt he was in a house that was burning down. The psychiatrist asked him what it brought to mind. The patient said, "it makes me think that I want to be with my wife."

Jeffrey left the room abruptly at that point. He later called me to apologize. When I met with him, I asked him what had happened. He cried profusely. Eventually, it became clear that he was in an unhappy marriage. Jeffrey came to terms with that situation and eventually became much more open and empathic with his patients.

In cases like Jeffrey's, the stressor that limits the physician emanates from outside of the work environment, but it affects profoundly the ability to connect with patients in a meaningful way. On this occasion, Dr. Weiner, who was there nominally and substantively to engage in the patients' psychological issues, understood full well that the encounters would redound upon the other clinicians.

Not all physicians are fortunate enough to have a pedagogical experience that aids in the identification and resolution of emotional problems. Many of them need professional help but never get it. In one national survey of more than 5,000 physicians, nearly 40% indicated reluctance to seek treatment for an emotional problem because they worried about the effect of doing that on their medical licensure.[18] When such problems are not addressed, it is hard for physicians to take on the social and emotional challenges of their patients, and it can affect the quality of health care more broadly.[19]

Fourth, while most physicians have some instruction in communication skills development, it is rarely framed, taught, or evaluated formally in ways that are likely to have enduring impact. Consequently, many practitioners have little preparation for, experience in, or comfort with engaging in difficult conversations.[20]

When I was a resident, one of my colleagues recounted an episode that occurred in the coronary care unit at UCLA. A patient who had had a heart attack was distressed about his situation and reluctant to agree with the plan for care after discharge. The cardiologist supervising his care was unwilling to engage him in an extended discussion about what he would need to do after his life-changing event, beyond the usual, formulaic recommendations.

He told his residents, "That is a conversation for the general internist."

A survey of radiology residents who were attending a communication workshop revealed that prior to the training, 65% were uncomfortable about conveying information about risks to patients, and 55% were reluctant to discuss unexpected or "bad news." Comfort improved in the daylong session, but most wanted additional training.[21]

Some reluctance to engage in difficult conversations amounts to negligent delegation of responsibility. A particularly unfortunate practice occurs at the fateful moment when it is time to limit care for someone who is dying. When the medical team has access to an advance directive (in which a patient has indicated their care preferences regarding life-sustaining treatment), it usually is not a problem. But such a document is not always available, and even when it is, circumstances may evolve during a hospitalization. When it becomes clear that there is no further treatment to offer with meaningful potential to increase the quality and quantity of life, the medical team needs to have a discussion with the patient and/or family about the option of limiting care.

Far too often, this task is assigned to an intern, the most junior of the physicians on a clinical team, who has little experience with death and dying or with such conversations. Of all the conversations one can have with the patient and family, this is one of the most nuanced and complex. Just as heart surgery should not be left to a neophyte, the most experienced physicians need to be involved in end-of-life discussions. It is not surprising that some patients are resistant to the recommendation of a junior physician.[22] Of note, African American and Latino patients are less likely to accept such recommendations (which usually come from white physicians).[23]

Similarly, some patients who are being evaluated for liver transplants may be transferred from the liver service to a general medical service when a decision has been made that they are not eligible for the transplant, *without anyone from the transplant team telling them that they will not be getting the transplant.* When that occurs, sharing the bad news is left to the medical team, which has not known the patient up to that point. Likewise, while many oncologists do a good job of providing cancer patients with all of the information that they want to receive about their prognosis, others do not and continue to offer treatment when it is futile. Such abandonment may at times reflect indifference. It also may be a result of competing economic interests (as in oncology, where chemotherapy is a major source of income). In

many cases, it most likely reflects a shying away from these most difficult of conversations.

Fifth, the socioeconomic, racial, ethnic, and cultural differences between practitioners and their patients present substantial challenges to
meaningful engagement. Many physicians are not imbued with a
strong ethic of moral and social responsibility to establish and maintain
the well-being of their patients and of society as a whole as their highest
priority (or, at the very least, on par with their own well-being). They may
not make every effort to understand the problems of the disadvantaged
and treat them comparably to other patients.[24] Even when physicians are
motivated to listen to patients and help them on their journey, sociocultural distance can be a major problem. It is difficult to understand the
perspective of someone whose background differs from your own.

Medical schools and the profession underrepresent minority groups
and those who come from disadvantaged backgrounds. Accordingly, communication with these groups is less than satisfactory much of the time,
which likely contributes to disparities in the quality of care that they receive. A study of diabetics in California found that people who perceived
themselves to be of lower social position reported poorer interpersonal
processes of care. These included measures of a how often their personal health care provider listened carefully, showed respect, explained
clearly, spent enough time, involved patients in decisions, elicited trust,
and put patients' needs first.[25] Likewise, women of lower socioeconomic
status with breast cancer were less satisfied with the communication and
decision-making, which more often was based on incomplete information, relative to women of higher socioeconomic status.[26]

Sixth, many physicians have difficulty dealing with ambiguity, and
that affects their willingness to be open to psychosocial complexity. Those
choosing surgical careers appear to have a lower tolerance for ambiguity
than those planning careers in internal medicine.[27] A greater tolerance
for ambiguity in medical trainees is associated with better emotional
well-being, which, as noted above, makes the prospective practitioner
more amenable to relationships of some depth with patients.[28]

Such skills are essential when patients have multiple demands, are dependent or hostile, or exhibit self-destructive behavior. The challenge of engaging with such patients, rather than dreading or despising them, requires self-reflection, which not all students or physicians are prepared to undertake.[29]

These issues profoundly affect the practice of medicine. They also have important implications for undergraduate and postgraduate medical education. I will revisit some of these issues in chapters 5 and 6, when we consider the adequacy of the ways in which we select applicants to medical school and prepare them for their professional work.

Donna Zulman and her colleagues reviewed literature, interviewed practitioners, and observed practices, then assembled an expert panel to analyze and draw inferences from the evidence regarding how to improve the human connection in medical care. They produced five sensible recommendations:

1. Prepare with intention (pause and focus on the visit).
2. Listen completely, intently, and without interruptions.
3. Focus on what matters most to the patient.
4. Connect to the patient's story by considering their personal circumstances and acknowledging their efforts.
5. Explore emotional cues by discerning both verbal and nonverbal communication and asking questions to elicit their emotions.

The panel acknowledged that system-level interventions would be needed "to create a supportive environment for implementation."[30] This is a wonderful treatise on how doctors could connect with their patients, but many practitioners are unable or unprepared (or both) to implement these strategies, and the health systems for which they work are unlikely to respond positively to attempts to do so. While a checklist of sorts might help clinicians implement these recommendations more consistently, the additional time and effort required to incorporate these essential components into clinical encounters should be compensated through payment reform.

What the Caring Physician Has to Offer

Can practicing physicians make a difference in ways that matter? Are they so lost in their commodified business of medicine that they cannot be retrieved for more humane and meaningful interactions with patients? In chapter 3, I described some physicians who were not that way at all and were committed to making the world a better place. It is important not to say reflexively that physicians have to get their act together. They are products of a society, a health care system, and (as discussed in chap. 3) an educational system that predictably produces physicians who act in the ways that they do.

Nonetheless, there are opportunities for physicians to make small (or large) differences for individual patients, *should they choose to do so*. That is more likely to happen if they have some insight that there are problems to be addressed. While I was not caught up in the careerism and calculatedness of so many medical students, I was not particularly well equipped to meet the needs of my patients. A few salient experiences had an enormous effect on me.

First, as I recounted previously, my father died when I was a medical student, in large part because his doctor failed to pay attention to what he, my mother, and my sister told him about his level of disability. I vowed that rather than ignore my patients' experiences, I would focus on what mattered to them.

Second, I had some lingering emotional problems and entered psychoanalysis for several years. It was a powerful experience for me. I ceased to be afraid of my own feelings. I was then able to welcome the opportunity to explore the emotional needs, experiences, and inner lives of my patients, and I did not interpret their behaviors as affronts to me.

Third, I treated a patient with psychotherapy, under the supervision of a psychiatrist. During the 18 months or so that I was doing that, I learned a lot about the doctor-patient relationship and about the limits of what the doctor can accomplish in it.

I came to realize that there are things that doctors can do to support their patients in their crises without opening the floodgates to spending endless hours with them or ordering all kinds of unnecessary medical services. Many people have needs that are primarily products of their medical conditions. Others have needs that represent an interplay between medical illnesses and other complexities in their lives. These represent wonderful opportunities for physicians and other medical providers really to make a difference in a positive way.

Here are examples of some things I have done to help patients along in their journeys. Many other doctors could describe similar situations. I treasured all of these encounters and expected nothing more in return for what I did. Being a physician is a privilege. We have the opportunity to improve people's lives. Doing so can consume considerable intellectual and emotional energy and lots of time. The skills involved are no less complex and no less vital than the ones involved in passing catheters into the heart, removing cataracts, or replacing knees. In this context, we ought to consider the personal characteristics of the physicians who should be attending to these situations, and the structure of the incentives, to encourage such engagement. In fee-for-service medicine, physicians are paid far more for technical acts than for actual caring.

"Rage against the Dying of the Light"
Dylan Thomas, "Do Not Go Gentle into That Good Night"

Tanya was a ballet dancer in her youth in Eastern Europe. When I met her, she was in her late fifties and in pretty good health. She called me "honey" and regaled me with stories of a life much more interesting than my own. Tanya showered me with gifts, cologne, and throw pillows that she knitted herself. The cologne had a nice bouquet, but I was not a cologne guy. Nonetheless, I dutifully expressed my appreciation each time she added to my stockpile.

One day, when I had been caring for her for about 10 years, I felt a mass in Tanya's lower abdomen. It turned out she had uterine cancer, and it was metastatic. She had a resection and chemotherapy but lived less than a year. Tanya was upbeat and determined to conquer it. Only in the last two weeks did she acknowledge the hopelessness of her situation. She then became hostile toward me, saying that her imminent death was my fault, and that she hated me and never wanted to talk to me again. From a distance, I helped her family manage her terminal care.

Our last words were not pleasant ones, yet my recollections of Tanya are only affectionate. She needed to be angry with someone, and I was the most reasonable target. In psychologic terms, such transference and countertransference (projection of emotions on another) occur to some degree in almost every medical encounter. Godspeed, Tanya.

I'm Not Crazy: Write It Down

Marlene, who was in her mid-forties, came to my clinic on a Friday afternoon complaining of a terrible headache. The nurse alerted me that her blood pressure was very high. When I measured it on a mercury sphygmomanometer, the systolic blood pressure (the top number) was more than the maximum reading of 308 mm on the device. The lower number was over 180 mm. This was a dangerous blood pressure level that could cause a catastrophic complication, like a brain hemorrhage, at any moment.

"You need to go to the hospital," I told her.

"I am not going to the hospital. I have been treated badly in the hospital," she responded.

"Your blood pressure is dangerously high; you could die."

"I will take pills. I won't go to the hospital."

The clinic staff gave Marlene medicine by mouth that lowered her blood pressure to under 200. I wrote a prescription and asked her to come back on Monday but implored her to take all of the pills that I prescribed.

"I can't afford the medicine. I don't have any money, and MediCal [California Medicaid] won't let me fill another prescription this month."

I walked her over to the pharmacy, paid for her prescription, and got her to agree to show up on Monday. When she did, her blood pressure was still elevated but improving. Over time, it became clear to me that something was a little off about Marlene. She asked me to give her a copy of everything that I had written down and to document in the chart that she was not crazy. I did that. She also told me that she thought that the real cause of her headaches was the neighbor emitting lasers that came in through the wall of her apartment and entered her head. I recognized this as a delusion and knew not to challenge it, since my priority was to keep her blood pressure down.

I never did control Marlene's blood pressure to my satisfaction. She took some of the medicine, but not all of it. Still, her blood pressure was only a little elevated most of the time. She missed most of her appointments. The clinic manager suggested that we dismiss her from the clinic because of her no-shows. I could not do it, knowing what the consequences would be. When she did show up, she often arrived late. She always asked for documentation that she was not crazy.

This went on for many years. Marlene constantly complained about her neighbor. When she once said that she would have to kill him, I called a police officer at the station near her home. (She had given me his name and number.) The police officer knew Marlene and referred to her as "the laser lady." He reassured me that she was harmless.

One day, she showed up in my clinic with a box. It was a gift for me, some shirts and ties.

"Why are you giving this to me?" I asked.

"Read the card."

It said that I had saved her life and kept her going for 25 years.

Marlene eventually died of complications of long-standing hypertension, but I felt like I had done a good thing, even though there was lots of frustration with her tardiness, noncompliance with appointments, and failure to adhere to her medicines. She had a chronic mental illness that limited her life. She came to me for support, not just treatment of her hypertension, and from her perspective, not really for that at all.

Medical Care Doesn't Help

Leonard was a 28-year-old man who came to me with chest pain and swelling in the lymph nodes in his neck. He was a political operative, energetic, intelligent, and apparently effective in his job. I obtained a chest x-ray that showed a large mass in his mediastinum, the space between the lungs that also holds the heart. I had a strong intuition as to what was wrong. A large mediastinal mass is a classical presentation of Hodgkin disease, a lymph cancer common in young adults. Additional tests identified some lesions in his pelvic bones, making him Stage 4A.

I referred Leonard to an excellent medical oncologist, who obtained the confirmatory biopsy and informed him of his situation. He needed two forms of treatment: radiation of the lesion in the chest and chemotherapy to eradicate the rest of the disease. Leonard's younger brother had died recently of complications of diabetes. He was terrified. He also had a high degree of skepticism about medical therapies and medical authorities, and he was articulate in explaining why they should not be trusted. He resolved to seek alternative forms of treatment for the disease. I worried that he would bolt.

Hodgkin disease is fatal if untreated, but a large proportion of cases can be cured, even at an advanced stage. I met with him to talk it over. Leonard was not going to be easy to convince. I found several articles on Hodgkin and its prognosis. We read them over together. I then took him to the pathology department, and we reviewed the slides from his lymph node biopsy with the pathologist.

Eventually, Leonard came to understand that although his situation was serious, he was likely to benefit enormously from the treatment. He negotiated. Why radiation and chemo? Because the chemo could not penetrate the large mass adequately. Why not just radiation? Because it would not get the other lesions. How much chemo? The recommendation was 12 months including two regimens.

Leonard was skeptical but he said that he would proceed. As his treatment went on, I phoned him frequently to see how it was going, and to make sure that he was not going to bail out. He had moments of uncertainty, but he persisted. Finally, he asked if he would need the full 12 months of chemo. I agreed that it would be reasonable to get a second opinion. He saw a doctor at another hospital, and she advised him that 8 or 9 months of treatment should be enough.

Leonard completed the course. Throughout his treatment, I had an initial visit with him, then a couple more of formal visits to talk things over, but most of the time that I spent with him—reading articles, reviewing slides, talking about sticking with the treatment, and so on—was not in visits for which I billed. The oncologist and radiation therapist charged for each visit, and their departments were paid for the treatments administered.

I did not consider myself to have been underpaid for what I did. I know that my interventions saved his life. The diagnosis was the easy part. Being there for him, understanding his anguish and doubt, supporting him until he had had enough treatment to maximize his chances of cure, all were essential. I felt gratified about what I had done. The system of reimbursement rewards the specialist substantially for what he or she does. I likely was paid one-tenth, or even less, of what the cancer doctors and their departments received.

Leonard was appreciative of my efforts. For the next 25 years, he called me from his new home in another city on the anniversary of the date of his diagnosis to thank me yet again. On those occasions, we talked at length about what he was doing with the life that medical treatment had helped to preserve. When he developed another malignancy and was dying in hospital, we spoke again, and he made a point of expressing his appreciation for the extra time that I had helped him obtain.

This man was terrified. He needed hope and comfort, but he also needed evidence, shared with him in a way that he could fully grasp, that he need not die as his brother had so recently. He also needed a physician who was willing to spend the time needed to accomplish that.

I Feel Like I Am Your Only Patient

I met Larry when he was 33. He was my first clinic patient with AIDS. Larry was referred relatively early in the epidemic by another doctor for fever and an abnormal chest x-ray, which revealed that he had pneumocystis pneumonia. Larry was gay and had had few sexual encounters in his life. He approached his situation with courage and determination to use his time well. Zidovudine (the first drug shown to improve survival in AIDS) had become available, so I prescribed it for him. Larry's condition worsened. Didanosine (DDI) was licensed. He took it but nearly died from pancreatitis. He developed a progressive myelopathy (disease of the spinal cord) that caused paralysis of his legs. All the while, he continued his work as a graduate student and successfully defended his PhD dissertation.

Larry lived three more years before dying quietly at home, surrounded by a loving community, many of whom were in a church choir with him. I felt so helpless when I saw him. It seemed wrong that there was not more that I could do. HIV became a major focus of my research, and I often thought about Larry when formulating research questions. I always enjoyed listening to stories about his life.

A friend of his later told me that when Larry was with me, he felt like he was my only patient. I am glad that he felt that way. It made me want to be more attentive to every patient. I went to Larry's funeral, a sad but wonderful event in which his fellow choir members poured out their hearts in loving song, and speakers talked about what a bright light he was in the world, right up to the end. It felt good to help.

Publish the Book Now

Eve and Dick had been married since just after college and now were in their seventies. She was a nurse and he was a professor. They had mostly minor health problems. One day, Dick mentioned that Eve was having some trouble with numbers, mixing them up. I did a cognitive assessment. She had other abnormalities on my screening test. I obtained a neurology consultation, and my colleague confirmed that Eve had frontal lobe dementia. It was not severe at that point, but it was not trivial either. I knew that Eve had been working on a memoir for a number of years. After discussing the diagnosis with her and Dick, and knowing the uncertainty of the time course ahead, I suggested that it would be good to wrap up the book soon. I continued to monitor her condition. When the manifestations of Eve's condition became more pronounced, I told them that she had to stop driving.

As symptoms continued to progress more rapidly than we had hoped, I had a conversation with Dick. I had just seen the film *Iris*, about the life of the writer Iris Murdoch, including her decline and eventual death from dementia. According to the film, when her final book was published and a box of copies arrived at her home, she opened the box and did not realize that they were copies of a book that she had written. I told Dick that it was urgent to publish the book while Eve still recognized the work as her own. They did that, and then threw a party to celebrate the self-publishing of the book. They gave me a signed copy. A couple of years later, when Eve was admitted to the hospital with a complication of dementia, I was able to talk to the family about appropriately limiting care. Dick was heartbroken to lose her, but they had achieved some closure.

In the introduction to her book, Eve acknowledges that she has "started to lose some memory" and states, "My life has been an amazing journey and I would like this memoir to be an acknowledgement of who I am and whom I have influenced, or impacted, in my lifetime."[31] In this case, the key intervention wasn't clinical. It was the application of a clinical insight, in the context of a progressive illness, in order to reframe the disease's progression and achieve an important, life-enhancing goal.

Pallbearer

Frank was in his early forties and lived with his mother. Curiously, he always wanted his mother to come into the examining room with him. He was obese and had high blood pressure but no other obvious problems. Frank had never had a job. He was a gentle soul. I tried unsuccessfully to get him to lose weight, but I was able to manage his blood pressure pretty well. My major accomplishment was something else. Eventually, I was able to help him to overcome his anxiety and come into the examining room with me while his mother stayed in the waiting room.

One day, I had a call from an emergency department. Frank had sustained a cardiac arrest and tragically had died. I felt terrible. I called his mother and went over to her place to pay condolences. I was surprised when she asked me to be a pallbearer at his funeral. They needed a full contingent because he was so heavy. I agreed to go. It was a small funeral, with just a few friends and relatives, but it was dignified, and everyone there cared deeply about Frank.

When I returned to work after the funeral, a resident who would go on to a career in cardiology commented on my attire, which was more formal than usual. I told him where I had been.

"A doctor should never go to a patient's funeral," he said. "We are supposed to keep our professional distance."

I told him that I strongly disagreed, that we have a responsibility to be available to patients and their families in times of need. A few years later, he contacted me when he saw an article about physicians attending funerals. He acknowledged that maybe I had a point.[32]

Home for Christmas

Raymond was a 65-year-old man who smoked and developed lung cancer. He was inoperable at diagnosis and received some radiation therapy. The disease began to progress, metastasizing to his brain, and it was clear that he would die soon. He wanted to be with his family. I arranged for him to receive care at home. Raymond was not too stable, so I visited him every other day for several weeks in a part of town that I had not visited before. His home was cluttered with the artifacts of his life, and I learned much more about him by visiting him there. His wife, kids, and grandkids were around. Raymond would smile at me, but he said little during my visits.

Eventually, as expected, he died at home, just before Christmas. I expressed my sympathy to the family and felt pretty good about what I had done to ensure a good death. The next year, on the anniversary of his passing, Raymond's wife called and told me how much it had meant to them for him to be able to die at home. She appreciated my efforts and my visits. Twenty years later, I saw her name on a hospital room door. I went in and reintroduced myself. We hugged. I cried.

At that moment, I realized that the process of getting Raymond home and facilitating that "good death" was profoundly important to me emotionally, just as it was to his wife. Often, medicine is practiced as though death is an enemy to be forever vanquished rather than an inevitable part of life. Although some doctors take the time to explore how individuals want their lives to end, many do not. Yes, there are the so-called goals of care conversations (discussed earlier in this chapter) in which patients may be asked whether they want cardiopulmonary resuscitation, long-term intubation, and other things that may be done to delay death when there is little hope. Such conversations can be rather artificial (even if not conducted by an intern who is meeting the patient for the first time). Engaging a patient in such a discussion is complex, and their feelings and thoughts about it may be multilayered.

A young physician who works at Memorial Sloan Kettering Cancer Center in New York recently undertook an effort to build a "values tab" in their electronic medical record. She consulted scores of medical providers and many patients and their families to learn about all the things that could be included, not just about preferences for cardiopulmonary resuscitation, but also information about their values, priorities, and much more.[33] What a wonderful mission! There is hope it will improve care by increasing awareness of the patients' perspectives among care providers and giving patients a more appropriate mix of what they want and what they need or, as my patient Eve wrote in her memoir, constituting an acknowledgment of who they are.

I Don't Want to Be in Pain

I saw Richard only about five times in my clinic. He was 37 years old, and our first visit was on the day before Thanksgiving. He had been throwing up and unable to keep down any solid foods for five days. On examination, I felt a mass in his upper abdomen. His pulse, blood pressure, and laboratory tests were normal, so he was not dehydrated. It was late in the afternoon, but I was able to arrange an emergency computed tomography (CT) scan. It showed what looked like a tumor in the duodenum, the first part of the small intestine. I called a surgeon, explaining the urgency. He agreed to see him on Monday. The diagnosis was not certain, so I cautiously told Richard that there was a problem in his small intestine and that he was going to see a surgeon about fixing it in five days.

I encouraged him to go home and enjoy Thanksgiving with his family, but restrict himself to fluids and come to the emergency department if he had trouble keeping fluids down. I saw him again before surgery, which found cancer in the duodenum and in one lymph node nearby. I saw him again a couple of times after he started his chemotherapy.

About a year later, Richard came to see me again. He had lost weight. He was in constant pain. He was continuing chemotherapy, but it was not helping. He loved his family, including three young children. He was struggling with his situation.

"What do you want to do?" I asked.

"I don't want to be in pain anymore."

I told him that he could get stronger medicine for pain, but he was on a great deal already, and Richard did not want to take anything else.

I advised Richard that if he felt that he had reached his limit of tolerance, it would be all right to stop his cancer treatment. He could get palliative treatment to keep him comfortable. He left without saying how he would proceed, but I learned that he did stop active cancer treatment and opted to receive palliative care at that point.

Much later, I happened to meet Richard's mother. She said that the last conversation I had with Richard was extremely helpful. His family had not wanted to see him suffer anymore, but he needed permission from a doctor whom he trusted to make the decision that he wanted to make.

A doctor does not get paid much for a handful of outpatient visits. This man's illness was heartbreaking. I earned far less than the surgeon who operated on him, the oncologist who gave him chemotherapy, or even the anesthesiologist who spent perhaps two hours with him in the operating room. Yet I felt amply recompensed for what I did. Getting Richard diagnosed rapidly, letting him spend a final Thanksgiving with his family before beginning his cancer treatment, and helping him make the decision that he needed to make at the end gave me a sense of doing my job. He knew that I cared, and he trusted me.

Few would argue that patients like this man need compassion and empathic treatment, but so do many people whose dis-eases are not primarily anatomic, physiologic, or biochemical disorders. The health care system does not reward compassion. It pays for procedures. It is true that the physician cannot fix individual social or broader societal problems, but the physician can always be a heart in a world that has dealt a bad hand to their patient. This is an imperative, whatever the reimbursement mechanism.

Shall We Dance?

Florence first came to my clinic during my fellowship when she was 66, and I cared for her for more than 25 years. She had osteoarthritis of both knees, hypertension, and mild congestive heart failure. I saw her through two knee replacements, a lumpectomy and treatment for breast cancer, a pacemaker, and a bad scare with weight loss and what appeared to be an irregular mass in her pancreas. (She declined surgery or biopsy and was resigned to her fate until the alleged mass disappeared.)

Florence came to clinic each time with a different grandchild. Her daughter, who used to bring her in, died of lung cancer. She told me that you never get over the loss of child. She had strong political views, and we talked about politics a lot. She asked me to help her stay alive so that she could vote for her candidate in the next federal election. She always asked about my kids, and I asked about her grandkids. Once, when she was ill and feeling weak, Florence seemed disheartened by her recent decline. I wanted to lift her spirits, so I offered to dance with her around the examining room. She accepted, and felt better after that. There isn't always something that can be done clinically to change the patient's course, but nonmedical procedures may make a difference. We had a good time whenever she gave me the gift of a visit to my office.

Let Him Stay There

Charles was a delight. In his early eighties, he had spent a lifetime working on passenger trains. He had great stories about his work. I always looked forward to seeing him. He had some medical problems fairly typical for a man in his early eighties: hypertension that was well controlled and a history of prostate and colon cancer that had not recurred. At one point, he lost several pounds, and I thought that I felt a solid mass in his abdomen. A scan was suspicious for a tumor. I suggested a biopsy, but Charles was apparently channeling the philosophy and wisdom of Archie Cochrane.

"You ain't cuttin' on me no more," he insisted, "so I don't need the test."

Well, that was clarifying. I enthusiastically supported his decision, and the mass never gave him any trouble (if it really was a mass). One complication was his adoring children. They were worried about Charles. A widower of late, he had been spending some time at the house of a woman friend. His kids called me up. They said that they felt that his health was precarious and that he should not be spending time with that woman. They worried it could be bad for his heart. I disappointed them. I conveyed my opinion that if visiting her is something Charles wanted to do, he should do it. I also told them that I did not think that visiting her would affect his heart any more than staying home. They accepted my judgment, and he continued to make those visits. As in this case, sometimes the most important things that a doctor can prescribe have nothing to do with disease at all.

The Best Materials

Marshall was in his mid-nineties when I became his physician. He was a distinguished individual in the university, and I had known him since my first year on the faculty. I was pleased that he had asked me to care for him. He had severe aortic valve stenosis, and the symptoms had progressed rapidly in the months before I took on his care. He was able to take only a few steps before sitting down. His echocardiogram showed "critical" stenosis. We discussed the possibility of replacing his aortic valve through a catheter inserted into an artery in his groin, and he was game.

We consulted a cardiologist. I accompanied Marshall to the visit, to make sure that he was presented with the information in an evenhanded way and was able to understand what was being communicated. The cardiologist was terrific. He strongly supported going ahead, but he explained the options and potential outcomes. Marshall opted to get it done, tolerated the procedure well, and returned home after a few days.

While his function improved, he could not be out of bed for more than a couple of hours a day. His mind was sharp. He took great interest in academics, in sports, and in politics. He was clear that he wanted no further procedures and really did not want to go into the hospital again.

I saw Marshall frequently at his home, which was in my neighborhood. It was too hard for him to get to the hospital clinic, even though he had full-time caregivers who could transport him. When I would go over to his place, I would encourage him to walk, sometimes dragging him out of bed. But we spent most of the time just talking: about the Dodgers, the presidential election, his family, the university, literature, and much more. We found that we both liked the poet-physician Oliver Wendell Holmes. (He had Holmes's complete works.) We talked about some of the poems. For both of us, "The Deacon's Masterpiece" was our favorite.

Marshall died peacefully at home. The university planned a memorial service for him, and I was surprised to be asked to be one of the speakers. At the event, several senior faculty members spoke about the great things he had done, and in some cases how he had influenced their careers. I talked about him as a person, speaking about his values, his dreams, and the choices that he had made along the way. As his physician, I had gotten to know Marshall in a special way. I talked about the Holmes poem that he loved, about a man who collects the best materials to build a carriage that lasts 100 years. I reworked the description in the poem to describe what I thought about this man, who was wonderful in so many ways. Being a physician who is present and attentive can be an opportunity to gain profound insights into the person behind the patient. It was a privilege to know him, to be his physician, and to talk about him as I knew him.

I cherished all of these patients, and I believe that I made a difference for each of them. It didn't always change their life trajectory, but it did make a difference regarding what happened along the way. I also feel that I became a better person by being their doctor, as imperfect as I was in some ways.

Many doctors try to be there for their patients in these ways. Why can't all physicians respond to their patients with compassion, and even with love, and address their concerns with empathy and not primarily with procedures? In chapters 5 and 6, we will explore how medical education is a deterrent to that.

Notes

1. Edelstein, Ludwig, trans., "Hippocratic Oath—Classical Version," in *The Hippocratic Oath: Text, Translation, and Interpretation* (Baltimore: Johns Hopkins Press, 1943).

2. "WMA Declaration of Geneva," World Medical Association, accessed October 22, 2021, https://www.wma.net/policies-post/wma-declaration-of-geneva/.

3. Ryan M. Antiel et al., "The Impact of Medical School Oaths and Other Professional Codes of Ethics: Results of a National Physician Survey," *Archives of Internal Medicine* 171, no. 5 (March 14, 2011): 469–71, https://doi.org/10.1001/archinternmed.2011.47.

4. Barbara M. Korsch, Ethel K. Gozzi, and Vida Francis, "Gaps in Doctor-Patient Communication: I. Doctor-Patient Interaction and Patient Satisfaction," *Pediatrics* 42, no. 5 (November 1968): 855–71, PMID 5685370.

5. Howard B. Beckman and Richard M. Frankel, "The Effect of Physician Behavior on the Collection of Data," *Annals of Internal Medicine* 101, no. 5 (November 1984): 692–96, https://doi.org/10.7326/0003-4819-101-5-692.

6. M. Kim Marvel et al., "Soliciting the Patient's Agenda: Have We Improved?," *JAMA* 281, no. 3 (January 1999): 283–87, https://doi.org/10.1001/jama.281.3.283.

7. Leon Eisenberg and Arthur Kleinman, "Clinical Social Science," in *The Relevance of Social Science for Medicine*, ed. Leon Eisenberg and Arthur Kleinman (Dordrecht: D. Reidel, 1981), 1–23; Hilary Daniel et al., "Addressing Social Determinants to Improve Patient Care and Improve Health Equity: An American College of Physicians Position Paper," *Annals of Internal Medicine* 168, no. 8 (April 17, 2018): 577–78, https://doi.org/10.7326/M17-2441.

8. Joel Braslow, *Mental Ills and Bodily Cures: Psychiatric Treatment in the First Half of the Twentieth Century* (Berkeley: University of California Press, 1997), 1–13, 171–75; Rebecca Lemov, "Brainwashing's Avatar: The Curious Career of Dr. Ewen

Cameron," *Grey Room* 45 (2011): 61–87, https://doi.org/10.1162/GREY_a_00050; Barron H. Lerner, "Last-Ditch Medical Therapy—Revisiting Lobotomy," *New England Journal of Medicine* 353, no. 2 (July 14, 2005): 119–21, https://doi.org/10.1056/NEJMp048349; Robert Freudenthal and Joanna Moncrieff, "'A Landmark in Psychiatric Progress'? The Role of Evidence in the Rise and Fall of Insulin Coma Therapy," *History of Psychiatry* 33, no. 1 (2022): 65–78, https://doi.org/10.1177/0957154X211062538.

9. George Weisz, *Divide and Conquer: A Comparative History of Medical Specialization* (Oxford: Oxford University Press, 2005), 20.

10. Bruce E. Landon et al., "Physician Specialization and Antiretroviral Therapy for HIV," *Journal of General Internal Medicine* 18, no. 4 (April 2003): 233–41, https://doi.org/10.1046/j.1525-1497.2003.20705.x; Bruce E. Landon et al., "Physician Specialization and the Quality of Care for Human Immunodeficiency Virus Infection," *Archives of Internal Medicine* 165, no. 10 (May 2005): 1133–39, https://doi.org/10.1001/archinte.165.10.1133.

11. Jodi Halpern, "What Is Clinical Empathy?," *Journal of General Internal Medicine* 18, no. 8 (August 2003): 670–74, https://doi.org/10.1046/j.1525-1497.2003.21017.x; Melanie Neumann et al., "Empathy Decline and Its Reasons: A Systematic Review of Studies with Medical Students and Residents," *Academic Medicine* 86, no. 8 (August 2011): 996–1009, https://doi.org/10.1097/ACM.0b013e318221e615; Daniel C. R. Chen et al., "Characterizing Changes in Student Empathy throughout Medical School," *Medical Teacher* 34, no. 4 (March 2012): 305–11, https://doi.org/10.3109/0142159x.2012.644600; Lisa M. Bellini and Judy A. Shea, "Mood Change and Empathy Decline Persist during Three Years of Internal Medicine Training," *Academic Medicine* 80, no. 2 (February 2005): 164–67, https://doi.org/10.1097/00001888-200502000-00013.

12. Max J. Romano, "White Privilege in a White Coat: How Racism Shaped My Medical Education," *Annals of Family Medicine* 16, no. 3 (May 2018): 261–63, https://doi.org/10.1370/afm.2231; Elizabeth N. Chapman, Anna Kaatz, and Molly Carnes, "Physicians and Implicit Bias: How Doctors May Unwittingly Perpetuate Health Care Disparities," *Journal of General Internal Medicine* 28, no. 11 (November 2013): 1504–10, https://doi.org/10.1007/s11606-013-2441-1.

13. Jodi Halpern, "Empathy and Patient-Physician Conflicts," *Journal of General Internal Medicine* 22, no. 5 (May 2007): 696–700, https://doi.org/10.1007/s11606-006-0102-3; Rita Charon, "The Patient-Physician Relationship. Narrative Medicine: A Model for Empathy, Reflection, Profession, and Trust," JAMA 286, no. 15 (October 2001): 1897–902, https://doi.org/10.1001/jama.286.15.1897.

14. Shailesh Kumar, "Burnout and Doctors: Prevalence, Prevention and Intervention," *Healthcare (Basel)* 4, no. 3 (June 30, 2016): 37, https://doi.org/10.3390/health care4030037.

15. Nurit El-Bar et al., "Compassion Fatigue, Burnout and Compassion Satisfaction among Family Physicians in the Negev Area—a Cross-Sectional Study," *Israel Journal of Health Policy Research* 2, no. 1 (August 2013): 31, https://doi.org/10.1186/2045

-4015-2-31; Seema Jilani, "Why So Many Doctors Treat Their Mental Health in Secret," *New York Times*, March 30, 2022, https://www.nytimes.com/2022/03/30 /opinion/doctors-mental-health-stigma.html.

16. Sean Stitham makes a related point, noting the reluctance of young physicians at times to take care of young patients who are seriously ill. "Merging Mortalities," *New England Journal of Medicine* 384, no. 22 (June 3, 2021): 2078–79, https://doi .org/10.1056/NEJMp2033580.

17. Marty Player et al., "The Role of Balint Group Training in the Professional and Personal Development of Family Medicine Residents," *International Journal of Psychiatry in Medicine* 53, no. 1–2 (January–March 2018): 24–38, https://doi.org/10 .1177/0091217417745289; Michael Balint, *The Doctor, His Patient and the Illness*, 2nd ed. (Edinburgh: Churchill Livingstone, 1964; repr., 1986).

18. Liselotte N. Dyrbye et al., "Medical Licensure Questions and Physician Reluctance to Seek Care for Mental Health Conditions," *Mayo Clinic Proceedings* 92, no. 10 (October 2017): 1486–93, https://doi.org/10.1016/j.mayocp.2017.06.020; Jilani, "Why So Many Doctors."

19. Jean E. Wallace, Jane B. Lemaire, and William A. Ghali, "Physician Wellness: A Missing Quality Indicator," *Lancet* 374, no. 9702 (November 14, 2009): 1714–21, https://doi.org/10.1016/S0140-6736(09)/61424-0.

20. Gregory Makoul, "Communication Skills Education in Medical School and Beyond," *JAMA* 289, no. 1 (January 1, 2003): 93, https://doi.org/10.1001/jama.289.1 .93; Charlotte Rees, Charlotte Sheard, and Susie Davies, "The Development of a Scale to Measure Medical Students' Attitudes toward Communication Skills Learning: The Communication Skills Attitude Scale (CSAS)," *Medical Education* 236, no. 2 (February 2002): 141–47, https://doi.org/10.1046/j.1365-2923.2002.01072.x; David M. Browning et al., "Difficult Conversations in Health Care: Cultivating Relational Learning to Address the Hidden Curriculum," *Academic Medicine* 82, no. 9 (September 2007): 905–13, https://doi.org/10.1097/ACM.0b013e31812f77b9; Elisabeth MacDonald, *Difficult Conversations in Medicine* (Oxford: Oxford University Press, 2004); Richard P. Gunderman and Peter R. Gunderman, "Forty Years Since 'Taking Care of the Hateful Patient,'" *AMA Journal of Ethics* 19, no. 4 (April 2017): 369–73, https://doi.org/10.1001/journalofethics.2017.19.4.nlit1-1704; Halpern, "Empathy and Patient-Physician Conflicts."

21. Stephen D. Brown et al., "Radiology Trainees' Comfort with Difficult Conversations and Attitudes about Error Disclosure: Effect of a Communication Skills Workshop," *Journal of the American College of Radiology* 11, no. 8 (August 2014): 781–87, https://doi.org/10.1016/j.jacr.2014.01.018.

22. Lorraine M. Stone and James A. Tulsky, "Discussing Code Status with Patients and Their Families," *Virtual Mentor* 8, no. 9 (September 2006): 559–63, https://doi.org/10.1001/virtualmentor.2006.8.9.ccas1-0609; Elizabeth Dzeng et al., "Influence of Institutional Culture and Policies on Do-Not-Resuscitate Decision Making at the End of Life," *JAMA Internal Medicine* 175, no. 5 (May 2015): 812–19, https://doi.org/10.1001/jamainternmed.2015.0295.

23. Laura B. Shepardson et al., "Racial Variation in the Use of Do-Not-Resuscitate Orders," *Journal of General Internal Medicine* 14, no. 1 (January 1999): 15–20, https://doi.org/10.1046/j.1525-1497.1999.00275.x.

24. Howard S. Becker and Blanche Geer, "The Fate of Idealism in Medical School," *American Sociological Review* 23, no. 1 (February 1958): 50–56; Catherine Thomasson, "Physicians' Social Responsibility," *Virtual Mentor* 16, no. 9 (September 2014): 753–57, https://doi.org/10.1001/virtualmentor.2014.16.09.oped1-1409; Christine Loignon et al., "Physicians' Social Competence in the Provision of Care to Persons Living in Poverty: Research Protocol," *BMC Health Services Research* 10 (2010): 79, https://doi.org/10.1186/1472-6963-10-79; Alicia Fernandez et al., "Physician Language Ability and Cultural Competence: An Exploratory Study of Communication with Spanish-Speaking Patients," *Journal of General Internal Medicine* 19, no. 2 (February 2004): 167–74, https://doi.org/10.1111/j.1525-1497.2004.30266.x; Els L. M. Maeckelberghe and Peter Schröder-Bäck, "Ethics in Public Health: Call for Shared Moral Public Health Literacy," *European Journal of Public Health* 27, suppl. 4 (October 10, 2017): 49–51, https://doi.org/10.1093/eurpub/ckx154; Barbara Herman, *Moral Literacy* (Cambridge, MA: Harvard University Press, 2007).

25. David Moskowitz et al., "Patient Reported Interpersonal Processes of Care and Perceived Social Position: The Diabetes Study of Northern California (DISTANCE)," *Patient Education and Counseling* 90, no. 3 (March 2013): 392–98, https://doi.org/10.1016/j.pec.2011.07.019.

26. Marie-Anne Durand et al., "What Matters Most: Protocol for a Randomized Controlled Trial of Breast Cancer Surgery Encounter Decision Aids across Socioeconomic Strata," *BMC Public Health* 18, no. 1 (February 2018): 241, https://doi.org/10.1186/s12889-018-5109-2.

27. Gail Geller, Ruth R. Faden, and David M. Levine, "Tolerance for Ambiguity among Medical Students: Implications for Their Selection, Training and Practice," *Social Science and Medicine* 31, no. 5 (1990): 619–24, https://doi.org/10.1016/0277-9536(90)90098-d; Jason Hancock et al., "Medical Student and Junior Doctors' Tolerance of Ambiguity: Development of a New Scale," *Advances in Health Sciences Education Theory and Practice* 20, no. 1 (2015): 113–30, https://doi.org/10.1007/s10459-014-9510-z.

28. Jason Hancock and Karen Mattick, "Tolerance of Ambiguity and Psychological Well-Being in Medical Training: A Systematic Review," *Medical Education* 54, no. 2 (February 2020): 125–37, https://doi.org/10.1111/medu.14031.

29. James E. Groves, "Taking Care of the Hateful Patient," *New England Journal of Medicine* 298, no. 16 (April 20, 1978): 883–87, https://doi.org/10.1056/NEJM197804202981605; S. Smith, "Dealing with the Difficult Patient," *Postgraduate Medical Journal* 71, no. 841 (November 1995): 653–57, https://doi.org/10.1136/pgmj.71.841.653.

30. Donna M. Zulman et al., "Practices to Foster Physician Presence and Connection with Patients in the Clinical Encounter," *JAMA* 323, no. 1 (January 2020): 70–81, https://doi.org/10.1001/jama.2019.19003.

31. Eva Molineux Sklar, *My Life* (New York: RJ Communications, 2002), 12. Cited and identified with permission of her husband.

32. Patrick Irvine, "The Attending at the Funeral," *New England Journal of Medicine* 312 (June 27, 1985): 1704–5, https://doi.org/10.1056/NEJM198506273122608.

33. Anjali V. Desai et al., "Needs and Perspectives of Cancer Center Stakeholders for Access to Patient Values in the Electronic Health Record," *JCO Oncology Practice* 17, no. 10 (October 2021): e1524–e1536, https://doi.org/10.1200/OP.20.00644; Anjali Desai et al., "Designing a 'Patient Values Tab' for the Electronic Medical Record (EHR): An Investigation of the Needs and Perspectives of Key Stakeholders at a Dedicated Cancer Center (FR461B)," *Journal of Pain and Symptom Management* 59, no. 2 (February 2020): 479, https://doi.org/10.1016/j.jpainsymman.2019.12.171.

| Dialogue #4 |

Student: You were right. There is more to it than just the money. I can see that doing things besides procedures with patients can be complicated and psychologically demanding. I had not thought about biological reductionism as a problem.

Professor (reading a document): We have learned about a number of factors that influence what physicians do (and don't do), and why. When these factors are in play, pulling a payment policy lever (or even waving a magic wand at one) won't necessarily change behaviors that meet other needs or reflect certain limitations of the physicians.

Student: You obviously enjoyed the things you did for your patients. Is it reasonable to expect other doctors to get involved like that?

Professor: Lots of doctors do, and they derive great joy from the privilege of playing such a role. It would be great if we could unlock the potential of others to do the same.

Student: Well, as long as they have the financial incentives that currently exist, they may prefer to throw away the key!

Professor: Don't be so pessimistic. We're still missing something that might illuminate doctor behavior.

Student: What do you have in mind?

Professor: What goes on in medical schools? You'd think they'd equip students with the skills to practice ethically sound medicine that is based on good evidence without bankrupting the country.

Student: Aha! I sense that you doubt that they are doing that. Still, the doctors are responsible for what they do. And if we scapegoat the medical schools, I worry that we may be diverting attention from the doctors and others who profit from the system.

Professor: I don't think we will. I would like to understand, as comprehensively as possible, why things work (or don't work) the way they do.

Student: Well, then, we also should take a look at who is getting into medical school. Maybe that is part of the problem.

Professor: That is an excellent point. Ready to attack this piece?

Student: Sure. I suppose that it may help us understand some of what we have seen so far.

5

Idealism on Life Support

Missed Opportunities in Medical Student Education

It is through the idealism of youth that man catches sight of truth, and in that idealism he possesses a wealth which he must never exchange for anything else.
—Albert Schweitzer, "On Maturity"

I met with my uncle Sam for dinner at a Spanish restaurant close to campus. I had graduated from university a few months earlier and was considering a number of possible careers ranging from journalism and law to medicine and business. Sipping sangria, I explained to him how, after much ambivalence, I had registered in and started first year of medical school.

He was a fiercely progressive man who did not pull his punches and could be intimidating. "It's good that you've chosen to go into medicine," he said." In most careers, you'd have to take whatever jobs were available. In medicine, you'll have choices. You can go out and make a lot of money, or you can choose to do something less lucrative that serves the needs of society. Based on the choice you make, we can judge your worth as a human being."

His words were intense. It certainly was not the reassurance that I had been seeking. But I came to recognize that it was a gift. Not a week has gone by in the interceding years that I have not thought about what he said and whether I am doing enough. As will become evident in this chapter, that kind of jolt out of complacency may be what many medical students today need but unfortunately never receive.

How doctors are selected into medical schools and the ways in which they are educated profoundly influence the roles that they come to play in the US health care system. A brief survey of the historical development of American medical education provides insight into the nature of some of its problems and how they came about.

Medical Education in the United States before 1900: A Less Elite Profession

Medical practice emerged in colonial America with practitioners who, for the most part, had less formal training than those throughout Western Europe. The earliest physicians in the colonies often had been ship surgeons, apothecaries, or people in other professions, such as ministers or even planters. Connecticut Governor John Winthrop the younger gave medical advice to persons in his colony. There was less emphasis on understanding the causes of diseases than in treating their manifestations.[1]

Doctors were mostly trained by apprenticeship, working under the tutelage of other physicians in the colonies. As such (and unlike in Britain, where surgeons and physicians were distinct), the great majority treated medical conditions such as fever outbreaks, performed surgeries, and dispensed medications. The early practitioners did not have university degrees. By the 1770s, only 200 of the 3,500 who were practicing medicine in the colonies held university degrees, generally from Edinburgh or another European school.[2] The doctors who received this training sought to limit practice to those with licenses and university degrees. This effort to create a more elite medical profession and end the "levelling of all kinds of practitioners," regardless of their formal education (or lack thereof),[3] failed, at least initially.

There were no medical schools in the colonies until 1765, with the opening of one at the College of Philadelphia (later merged into the University of Pennsylvania). This soon was followed by the establishment of a medical school in King's College in New York (later Columbia University), then of Harvard's medical school in Boston in 1783. By the early 1800s, all of these university-based programs were requiring premedical education and granted an MD degree.[4] This model, which was different from those in most European countries, where students entered medical schools without prior university education, reflected elite institutions' interest in creating a more elite and prestigious profession. Most practitioners continued to train through apprenticeship, however, and there were no obvious distinctions (other than prestige) between them and the great majority of doctors, who lacked elite education but took care of the bulk of the population. As Rosemary Stevens notes, "Attempted distinctions between one doctor and another had to be molded out of the educational backgrounds instead of functional differences—that is between those trained wholly by domestic apprenticeship and the small but influential group of practitioners who, by the outbreak of the revolutionary war, were receiving some kind of university education."[5]

After 1800 (when there were only 4 operational medical schools), the number of schools began to grow: 14 new ones emerged by 1825, 26 more by 1840, another 47 by 1876, and an additional 114 by 1890. By one estimate, 400 medical schools were established at various times during the nineteenth century, many of which failed, lacking support from universities or other institutions. Some were affiliated with existing colleges, but many others were not. Beginning in the 1760s, state governments or state medical boards acquired the authority to license practitioners. By 1830, all states had such requirements. States allowed graduates of any chartered medical school to get a license. These nonaffiliated for-profit ("proprietary") medical schools came to outnumber the ones that were affiliated with universities.

Like the apprenticeship system of which they were an outgrowth, these proprietary institutions played an important societal role, caring for groups such as pioneers, who would not have had access to the elite physicians. Nonetheless, the increasing numbers of graduates of these schools were perceived as a threat by those trained in the elite medical schools, who viewed them as charlatans. There is no doubt that proprietary institutions undermined the prestige of the medical profession and the status which the elite doctors sought. They did, however, take care of a broad cross-section of the population, something that relatively few of our university-trained physicians did or even do today.[6]

Flexner, Carnegie, and the Emergence of Elitist, Science-Based Medical Education

The American Medical Association (AMA), which was founded in 1847, was interested in developing national standards for medical practice and education. It had little influence until 1902, when it succeeded in creating a national hierarchy of local, county, and state organizations.[7] In that year, they established a Council on Medical Education, which was concerned about the quality of the plethora of medical schools. They surveyed 160 schools in 1906–7 and judged only half of them to be "acceptable" (the rest being "doubtful "or "unacceptable"). They did not publish the names of the offending institutions but informed each school of its ranking. The Carnegie Foundation for the Advancement of Teaching became actively involved with this issue and joined forces with the AMA. Subsequently, Abraham Flexner of the foundation visited every medical school with Nathan Colwell of the Council on Medical Education.

The result of this was the Flexner report, published in 1910, which had a profound and enduring impact upon American medical education. It gave a top rating to only three medical schools. Some of the schools were judged to be mediocre. Many others were considered to be beyond the pale, with such descriptors as "utterly wretched," "dirty," and "miserable" applied liberally. The document was made public. The proprietary schools received the worst reviews, and the report endorsed university-based medical education with a four-year curriculum. The report concluded that all medical students should have a solid foundation of knowledge about the sciences.[8]

Since much of medical education and practice had been functional up to that point (teaching about how to care for the sick), this was a radical break, and it is credited with laying the "scientific foundations for medical practice." The report recommended slashing the number of medical schools in the country to 31, strictly limiting the number of graduates each year (and hence the number of practicing doctors). Radical transformation followed. Some schools closed in order not to be named in the report.

Carnegie Foundation president Henry S. Pritchett did not shy away from ideological considerations in his introduction to the report:

> the existence of many of these unnecessary and inadequate schools has been defended by the argument that a poor medical school is justified in the interest of a poor boy. It is clear that the poor boy has no right to go into any profession for which he is not willing to obtain proper preparation . . . Progress for the future would seem to require a very much smaller number of medical schools, better equipped and better conducted than our schools as a rule now are; and the needs of the public would require that we have fewer physicians graduated each year, but that these should be better educated and better trained.[9]

Although Flexner's target reduction to 31 medical schools was never achieved, a large proportion did close. The number of medical schools fell to 95 by 1915, and only 85 remained in 1920. Whereas 5 schools required college premedical coursework in 1905, by 1932 all required at least two years of such education.[10] The Carnegie Foundation and the Rockefeller Foundation (for whom Flexner also worked) ensured the success of this model by pouring substantial funding for research and education into the elite medical schools over the ensuing 30 years. Flexner became the Rockefeller philanthropy's director of their medical education programs.

The research programs targeted the pure sciences and biological reductionism, ignoring societal problems that had captured the attention of distinguished clinician scholars like Rudolf Virchow in Germany and Louis René Villermé in France.[11] The socioeconomic status of the medical profession was indeed elevated. "Poor boys" ceased to have many opportunities to go to medical school. Flexner, who was less interested in improving medical care than in securing an elite, well-educated medical profession that was much smaller in numbers, had complained that "a mass of unprepared youth" were being "drawn out of industrial occupations into the study of medicine."[12] That problem went away.

The resulting evolution of medical education reflected the socioeconomic evolution of the United States. The industrial revolution and the triumph of the North in the Civil War prompted a shift away from a slave-based economy in the South and a relatively free enterprise economy in the North to a system in which large monopolies began to control greater swaths of production in the context of rapid industrialization. The Carnegie and Rockefeller Foundations understood these trends well. They promoted development of the health system as a manifestation of the new economy: big medicine, based in hospitals, and with elite educational institutions defining the ethos and nature of practice. Interestingly, much less attention has been given to Flexner's views of physicians' responsibilities to society and the value of collaboration between academic medical institutions and public health practitioners. He argued that physicians have societal obligations to promote health and prevent disease, and medical training should include the range of knowledge that they would need to fulfill those obligations.[13]

Philanthropies recognized the goal of creating scientific medical institutions as a necessary tool to enforce the ideology and goals of industrial capitalism. As William H. Welch, who was chosen to lead the Rockefeller-funded first US school of public health at Johns Hopkins University, said, scientific medicine made possible "great industrial activities of modern times, efforts to reclaim for civilization vast tropical regions, and the immense undertaking to construct the Panama Canal."[14]

Undergraduate Medical Education and Its Failures: Getting In

After the Flexner report was issued, science and mathematics requirements became standard prerequisites for medical schools. In addition, preadmission testing was introduced in 1928. The Moss Test was the first standardized test to be administered widely to medical school applicants.

It included components relating to visual and content memory, scientific vocabulary and definitions, understanding printed material, premedical information, and logical reasoning. The content of the test and its successors changed somewhat over the years but continues to prioritize preparation in the sciences. It clearly reflects some notions of what knowledge entering students should possess but does not address in a serious way the applicants' values and capabilities as future physicians.

It was replaced in 1946 by a test that became known as the Medical College Admission Test (MCAT), which included four components: verbal ability, quantitative ability, scientific achievement, and understanding modern society. Each component received a separate score, and they were integrated into an overall score. Reportedly, medical schools placed much less emphasis on the component related to understanding modern society, which covered topics in the social sciences in which liberal arts students might excel.

After 1962, the fourth section was renamed "general information," but the test continued to emphasize academic achievement and did not focus on the characteristics, interests, values, or ethics of the applicants. In 1977, the general information section was eliminated. The four sections going forward were scientific knowledge, science problems, reading skills analysis, and quantitative skills analysis. It was intended to assess "information gathering and analysis, discerning and formulating relationships, and other problem-solving skills."

The test changed again in 1991. The new sections were verbal reasoning, biological sciences, physical sciences, and a writing sample.[15] The next revision, in 2015, eliminated the writing sample (to which admissions committees had not paid much attention) and added sections dealing with biochemistry, psychology, and sociology.[16]

The introduction of the test did coincide with a decrease in the proportion of students who dropped out of medical school (from about 20% to 7% in the period before World War II). It is not clear whether the trend can be attributed to the introduction of the test, although it may well have screened out students who were unable to assimilate knowledge that they might need in their medical school courses. The argument in favor of the MCAT is that it ensures students who enter medical school are better prepared. We might reasonably ask, "Prepared for what?" Such a test is a poor tool for distinguishing among applicants who are well qualified, and while it can predict academic grades and performance on licensing examinations, it does not assess some crucial issues in the selection of medical students, such as ability to empathize, interpersonal skills, and social values.[17]

Overwhelmingly, medical schools use grade point average (GPA) and MCAT scores to screen applicants. If the scores do not meet the threshold at that school, the student does not get interviewed. What is the impact of this structure on the admissions process? First, premedical students are focused on taking courses in which they can get an A. If a professor has a reputation for grading more stringently, many premedical students will avoid that class. Given the structure of the test, it is highly advantageous to major in one of the science fields that is tested in the MCAT. Students who have deviated from the sciences often pursue a postbaccalaureate course that exposes them to the required science courses over a period of a year or more.

In addition to curating their course list to get high grades, students also often pay for expensive test preparation courses. There is no doubt that these courses are effective. The largest test preparatory program is offered by Kaplan Testing Service, whose website promises improved test scores or your money back. It also explains the value of their preparatory course: "The MCAT covers a lot of content, and asks you to use what you know in new or unfamiliar contexts. The length of the MCAT is also a test of your stamina. As you get to know the MCAT's content in your prep course, you'll also learn strategies for conquering the test."[18]

Students who can afford a preparatory course have an advantage, possibly augmented by not needing to work at jobs while preparing. The emphasis in the selection process on the combination of MCAT scores and GPAs inevitably produces a crop of applying and entering medical students who excel in scientific subjects, who lack personal distractions affecting their grades, and who have the resources to maximize their preparation. They also may be able to afford help preparing medical school applications, enabling them to submit essays that attract the interest of the admissions committees. One company that assists with the personal statement portion of the application offers unlimited rounds of editing and doctor advisors to discuss the content for $999.[19]

I was ambivalent about going to medical school, and I applied at a time when it was somewhat less competitive. Accordingly, I did not take a test prep course or get professional help with my essay. As a junior faculty member at UCLA, I attended a conference at Asilomar, near Monterey, California, sponsored by the Association of American Medical Colleges, which sanctions the MCAT. I arrived a little late and sat down next to an elderly man. I introduced myself and told him what I do. He told me that his name was Stanley Kaplan. I asked him what he did. He graciously did not mock my ignorance, telling me that he ran a preparation program for the MCAT and other tests.

Kaplan started his testing programs in the late 1930s. His major product was a preparatory course for the Scholastic Aptitude Test (used for college admissions), but courses to prepare for the MCAT and the Law School Admission Test, and one for pre-kindergarten applicants, followed. He sold the business to the Washington Post in 1984 for $45 million. By 2008, the company was producing $2.3 billion of revenue annually from 1 million students.[20]

Why are medical schools so tied to these scores (and GPAs) that can be gamed? In the 2020 ratings of medical schools, published annually by U.S. News and World Report and which matter a great deal to medical schools, 13% of the score for the "research" rating of medical schools and 9.75% of their "primary care" rating score was based on the median MCAT score of entering medical students, and another 6% (research ranking) and 4.5% (primary care ranking) was based on undergraduate median GPA. Taking account also of the acceptance rate, the overall category of "student selectivity" contributes 20% of the score in the research model and 15% in the primary care model. None of this accounts for such factors as empathy, altruism, or creativity, which are extremely relevant to who should enter the medical profession.[21]

The latter constructs are complex and would be extremely difficult to measure on a standardized test in a way that would provide confidence in the validity of the results, but by depending on a test that doesn't address such concepts, medical schools legitimize its validity as a measure of students' appropriateness for entry into medical school. Having the MCAT scores and GPAs be so important in the medical school rankings has an insidious effect on student selection. Medical schools care about their rankings, and those whose students perform best in these metrics are not shy about sharing that information.

The tragedy of the commons holds that when people in medieval England did not equitably share the common grazing grounds, their competition in the end benefitted no one and led to the enclosure of those lands. The analogy is sometimes made to people in an auditorium or stadium standing to get a better view. Then everyone stands, and no one sees better.[22] The MCAT and similar tests are the tragedy of the commons magnified: not everyone can afford to stand up and do better. The result is that the advantage goes to the advantaged.[23]

Medical schools do not admit to being complicit in such biased selection procedures. They pride themselves on the diversity of their students and claim to judge applicants by "holistic" criteria, in search of as many as 15 core competencies, including cultural competence, social skills, service orientation, ethical responsibility to self and others, and capacity for improvement. At the margin, they consider these matters, but no one even gets interviewed if their grades and test scores fall short.[24]

As noted, the pursuit of the irresistibly high grade point average is part of the premedical journey. A consequence is narrowness in the premedical curriculum of most students. It is rare to see premedical students majoring in philosophy, literature, and the like, disciplines in which the professors do not administer "objective" tests but rather assess thinking in depth through essays and written examinations. "I can't afford a B" long has been a common refrain.[25] A grade of B in some advanced course on the latest developments in molecular genetics might be forgivable. Such a grade in a course on Kant and Hegel, or on theories of social justice, would likely be an indelible wound. In 1978, the eminent clinician scientist and former medical school dean Lewis Thomas eloquently proposed to dispense with admissions testing and with science courses as prerequisites for admission and to give highest priority to students who have studied the humanities as preparation for caring for and relating to human beings as patients. Three decades later, 56% of matriculating medical students had majored in the biological sciences, 13% in the physical sciences, and only 4% in the humanities.[26]

There is a story of a student coming to his philosophy professor, Herbert Marcuse, and complaining that he was spending 45 minutes reading each page of an assigned writing by Hegel but still did not understand the text.

Marcuse responded, "Forty-five minutes a page for Hegel? That's nothing!"

Wouldn't it be wonderful if medical schools did not discourage learning about complexity and society and culture in this way? It also might facilitate students being able to deal with nonlinear issues that require reasoned judgment that cannot be memorized from a book, and that give them some humility about the complexity of the world and the consequences of their and their patients' behavior within it. Some professors and occasional programs have that goal, but they should be central, not incidental, elements of medical education.

White Coats, White Students

As discussed above, once the students arrive in medical school, their socialization into the profession begins. Since the 1990s, almost all medical schools have held a white coat ceremony for the entering students. The foundation that promotes the ceremony states, "The iconic ritual provides an important emphasis on compassionate, collaborative, scientifically excellent care from the very first day of training."[27] This formal agenda is admirable, but it belies the atmospherics and hidden curriculum of the event. It is primarily an act of socialization.

As they don their white coats, entering medical students are separating themselves from other elements of society. The white coat—which replaced black attire and became common late in the nineteenth century, coinciding with the widespread acceptance of the need for antisepsis and cleanliness in clinical settings—is frequently associated with the medical profession.[28] Its whiteness can be a symbol of purity as well of cleanliness, but it is also a cultural symbol of power and authority.[29]

These newly minted medical students have accomplished nothing other than good GPAs and test scores, but the inherent message is that they have arrived and are not just starting a journey. Why socialize them and imbue them with a status that effectively communicates that they are part of the elite? I would argue that doctors should not have such status at all. At the very least, shouldn't they earn it by appropriating their medical skills for the greater good? When I graduated from medical school, three of us wrote a manifesto that we distributed at our graduation ceremony, denouncing the position that the medical profession had come to occupy in society. We also pledged not to wear white coats or use the title of doctor, until they came to represent something more healing in society. (Two of us largely adhered to that pledge. I lost touch with the third, but eventually saw him doing infomercials on late-night television for cosmetic procedures—wearing a white coat!)

Medical schools do pride themselves on attracting exceptional candidates and are not averse to taking students from diverse disciplines (providing their grades and test scores are good enough). Interviews have long been part of the process. Lately, many schools break down these interviews into a series of brief interactions ("multiple mini-interviews," which are semi-structured), in which the students are expected to react to a range of situations or challenges. These are more standardized than free-form interviews, but these, too, can be prepped, and prep companies do provide that service. Like traditional interviews, they are subject to the implicit biases of the interviewers. Often the interviewers are trained in an effort to offset such bias.[30]

The students, understandably, structure their applications to fulfill what they believe are the expectations of the selection committees. Prospective medical students carefully craft their applications with evidence not only of great grades and test scores, but also of social commitment: building homes in Central America, installing irrigation systems in Africa, and so on. Gauging the sincerity of such commitments is challenging, as is the assessment of other personal qualities in the application process. Not all students are in a position to demonstrate their supposed social commitment in these ways, often lacking financial resources to travel or even the time for local projects because they need to work to support their families or their studies.[31]

For a variety of reasons, whatever idealism is present upon admission dissipates rapidly in medical school, where any genuine longing for social justice soon is superseded by acute awareness of the economics of the medical profession. In one study, by the second year of medical school, idealism had declined in favor of concerns with income, status, and lifestyle.[32] By the time they arrive, many are aspiring to careers in orthopedics or other high-paying fields. As one senior educator commented to me recently, "Medical school applicants are very good at misrepresenting their motivations." Actually, their primary motivation is clear: get into medical school. What their professions of social commitment often do obscure are their personalities and true values.

Another consequence of the ways in which students are selected for medical school is an astonishing lack of diversity in the student body. For many years, women were seriously underrepresented. That situation began to improve gradually in the early 1970s (when my medical school class had 18 women among 135 students) to the point where now about half of entering medical students are women. This has been an extremely important change from the late nineteenth century, when medical icon William Osler was unhappy about the requirement for medical schools such as Johns Hopkins to admit women and said that only the larger cities could support even one female physician.[33]

Other disparities have not improved much. In 2007, only 4% of entering medical students in the United States came from households in the lowest 20% of household income, and 60% came from the top 20%. Despite strenuous efforts to diversify student bodies after that, by 2017, the respective percentages were 5% and 51%. In 2017, students in the top 5% of family income distribution (28% of the entering class) were 17 times as likely, as a share of the population, to be admitted as those with family incomes in the lowest 40% (13% of the class).[34] Pritchett's admonition that most "poor boys" do not belong in the medical school classroom remains the reality more than a century later.

Racial and ethnic minorities, such as African Americans and Latinos, who are underrepresented in other parts of US society, are also underrepresented in medical schools. In 2019, only 3.6% of medical school faculty were African American, and 5.5% were Hispanic. Between 1980 and 2016, the proportion of medical school applicants who were African American increased from 7% to 8.2%; the proportion of African Americans among entering medical students increased from 6% to 7.1%. Hispanics comprised 5% of applicants in 1980, increasing to 6.1% in 2016, while among entering medical students, 4.9% were Hispanic in 1980 and 6.3% in 2016.[35] These rates compare to census data that 13.4% of the US population in 2019 were African American and 18.5% were Hispanic.[36]

While the acceptance rate is somewhat lower for African Americans relative to their numbers in the applicant pool, the fundamental problem is that fewer minority group members are applying to medical school. There is a similar pattern for individuals from low-income families. One of the barriers that disadvantaged individuals face in applying is the cost of medical school education (which can range from about $150,000 at an instate public medical school to $250,000 out of state or at a private university or medical school). While loan programs and scholarships can help, in many families it is unimaginable to take on expenses of that magnitude.[37] Even applying for medical school can be an expense that is out of reach. The total cost of applying can easily reach $10,000, including the costs of multiple applications, test preparation courses, MCAT registration, and visits for interviews; scholarships do not cover these expenses.[38]

There have been extensive efforts to address racial, ethnic, and socioeconomic disparities, including efforts to increase applications and to increase readiness to apply.[39] But underlying the problems of minorities and the poor is that the application process is structured to reward the high-achieving student who consistently does well and who has substantial support in the application and testing process.

Scientific Prerequisites and the Medical School Curriculum

Do we really need medical students to be demonstrably outstanding in the physical and biological sciences and mathematics? There is no doubt that some knowledge of aspects of the sciences and mathematics is relevant to the practice of medicine, but the level of such knowledge that is required is not comparable to that needed by someone who is engaged in scientific research in those disciplines, or in product development that applies such knowledge. Some medical students choose to pursue careers in those fields, and such individuals should be identified and nurtured. They are a small minority of those who go to medical school, however. As for the rest, there is no doubt that they can acquire the needed knowledge when in medical school, as happens in most European countries, where students enter medical school without any prior university preparation.

I was far from committed to a medical career as a university undergraduate. Accordingly, I took the bare minimum courses required for medical school entry, including only one introductory course in biology. In that course, I had my poorest undergraduate grade. It being a less brutal era for applying to medical school, I was accepted despite that transgression. With only decent grades, I doubt that I even would be granted an interview today. Once I was in medical school, it certainly was more challenging to negotiate the curriculum in the courses in biochemistry and physiology than it had been for my classmates who had majored in those fields.

I only had the vaguest notions about some body parts, such as the hypophysis (which turns out to be the pituitary gland). Not having read ahead, I endured an entire lecture on the histology of the hypophysis without having the slightest idea what part of the body the professor was talking about. I might have mistaken the Krebs cycle for a piece of exercise equipment, the solar plexus for an astronomical phenomenon, and the parasympathetic nervous system for a way of communicating with the dead.

I did not excel in those classes, but I did muddle through. My bare-bones preparation for those classes did not impair my ability to practice and teach medicine later on. That is not to say that science should be missing from the curriculum. It is necessary at some level, but it is far from sufficient as a criterion for who should go to medical school, or for what should comprise the curriculum of the medical school, as I discuss later in this chapter.

While there have always been some medical students who majored in history, in other social sciences and in the humanities, acceptance to medical school requires them to score well on an admission test, which is mostly composed of math and science. The students who get in are good test-takers and good grade-getters. Does that make them educated, wise, or worldly? Not at all. The emphasis is on a limited definition of accomplishment.

I have never ceased to be amazed at the pervasive ignorance of many students at excellent medical schools, and in highly competitive residencies, about things in the world that matter and are relevant to what doctors do, or should do. There are lots of factors contributing to the narrowness and paucity of socially responsible values and to the predisposition to entering technical fields among physicians. Although certainly not the only factor, the domination of premedical and medical curricula by basic sciences, which has not diminished much, certainly does not help.

Does the strong emphasis on science among medical school prerequisites and in the first- and second-year curriculum in medical school matter? If a doctor knows which drug to give for pneumonia, what adverse reactions and interactions to watch out for, and how to manage complications, isn't that enough? Do they also need to know about the conditions in which people live? How relevant can it possibly be for the doctor to be an excellent communicator, and to be aware of philosophic arguments about social responsibilities, ethical obligations, nuances of debates about health and social policy, literature, current affairs, and the like?

While there is a modicum of curriculum content directed to such matters in most medical schools, it is not a particularly high priority in many of them, and it is not decisive in medical residency applications. Many schools offer a course in the medical humanities, a program of visits to art museums, or even a track in the medical humanities.[40] These courses are usually elective, and many students do not take them.

Even when humanities courses are required, they are not regarded as core elements. Performance on them is far less important to academic progress than other curricular components. There is some evidence that such courses can have salutary effects: in one school, taking a medical humanities course was associated with a more positive trajectory in empathy scores afterward (compared to their scores before taking the course) than was seen in students not enrolled, but only 25 of 68 students took the course.[41]

I think that humanities education is highly relevant to being a physician.[42] The future doctor has to build relationships with patients, make choices about caring for populations, and decide whether his or her priority is to serve society or pursue personal gain and a comfortable lifestyle. At the same time, physicians need to be able to relate to people at critical junctures in their lives, and to be empathic while having difficult conversations. These are tasks, responsibilities, and opportunities in the face of which too many modern physicians frequently fail to do the right thing.

As I try to imagine a curriculum that would be richer in values, empathy, compassion, and social responsibility, it certainly seems as though complementing the scientific content with generous helpings of sociology, philosophy, ethics, anthropology, literature, and history could not hurt. Why not give students who are interested an opportunity to spend a semester studying philosophical arguments about the individual in society as they pertain to health and medicine? Why not do more to improve the ability of students to express their feelings and deal with emotionally charged situations? Almost all schools have lectures on such topics. Extensive work in small groups and role-playing, which is done in some programs, needs to extend throughout training, to build up and reinforce competence as well as a reasonable balance of humility and confidence. Such an approach might prepare future physicians to be able to talk effectively to patients about sexuality, suicidal feelings, and end-of-life decision-making.

Why not spend more than 45 minutes per page trying to understand what a philosopher is getting at, or studying serious fiction in order to identify the literary devices used to communicate concepts that are not explicit in the text?[43] Such efforts might lead to a deeper appreciation of the importance and context of every word in a medical history, and to better communication with and greater empathy for patients, which has been shown to decrease errors, increase satisfaction, and even improve patient health.[44] Why not value and promote human relationships as the core of medical education? That might well lead to thinking about the selection of medical students in a different way, and to giving far more weight to evidence of empathy and of communication and listening skills.

Perhaps I was taking this point of view too far when I told my distinguished histology professor, Charles Leblond (histology is the study of tissues and cells), that he should make his course more socially relevant. In response, he related our conversation to the class at the beginning of a lecture on the histology of the large intestine. He then proceeded to tell us about his experience as an army doctor in India during World War II. He had been called to examine a sick elephant. His advice to us was, "If you are ever asked to examine a sick elephant, wear hip boots!" This was a gentle put-down of me, and he did not identify me to the class, but it would be nice if professors in the science courses could refer to values and social context once in a while.

Connecting Students with Patients' Values and Experiences

I often look for ways in my teaching to highlight human dimensions of patient care that are not represented by scientific formulas or sets of technical prescriptions. In an effort to accomplish that, I sometimes bring to hospital rounds poems that are relevant to people's profound experiences in medicine and share them with the residents and students. These efforts on my part reflect the fine programs on medicine and literature that have been developed in some medical schools. On one occasion, I was notified during the night by an on-call physician that a woman on our ward had died. She was a Holocaust survivor who had no remaining family. As we began our rounds the next morning, I asked how the patients were doing. I was told that everyone was stable.

"What about Mrs. Goldstein?" I asked.

"She coded during the night," the resident responded. "Coded" refers to code blue, which implies a cardiac arrest and an effort to attempt resuscitation. In this instance, the patient had indicated previously that she did not want cardiopulmonary resuscitation. He said "coded" because he was uncomfortable using the word "died."

I suggested that this woman, who lived a tough life after the war and had spent her final days alone, deserved a little reflection on her life and challenges. We sat down at the end of rounds to do that. We talked about her and took turns reading poems that reflected on death and illness. The students, residents, and I spoke of any personal experiences that we had had with the death of someone close to us. (For most of the trainees, it was a grandparent who had died.) The poems that we read were by Robert Browning ("Prospice"), Dylan Thomas ("Do Not Go Gently"), Oliver Wendell Holmes ("The Deacon's Masterpiece"), and W. H. Auden ("Surgical Ward"). When I read one of them, tears streamed down my cheeks. Afterward, the resident told me that the students thought I had a cold.

People at the end of life would benefit from having doctors who could let down their defenses and embrace the often intensely emotional context of medical care. For that to happen, we would need to recruit students who are inclined to do this, and we would need to give them the tools and support systems to make sure that they could accomplish it without being emotionally depleted themselves. Despite sporadic efforts to provide such training, the challenge of connecting medical students with the life experiences of their patients, and even with their own inner lives, is enormous.

Feeling Their Pain?

At one medical school, the first-year class was broken down into smaller groups for some interactive sessions. On one occasion, the topic of the day was grief. A group that worked with grieving family members gave a PowerPoint presentation. Then they introduced a woman in her forties whose husband of a similar age had died recently of cancer. She talked about her pain and anguish. A number of students got up and left the room while she was talking; some sobbed in the hallway. Several complained that they should not have been subjected to the presentation and that they should be allowed to skip such sessions.

The administration did not concur. But they did consent to provide students advanced word/warning of the subjects to be covered in such sessions. That's reasonable. It allows students to prepare emotionally and cognitively for classes with intense emotional content. Letting them opt out altogether, however, would not be appropriate. Physicians need to be able and willing to relate effectively to grieving patients and their families. If students are not willing to acquire the ability to do that, they shouldn't be in medical school. Their teachers need to convey this basic truth, even as they acknowledge and manage students' emotional reactions.

In reality, while some medical students want to be able to work effectively with patients, others have little or no interest in acquiring the skills needed to have difficult conversations, or to deal with situations that are emotionally challenging to them. They prefer procedural fields, in which the extent and complexity of interaction with patients is less, where doctors are often much less connected to the patients and may never talk to or see them again after the procedure is completed. All the better, from their perspective, that doctors in such fields make so much more money than the ones who build relationships with patients.

There is some evidence that female medical students are more empathic and communication minded than their male counterparts.[45] Accordingly, many procedural fields such as orthopedics, neurological and thoracic surgery, and interventional radiology are overwhelmingly male dominated, while fields like pediatrics and hospice and palliative medicine attract far more women.[46]

A director of medical education at one medical school recently lamented to me that many medical students tend not to want to figure things out: they expect to have everything handed to them in the most convenient way. They don't want to be criticized, challenged, or made uncomfortable. While this certainly is not true of all American medical students, many do feel entitled: to an easy time in medical school, to an easy life, and to lots of income.

Socialization

When I was early in my second year as a medical student at McGill University in Montreal, the Quebec government implemented the government-sponsored single-payer universal health insurance system that was being adopted across Canada. Quebec was one of the last provinces to sign up. There was acceptance of the new law among the general practitioners, but the medical specialists were prepared to fight it and even briefly went on strike.[47] For students in our medical school, this was of great interest. A large meeting was held in the main lecture hall to discuss the issue.

Some students were clearly aligned with each side. What astonished me at the time was that the students in the first two years were largely supportive of the new program, but those present from the upper years were strongly opposed. Obviously, this was not a scientific survey, and many students were not there, but it seemed clear that the upper-year students identified with the specialists, who feared that their freedom and income would be compromised, while my cohort identified more with Canadians outside of the medical profession, most of whom favored the new system.

Many students enter medical school professing idealism and social commitment. For some, these values persist; for others, the sentiments fade as they progress through their medical training. Some schools maintain programs intended to reinforce such values (such as free clinics where the students could volunteer, courses on ethics, etc.), but the level of exposure to such programs is insufficient for many students to overcome other influences.

Absent from most medical curricula is teaching about the grand tradition of physicians who were on the front lines of social activism because they saw it as directly relevant to their professional mission. Rudolf Virchow, to take one example, was a great German physician, scientist, and social activist. Concerned with the social determinants of much disease, he argued that "medicine is a social science and politics is nothing else but medicine on a large scale."[48] Not only did he write extensively about these matters, but he also joined the revolutionaries at the barricades in Berlin's Friedrichstrasse in March 1848. Similarly, Norman Bethune, a Canadian thoracic surgeon, offered his services to the Republicans in Spain in the 1930s along with many American physicians fighting Franco's fascists. He established a mobile blood transfusion service at the front. He died in China in 1939, where he had joined Mao's army in the struggle against the invading Japanese empire while providing medical care in rural areas.[49]

Obviously, we can't expect many medical students to meet such standards of putting their lives on the line for justice. At the same time, medical schools should want their graduates to act in ways that promote the well-being of the population as a whole (or, at the very least, do not undermine it). As we've seen, many schools seek to sensitize students to or reinforce values, but too often, it amounts to little more than an occasional lecture by a social scientist on social aspects of medicine as part of a course on "doctoring." We will consider the implications of these offerings, but they are not nearly enough. The four years of curricular time includes substantial periods of electives. Surely some of that time could be allocating to the task of trying to imbue the future doctors with good values.

Apart from what they are exposed to in these doctoring courses, students do get considerable education about societal values and the role of the physician during their clinical training. It's just the *wrong* education. It is crucial to find ways to neutralize the negative socialization of students that occurs when they are immersed in the culture of clinical medicine. Any impact of the token offerings in doctoring curricula, wedged as they are among the basic science courses, is washed away in the clinical years.

Required courses in empathy and effective communication,[50] social responsibility, and broader disciplines of the social sciences and humanities—including literature, philosophy, history, economics, and sociology—certainly could enrich medical school education. For such courses to have much impact on the students would require that letters of recommendation for residencies give performance in humanities courses as much emphasis as that in basic science and clinical courses, and that there be ongoing formal and informal support for students to reinforce positive societal values and interests.

Doing Well or Doing Good? Choice of Specialties

Why is it that students get socialized into conservative and less altruistic values in their clinical training? The second-century Greek physician Galen famously encouraged his disciples to "see for yourself." They dutifully learned not from what they saw, but rather what they read from Galen regarding human anatomy, which Galen had based upon dissections of animals. It was not until the sixteenth century that the Flemish anatomist and physician Andreas Vesalius, working in Padua, dissected a human cadaver and disproved key findings of Galen.

Medical students today do see for themselves and are keenly perceptive, if not about the society around them, then certainly about what doctors in the various specialties earn. During the long hours of clinical learning, they absorb the values of doctors they hope to emulate. Their expectations for income and lifestyle are influenced by what they observe. Websites keep them fully informed in this regard.[51] Students are cognizant of these income differences and are unburdened by any of the idealism or selflessness that suffused their medical school applications.

In one study, second-year medical students wrote essays about their motivations in choosing a specialty. Their reasons for valuing income included freedom and flexibility, belief that physicians are entitled to high incomes, financial security, prestige that comes with high income, and the opportunity to use some of that income to do good in the world. All students cared about financial security. A few felt that all specialty incomes are sufficient to achieve that, but most took potential earnings into account when choosing a specialty. Some talked of the prestige of the specialty as a factor and related that to the level competitiveness of the application process for that specialty, to the intellectual challenge of the field, or to the power or autonomy of those who practice in that area.[52]

There are other ways that students can gain insight into the income implications of specialty choices. What kinds of cars do their professors drive? Where do they live? At the University of California, with six public medical schools, information on faculty salaries is available online.[53] Any student exploring that database can see that a large number of faculty earn seven-figure incomes, with numerous assistant professors barely finished with their training earning $800,000 to $1 million, and many faculty earn in excess of $700,000, substantially more than the president of the university. Almost all of these are in specialties that do procedures or earn money by selling chemotherapy drugs to patients. It is hard for the students not to notice.[54]

What are the implications of this imbalance in professional income, other than making some physicians more economically prosperous than others? First, medical students clamor to get into the high-paying procedural fields. Whereas 40 years ago many of the best students went into a field like internal medicine or pediatrics, as we saw in chapter 3, the procedural specialties are much more popular today, and even among those entering internal medicine, many have their eyes set upon subspecializing in cardiology and other procedural disciplines, in which the incomes are twice as high as in general internal medicine, rheumatology, and infectious diseases. It has been well documented that the proportion of residency slots filled by US medical graduates, a measure of the competitiveness of the specialties, is highly correlated with specialty income. In the match for slots in the spring of 2021, only 33% of positions in family medicine and 39% in internal medicine were filled by

US medical graduates, compared to 80% or more in multiple procedural fields.[55]

The income disparities between specialists and generalists are now greater in the United States than in some countries with advanced economies, such as Germany and the United Kingdom.[56] What is the rationale for these differences? Some specialties require additional training. For example, a cardiologist or gastroenterologist may train for two or more additional years compared to a general internist or a primary care physician. As noted previously, however, rheumatologists and infectious diseases specialists, who do few procedures, also may have two or more years of additional training, and they do not derive the same amount of income benefit from this training, if any.

The additional training in a procedural field can mean millions of dollars in additional lifetime earnings in exchange for two or three additional years of training. In a nonprocedural field, the additional training time may be associated with loss of lifetime earning potential. This was demonstrated nicely by a study that compared the cost-effectiveness of medical subspecialty training in gastroenterology (a procedural field) and rheumatology (a subspecialty with few procedures). The choice between these two subspecialties had seven-figure implications for lifetime earnings. When the implications are so stark, it is not at all surprising which specialties are most competitive.[57]

If we were to stipulate that three years of additional training in subspecialties could be "repaid" by an income 10% or even 20% greater over a 30-year career, that would be much less of a disparity than we currently observe. Even such trimming of procedural incomes would not address societal priorities (such as the need for more primary care providers) or the performance of unnecessary procedures. Some specialties, such as dermatology, radiology, and anesthesiology, typically have only one year of additional training, compared to generalist physicians in internal medicine, pediatrics, or family medicine. Yet incomes in those specialties are often twice those of primary care physicians. There is an enormous "penalty" for going into primary care. Even medical students, who arrived in medical school professing their altruism or social awareness, may find the attraction of far superior income to be irresistible.

A factor sometimes blamed for the preference of medical students for high-paying procedural fields is their burden of student debt, although it is far from the only factor. Women and minority medical students are less likely to choose procedural fields.[58] Students with six-figure debts often express the view that they need to go into specialties that earn enough money to pay off their loans. This is tenuous logic, given that lifetime increased earnings in procedural fields, relative to generalist fields, will be several-fold greater than their student debts. And non-proceduralists do not go hungry or homeless! Objectively, student debt for many is more of a rationalization for making lucrative choices.

Nonetheless, steps have been taken to lighten that burden, in the hope that students may increasingly choose such fields as primary care. In 2018, New York University pledged to eliminate tuition for their medical students. Other schools, such as Cornell, developed plans to reduce student debt.[59]

Will these initiatives change specialty choice? It is far from clear that they will. In 2017, student debt averaged $192,000 among the 75% who had debt, and studies have found that doctors with debt in this range pay it off easily.[60] It would be surprising if tuition waiver programs induce a shift away from the highest-paying fields, given the magnitude of specialty income differences. There are public programs that will pay off portions in the military or in medical research, but most students do not pursue these options. Training in a lucrative field can cover the debts much more efficiently.[61]

Undoubtedly, income is not the only factor driving students toward specialties. As in any profession, many are attracted by the technical and intellectual challenges in the fields. They also are attracted to the prestige that is associated with holding exclusive jurisdiction over an area of competency.[62] At the same time, financial rewards are irresistible to many and tenaciously defended by their professional societies.

Lack of Positive Experiences with Longitudinal Care

Medical students' relative lack of interest in fields that provide longitudinal relationships may well be driven largely by economics. At the same time, it is difficult for them to gain an appreciation for what such longitudinal relationships would be like. A medical student should get to know the joy of seeing someone resume their life after a serious illness, the sense of accomplishment of helping a patient take charge of their health and do things to promote health and longevity, the poignance of being a source of comfort for someone going through hard times, the personal sadness of bearing witness when someone for whom you have cared develops a serious or fatal illness.

I won't propose any simple solutions here, but I am confident that brilliant minds could come up with approaches that would immerse students deeply in these textured and meaningful components of the doctor-patient relationship far more consistently than occurs at present. Certainly, some students do enter medical school with genuine ideals and aspirations to be doctors caring for people on an ongoing basis. Passionate teachers can reinforce those inclinations or even generate a spark of joy for the doctor-patient relationship in other students. Those of us who have done that know that it is a wonder and an extraordinary privilege to be let into people's lives, to share with them some of their most profound moments, both positive and negative.

Yet the educational experiences in outpatient care are far from optimal. Things are rushed. Patients are complicated. There is little continuity. The student may not even know what the outcome of a patient encounter was. It has been noted that we could not design a system more efficient at discouraging interest in outpatient care. The students see many faculty members and residents who are stressed and unhappy, who earn less than other specialists, and who work long hours. That is not a pretty picture.[63]

At times, medical schools have assigned students a family to follow throughout medical school, and that can be meaningful. But there is more to the experience than that. In the inpatient setting, time is compressed, and stuff is happening all the time. It is dramatic. It is exciting. In out-patient care, the pace is slower. Things do happen, but often more sub-tly. It is a chance to relate to patients more humanely and to help them become more active participants in their care and masters of their fates. It is a chance to get to know them as people. Medical schools would have to radically change what they do to convey that effectively. It does not fit into the world of relative value units that measure so-called clinical productivity.

The Organization of the Learning Environment

The *structure of pedagogy*, both in preclinical classes and in clinical set-tings, affects the attitudes, priorities, and personal styles of the students. With the exception of courses on doctoring and behavioral medicine, much of the learning in medical school is didactic (lectures), formulaic (memorizing lists, formulae, differential diagnoses, and treatments), or both. Such courses do not teach students how to think critically. Many doctors would disagree and would contend that learning about different diagnoses promotes critical thinking. That is true in a narrow sense, but not in relation to pondering the totality of the human being in front of the student or physician. To some extent, the current models for learning ignore that totality and install doctors as authorities with exclusive knowl-edge who are superior to patients. It contributes to a kind of profes-sional dominance (in lieu of collaborative decision-making) that is not inevitable.[64]

Ironically, the circumstance in which this dominance may fade is when patients or families want care that is either ineffective or inappropriate. This may occur in situations where there is no measurable benefit. It may also occur when someone who has difficulty obtaining care in the health care system, or who does not trust a clinician who is of a different race or does not speak their language, sees any limitation in care for them or their family as a potential form of discrimination. Would more dynamic educa-tion, less singularly focused upon facts and more on processes and rela-tionships, change anything? There is at least the prospect that it might produce doctors better able to enter relationships with patients in ways that produced different authority structures, processes, and outcomes.

The doctoring and behavioral medicine courses are intended to generate a counterpoint to this. In some respects, they succeed. Meeting in small groups encourages the students to participate more actively in discussions of critical issues. For example, teaching about sharing decision-making with the patient produces more positive attitudes toward doing so, as well as skills in this area.[65] Objective structured clinical examinations (OSCEs, often with actors as patients who can give feedback) can be used to assess communication skills of the student.[66]

The environment in which students and residents learn clinical medicine is hierarchical. The faculty member is in charge of major decisions. The senior resident handles operations and most communication with the boss. Interns are next on the ladder of authority, followed by fourth-year medical students (subinterns), then other medical students. The environment is very top-down. Although there are exceptions, speaking up and challenging the judgments and decisions of those more senior is rarely acceptable.

Students defer to the interns and interns to the residents. Challenging the supervising faculty member (the attending physician) is generally beyond the pale for the students, whatever they may think about the instructor's behavior. Recently developed programs promote "speaking-up behavior" by lower-ranking staff in crucial situations like the operating room, in the hope of averting critical errors. They have a steep hill to climb.[67]

The challenge of engaging in speaking-up behavior was evident to me early in my clinical training. I was taken into a room by a faculty member along with three or four other students. He told us to perform rectal examinations on a man who had advanced prostate cancer. One student examined him, and the patient howled in pain. The faculty member told the rest of us to follow suit. Although we recognized the situation and wanted to avoid inflicting pain, we all did examine him. To this day, I continue to regret my failure to decline to perform the procedure. I caused pain to a dying man in order to avoid inconveniencing myself by earning the displeasure of my supervisor.

Although that episode was a more dramatic moment than many, it reflects the structure of training. While there are numerous wonderful, open, empathic surgeons, surgical residency programs often have been described as even more authoritarian than those in other disciplines. Thus the movement toward "evidence-based" decision-making has lagged in surgery, where many practitioners do not welcome challenges by trainees or skepticism from patients.[68]

To be clear, such an authoritarian relationship has two participants: one who seeks to dominate and one who willingly submits.[69] Much of medical care has an authoritarian character, well beyond the time of training.[70] Most important, the patient is often subjected to the authority of the physician in situations in which the relationship could be more egalitarian.[71]

Szasz and Hollander, in their classic paper on the doctor-patient relationship, noted that there were three models of such interaction: activity-passivity, guidance-cooperation, and mutual participation. They contended that although the nature of the interaction inevitably varies when the patient is too sick to fully participate in decision-making, mutual participation is the desired mode, and it tends to occur when the sociocultural distance between doctor and patient is least (same socioeconomic class, education level, language, religion, national background, etc.). They also observed that activity-passivity (which is only appropriate when the patient is unconscious or otherwise unable to communicate at all) is common when the sociocultural distance is greatest.[72] Close to 90% of medical students come from families above the median income, so the sociocultural distance from patients of lower socioeconomic strata or different cultural backgrounds is often substantial. It is possible, with effort, for a clinician to diminish their sociocultural distance from a patient, but not nearly to the extent of someone who is familiar with and comfortable in the patient's culture and socioeconomic circumstances.

Narrowing of Vision and of Intellectual Domain

The scramble for procedural specialties also affects the students' approach to learning. This is reinforced by clinical teachers, many of whom are in those roles because they have excelled at their own forms of specialization. Specialization by its nature leads many (although not all) practitioners to consider less than the whole. A specialty in medicine survives if it controls a component of care. To do so, it may require rules (as to who can do certain acts) and specialized skills and knowledge. Thus the strategy for establishing the intellectual domain and functional turf of the specialty may be to limit the access of others (outside the specialty) to the knowledge, skills, and practice opportunities needed to achieve and maintain competency in a clinical area.

As a young faculty member in internal medicine, if one of my hospitalized patients required intensive care, my team and I followed our patient into the intensive care unit (ICU) and we were responsible for the care there. Pulmonary specialists, however, who managed ICU patients with critical lung diseases, particularly those who need to be on ventilators, soon claimed the ICU as their turf. They were most knowledgeable about acute problems of the lungs, but lots of other problems could bring a patient to the ICU. Nonetheless, it became their domain. They even rebranded the specialty and "pulmonary and critical care," with a new subspecialty certification examination established for the latter.

Soon enough, other doctors like me ceased to be up to date about the latest drugs and protocols in the ICU. We were outsiders, supplicants who depended on them to provide the expertise that was needed to care for our former patients. Were there benefits to such transfers of care? There often were, but the transfer of care also created discontinuity for patients and their families. Many times, the ICU team continued to manage the patient after the situation no longer required being in the ICU, so our relationship with that patient not infrequently ended with the transfer.

This specialization of knowledge, skill, and experience shapes medical practice, and it can become a slippery slope. Increasingly specialized knowledge leads to even more exclusivity of the domain. The cardiologist who understands the minutiae of the echocardiogram or details of the physiology of the cardiac myocyte (muscle cell) and electrical activity in the heart becomes the sub-subspecialist in echocardiography or cardiac electrophysiology. That doctor may limit his or her practice to application of certain technologies. Such super-subspecialization drives clinical practice toward biological and asocial framing of problems through their influence on future practitioners, whom they teach and supervise in academic hospitals. It is sometimes said that the generalist knows less and less about more and more, while the specialist knows more and more about less and less. Medical trainees cannot help but be awed by the technical wizardry and precise knowledge of the sub-subspecialist and may aspire to similar mastery of a narrow field.

This compartmentalization of practice also can propel science toward interest in the molecular and away from broader concerns, particularly if the people writing grant proposals and those reviewing them have intellectual interests that align with the technologies that they apply in their clinical work. None of this is to say that these technologies aren't useful (or that having people who are really experienced in their application is bad). At the same time, excessive attentiveness toward these lucrative procedures may crowd out awareness of matters larger than a cell, a current, or a device. These include subjects no less vital, such as getting to know patients in sufficient depth to be able to help them, in the context of their often complex social and emotional circumstances, to address disease risks or to adhere to treatments for diseases that are less complex to diagnose and treat.

When students enter medical careers already knowing that they want to be orthopedic surgeons or "invasive" cardiologists (who insert catheters into arteries), they are less likely to be humbled by (or even interested in) the enormity of the task of embracing and encountering their patients' humanity as they navigate important moments in their lives. Keen observers of the medical scene, they learn not to feel compelled to regard social and psychological circumstances of their patients as areas in which they need be expert. They are more likely to focus upon these issues when the patients are disruptive. Even then, the reaction may be to discard or avoid patients with such problems as dominating concerns. This disconnect from what they should be doing can be chilling. I have heard resident physicians say such deplorable things as "discharge that patient. I am not learning anything from him anymore."

There is little sense of the relevance of history, literature, and even psychology to the technical tasks at hand. Students may feel that only the clinical management task—and not the patient's experience of their illness or of the care that they are receiving—is important.

I learned a valuable lesson from Lloyd MacLean, the chief of surgery at my medical school, when I was a fourth-year student. It was a Friday afternoon, and I was wandering around the operating rooms area looking for one more case in which to participate before the end of the day. I saw him scrubbing in.

"What is the case? I asked.

"Hemorrhoids."

I laughed. He then said, "It may not seem like much to you, but for this patient, it may be the biggest thing that happens to him all year."

Notwithstanding the hint of surgical grandiosity, he had a point. I needed to immerse myself in the patient's perspective if I was going to be a good doctor.

But many medical students do not see the patient's experience, context, needs, or life as what they must master. Rather, it is the technical knowledge base that will get them good evaluations and the training program that they seek. The admissions process, much of the preclinical curriculum, and many of the clinicians and trainees whom they encounter in their clinical rotations promote intellectual narrowness. For most, little happens in graduate medical education to change that. Occasional cataclysmic events in society may get students' attention for a while about Black lives or medical care disparities during a pandemic. In the past, such insights faded for most pretty quickly, along with the societal concerns that they brought to admission interviews.

The alienation of trainees from the patient can manifest in many ways. One is the fascination with the interesting or unusual case, and the search for it. That gets many physicians-in-training more jazzed up than they are or would be by helping the more mundane patient plan the next steps in their lives. Another expression of such alienation (and one linked to biological reductionism in some ways) is discomfort in dealing with uncertainty. They want to know the answer to the clinical question, whatever the cost to the patient and to society, so they spare no expense in ordering tests. Many patients are anxious and want certainty as well, but part of good clinical skill is helping patients understand risk and probability, and helping them be or become comfortable with some level of uncertainty. This requires nuanced, textured conversations with patients about prognosis and risk. For example, it takes a while to explain to a patient that a cardiac stress test in an asymptomatic individual produces more false-positive than true-positive results and may lead to other unnecessary tests that can harm them.

Today, many patients understandably want as much information as possible about their prognosis. Such information is far from perfect. Camus talks about the inability to know when you will die in L'Étranger. He says that only one who is condemned to die possesses that information with certainty.[73] It also is not unreasonable to want to be able to undertake measures to fend off one's demise. (I am reminded of the man playing chess with Death in Ingmar Bergman's film The Seventh Seal.) That option is not always available. When a patient is near death, what is called for is something more than a "goals of care" conversation. Wouldn't it be enriching to have a physician present who could bring philosophical, religious, or cultural perspectives to bear in such situations, involving ethicists, clergy, or others as appropriate? But how prominent is that in the education of the physician?

When our mother was dying, I learned an important lesson, thanks to my sister, Laurie. A rabbi friend of hers had suggested we recite a Jewish prayer (The Shema) that traditionally should be said as someone breathes their last breath. Not being religious, I was skeptical, but the preparation for that task and beginning our recitation in anticipation of that moment gave us great calm and focus. I realized that such rituals, whether they be reciting prayers, reading poems, singing songs, or playing music, can transform those often-stressful experiences. I was able to recommend that approach to families in similar situations. I wished that someone had shared that insight with me sooner in my career.[74]

All medical schools have at least some curricula on death and dying, but students do not enter residency equipped to lead such discussions. They often do not possess the vocabulary, the multidisciplinary knowledge, or the life experience to know how to proceed. Some humanities in medicine programs bring illuminating perspectives to the physician's task therein. Rita Charon of Columbia University and Danielle Ofri of New York University use literature to enrich those moments.[75] I will say it again: such courses should be considered no less critical than other material that is required and that occupies considerable curricular time.

If medical schools selected on the basis of broad intellectual curiosity, at least on par with the ability to perform well on a standardized test, their students might be more likely to recognize the importance of such perspectives to their work as clinicians. It might also enrich the future doctors' conversations with patients in life's most poignant moments.

In chapter 6, we will explore the hospital environments in which these young medical graduates pursue their training in medical specialties and subspecialties. Do those experiences compensate for the missed opportunities in undergraduate medical education?

Notes

1. Rosemary Stevens, *American Medicine and the Public Interest* (Berkeley: University of California Press, 1998), 11–13; Henry R. Viets, *A Brief History of Medicine in Massachusetts* (Boston: Houghton Mifflin, 1930), 27.

2. Stevens, *American Medicine*, 11–16.

3. John Morgan, *A Discourse upon the Institution of Medical Schools in America* (Philadelphia: William Bradford, 1765; repr., Baltimore, 1937), vi, quoted in Stevens, *American Medicine*, 17.

4. Stevens, *American Medicine*, 18–19.

5. Stevens, *American Medicine*, 22–23.

6. Stevens, *American Medicine*, 24–33.

7. Stevens, *American Medicine*, 28–29.

8. Abraham Flexner, *Medical Education in the United States and Canada: A Report to the Carnegie Foundation for the Advancement of Teaching*, Bulletin No. 4 (New York: Carnegie Foundation for the Advancement of Teaching, 1910).

9. Flexner, *Medical Education*, xi.

10. Stevens, *American Medicine*, 55–74.

11. E. Richard Brown, *Rockefeller Medicine Men: Medicine and Capitalism in America* (Berkeley: University of California Press, 1979), 98–134.

12. Flexner, *Medical Education*, 18–19.

13. Rika Maeshiro et al., "Medical Education for a Healthier Population: Reflections on the Flexner Report from a Public Health Perspective," *Academic Medicine* 85, no. 2 (February 2010): 211–19, https://doi.org/10.1097/ACM .0b013e3181c885d8.

14. William H. Welch, "The Benefits of the Endowment of Medical Research," in *Addresses Delivered at the Opening of the Laboratories in New York City, May 11, 1906* (New York: Rockefeller Institute for Medical Research, 1906), 32, quoted in Brown, *Rockefeller Medicine Men*, 118–19.

15. William C. McGaghie, "Assessing Readiness for Medical Education: Evolution of the Medical College Admission Test," *JAMA* 288, no. 9 (September 4, 2002): 1085–90, https://doi.org/10.1001/jama.288.9.1085.

16. Darrell G. Kirch, Karen Mitchell, and Cori Ast, "The New 2015 MCAT: Testing Competencies," *JAMA* 310, no. 21 (December 2013): 2243–44, https://doi.org/10.1001 /jama.2013.282093.

17. Institute of Medicine (US) Committee on Institutional and Policy-Level Strategies for Increasing the Diversity of the U.S. Health Care Workforce, "Reconceptualizing Admissions Policies and Practices," in *In the Nation's Compelling Interest: Ensuring Diversity in the Health-Care Workforce*, ed. Brian D. Smedley, Adrienne Stith Butler, and Lonnie R. Bristow, chap. 2 (Washington, DC: National Academies Press, 2004), https://www.ncbi.nlm.nih.gov/books/NBK216012/; https://doi.org/10.17226 /10885.

18. "A Strong Score Requires Serious Prep," Kaplan MCAT Prep, accessed March 22, 2020, https://www.kaptest.com/mcat.

19. "Medical School Personal Statement Editing," Med School Insiders, accessed October 23, 2021, https://medschoolinsiders.com/services/personal-statement -editing/?gclid=Cj0KCQjwmdzzBRC7ARIsANdqRRlX_gtlzKb-puLVh-gGHo_aXcZDj MUC07PzgUiPQoFJhjNgMLS7PlEaAioiEALw_wcB.

20. Wikipedia, s.v. "Stanley Kaplan," accessed March 22, 2020, https://en .wikipedia.org/wiki/Stanley_Kaplan; Patricia Sullivan, "Test-Prep Pioneer Stanley H. Kaplan Dies at 90," *Washington Post*, August 25, 2009, https://www.washington post.com/wp-dyn/content/article/2009/08/24/AR2009082402105.html.

21. Robert Morse et al., "Methodology: 2021 Best Medical School Rankings," *U.S. News and World Report*, March 16, 2020, https://www.usnews.com/education/best -graduate-schools/articles/medical-schools-methodology.

22. Garrett Hardin, "The Tragedy of the Commons," *Science* 162, no. 3859 (December 12, 1968): 1243–48.

23. Daniel Markovits, *The Meritocracy Trap: How America's Foundational Myth Feeds Inequality, Dismantles the Middle Class, and Devours the Elite* (New York: Penguin Press, 2019), 124–56; Carol A. Terregino et al., "The Diversity and Success of Medical School Applicants with Scores in the Middle Third of the MCAT Score Scale,"

Academic Medicine 95, no. 3 (March 2020): 344–50, https://doi.org/10.1097 /ACM0000000000002941; Jorge A. Girotti et al., "Investigating Group Differences in Examinees' Preparation for and Performance on the New MCAT Exam," *Academic Medicine* 95, no. 3 (March 2020): 365–74, https://doi.org/10.1097/ACM .0000000000002940; Peter Gliatto, I. Michael Leitman, and David Muller, "Scylla and Charybdis: The MCAT, USMLE, and Degrees of Freedom in Undergraduate Medical Education," *Academic Medicine* 91, no. 11 (November 2016): 1498–500, https://doi.org/10.1097/ACM.0000000000001247.

24. "What Medical Schools Are Looking For: Understanding the 15 Core Competencies," Association of American Medical Colleges, accessed May 23, 2020, https://students-residents.aamc.org/applying-medical-school/article/med-schools -looking-for-15-competencies/.

25. Stewart G. Wolf, "I Can't Afford a B," *New England Journal of Medicine* 299, no. 17 (October 26, 1978): 949–50, https://doi.org/10.1056/nejm197810262991711.

26. Lewis Thomas, "Notes of a Biology-Watcher: How to Fix the Premedical Curriculum," *New England Journal of Medicine* 298, no. 21 (May 25, 1978): 1180–81, https://doi.org/10.1056/NEJM197805252982106; Richard B. Gunderman and Steven L. Kanter, "Perspective: 'How to Fix the Premedical Curriculum' Revisited," *Academic Medicine* 83, no. 12 (December 2008): 1158–61, https://doi.org/10.1097/ACM .0b013e31818c6515.

27. "White Coat Ceremony," Gold Foundation, accessed March 28, 2020, https://www.gold-foundation.org/programs/white-coat-ceremony/.

28. Mark S. Hochberg, "The Doctor's White Coat: An Historical Perspective," *Virtual Mentor* 9, no. 4 (April 1, 2007): 310–14, https://doi.org/10.1001/virtualmentor .2007.9.4.mhst1-0704.

29. Dan W. Blumhagen, "The Doctor's White Coat: The Image of the Physician in Modern America," *Annals of Internal Medicine* 91, no. 1 (July 1979): 111–16, https://doi .org/10.7326/0003-4819-91-1-111; Sarah Mahoney, "The White Coat: Symbol of Professionalism or Hierarchical Elitism?," *Association of American Medical Colleges News and Insights*, July 31, 2018, https://www.aamc.org/news-insights/white-coat -symbol-professionalism-or-hierarchical-elitism.

30. Mark C. Henderson et al., "Medical School Applicant Characteristics Associated with Performance in Multiple Mini-Interviews versus Traditional Interviews: A Multi-Institutional Study," *Academic Medicine* 93, no.7 (July 2018): 1029–34, https://doi.org/10.1097/ACM.0000000000002041.

31. Mark A. Albanese et al., "Assessing Personal Qualities in Medical School Admissions," *Academic Medicine* 78, no. 3 (March 2003): 313–21, https://doi.org/10 .1097/00001888-200303000-00016; Emily M. Mader, Carrie Roseamelia, and Christopher P. Morley, "The Temporal Decline of Idealism in Two Cohorts of Medical Students at One Institution," *BMC Medical Education* 14, no. 58 (2014), https://doi.org/10.1186/1472-6920-14-58.

32. Christopher P. Morley et al., "Decline of Medical Student Idealism in the First and Second Year of Medical School: A Survey of Pre-Clinical Medical Students at One Institution," *Medical Education Online* 18 (August 2013): 21194, https://doi.org

/10.3402/meo.v18io.21194. Howard S. Becker and Blanche Geer argue that while cynicism grows in medical school, it never entirely displaces idealism, which reemerges as they approach graduation and "again worry about maintaining their integrity, this time in actual medical practice." "The Fate of Idealism in Medical School," *American Sociological Review* 23, no. 1 (February 1958): 50–56; Jack Haas and William Shaffir, "The 'Fate of Idealism' Revisited," *Journal of Contemporary Ethnography* 13 (1984): 63–81, https://doi.org/10.1177/0098303984013001004.

33. Neil McIntyre, "Was Osler Opposed to Women Becoming Doctors?," *Journal of Medical Biography* 15, suppl. 1 (2007): 22–27, https://doi.org/10.1258/j.jmb.2007.s-1 -06-05.

34. "An Updated Look at the Economic Diversity of U.S. Medical Students," *AAMC Analysis in Brief* 18, no. 5 (October 2018): https://www.aamc.org/system/files /reports/1/october2018anupdatedlookattheeconomicdiversityofu.s.medicalstud .pdf. The situation in American law schools is similar, with only 16% of students coming for the lowest half of the socioeconomic distribution, and even fewer (5%) in the 10 top-rated law schools. Richard H. Sander, "Class in American Legal Education," *Denver University Law Review* 88, no. 4 (2011): 631–82.

35. James P. Guevara, Roy Wade, and Jaya Aysola, "Racial and Ethnic Diversity at Medical Schools—Why Aren't We There Yet?," *New England Journal of Medicine* 385, no. 19 (November 4, 2021): 1732–34, https://www.doi.org/10.1056/NEJMp2105578; "Trends in Racial and Ethnic Minority Applicants and Matriculants to U.S. Medical Schools, 1980–2016," *AAMC Analysis in Brief* 17, no. 3 (November 2017): https://www .aamc.org/system/files/reports/1/november2017trendsinracialandethnicminorityap plicantsandmatricu.pdf.

36. "Population Estimates, July 1, 2019," US Census Bureau Quick Facts, accessed March 23, 2020, https://www.census.gov/quickfacts/fact/table/US/PST045218.

37. "How Much Does Medical School Cost? Average Medical Degree Tuition & Costs," College Ave Student Loans, April 9, 2020, https://www .collegeavestudentloans.com/blog/how-much-does-medical-school-cost-average -medical-degree-tuition-costs/; Michael R. Bloomberg et al., "To Save Black Lives, We Need More Black Doctors," CNN Opinion, September 3, 2020, https://www.cnn .com/2020/09/03/opinions/black-doctors-medical-school-debt-bloomberg-frederick -carlisle-rice-hildreth/index.html.

38. Most students apply to many medical schools (15 to 30 is common). The application costs $170 for the first school to which a student applies and $40 to forward their general application to each additional one. The schools also charge a fee directly. In addition, students need to pay for the MCAT test ($315) and generally a test preparation course ($2,500). Finally, if they are selected for an interview, they need to travel to the school to be interviewed. Mallika Mitra, "Here's How Much Medical Students Are Paying Just to Get into School," CNBC Personal Finance, October 4, 2019, https://www.cnbc.com/2019/10/04/it-can-cost-10000-to-apply-for -medical-school.html.

39. "Increasing Minorities in Medical Schools: Programs Alter the Pipeline," American Medical Association Medical School Diversity, February 11, 2016,

https://www.ama-assn.org/education/medical-school-diversity/increasing
-minorities-medical-schools-programs-alter-pipeline; Robin Warshaw, "Priming
the Medical School Pipeline: Schools Reach Out to Teens in Minority and Underserved Communities," AAMC Diversity and Inclusion, September 29, 2016, https://
www.aamc.org/news-insights/priming-medical-school-pipeline-schools-reach-out
-teens-minority-and-underserved-communities.

40. "Medical Humanities: Deeper Understanding," University of Michigan Medical
School, accessed August 26, 2020, https://medicine.umich.edu/medschool/education
/md-program/curriculum/impact-curriculum/paths-excellence/medical-humanities.

41. Jeremy Graham et al., "Medical Humanities Coursework Is Associated with
Greater Measured Empathy in Medical Students," *American Journal of Medicine* 129,
no. 12 (December 2016): 1334–37, https://doi.org/10.1016/j.amjmed.2016.08.005.

42. Mary E. Kollmer Horton, "The Orphan Child: Humanities in Modern
Medical Education," *Philosophy, Ethics, and Humanities in Medicine* 14, no. 1 (January 4, 2019): https://doi.org/10.1186/s13010-018-0067-y.

43. Marguerite Holloway, "When Medicine Meets Literature," *Scientific American*,
May 1, 2005, https://www.scientificamerican.com/article/when-medicine-meets-liter/.

44. Richard L. Street Jr. et al., "How Does Communication Heal? Pathways
Linking Clinician-Patient Communication to Health Outcomes," *Patient Education and
Counseling* 74, no. 3 (March 2009): 295–301, https://doi.org/10.1016/j.pec.2008.11.015.

45. Daniel C. R. Chen et al., "Characterizing Changes in Student Empathy
throughout Medical School," *Medical Teacher* 34, no. 4 (March 28, 2012): 305–11,
https://doi.org/10.3109/0142159X.2012.644600.

46. Brendan Murphy, "These Medical Specialties Have the Biggest Gender
Imbalances," American Medical Association Specialty Profiles, October 1, 2019,
https://www.ama-assn.org/residents-students/specialty-profiles/these-medical
-specialties-have-biggest-gender-imbalances.

47. "Making Medicare: The History of Health Care in Canada, 1914–2007: Quebec
and Medicare," Canadian Museum of History, accessed March 28, 2020, https://www
.historymuseum.ca/cmc/exhibitions/hist/medicare/medic-6h03e.html.

48. Rudolf Virchow, "Der Armenarzt" [The poor doctor], *Die Medizinische Reform*
18 (November 3, 1848): 125–27.

49. Ted Allen and Sydney Gordon, *The Scalpel, The Sword: The Story of Dr. Norman
Bethune* (Toronto: McClelland and Stewart, 1989); Martin F. Shapiro, "Medical Aid to
the Spanish Republic during the Civil War, 1936–1939," *Annals of Internal Medicine* 97,
no. 1 (July 1982): 119–24, https://doi.org/10.7326/0003-4819-97-1-119.

50. Elizabeth A. Rider, Margaret M. Hinrichs, and Beth A. Lown, "A Model for
Communication Skills Assessment across the Undergraduate Curriculum," *Medical
Teacher* 28, no. 5 (August 2006): e127–e134, https://doi.org/10.1080
/01421590600726540.

51. See, e.g., "Physician Starting Salaries by Specialty: 2018 vs. 2017," Merritt
Hawkins, November 19, 2018, https://www.merritthawkins.com/news-and-insights
/blog/job-search-advice/physician-starting-salaries-by-specialty-2018-vs-2017/.

52. Julie P. Phillips et al., "Specialty Income and Career Decision Making: A Qualitative Study of Medical Student Perceptions," *Medical Education* 53, no. 6 (June 2019): 593–604, https://doi.org/10.1111/medu.13820.

53. "2019 Salaries for University of California," Transparent California, accessed July 30, 2021, https://transparentcalifornia.com/salaries/2019/university-of -california/.

54. Ironically, the enormous disparities in income do not correlate clearly with job satisfaction, which is more closely related to lifestyle. In some studies, physicians in some of the highest-paying specialties are the least satisfied. J. Paul Leigh et al., "Physician Career Satisfaction across Specialties," *Archives of Internal Medicine* 162, no. 14 (July 22, 2002): 1577–84, https://doi.org/10.1001/archinte.162.14.1577; J. Paul Leigh, Daniel J. Trancredi, and Richard L. Kravitz, "Physician Career Satisfaction within Specialties," *BMC Health Services Research* 9 (September 16, 2009): 166, https://doi.org/10.1186/1472-6963-9-166.

55. US medical school graduates filled 94% of slots in thoracic surgery, 89% in plastic surgery and otolaryngology, 85% in neurological surgery, 82% in vascular surgery, 81% in orthopedic surgery, and 80% in dermatology and interventional radiology. Rates were 75% in obstetrics-gynecology, 66% in general surgery, 63% in psychiatry, and 60% in pediatrics. National Resident Matching Program, "Table 8: Positions Offered and Percent Filled by MD Seniors and All Applicants, 2017–2021," in *The Match: Results and Data 2021 Main Residency Match*: 25 (Washington, DC: National Resident Matching Program, May 2021), https://mkonrmp3oyqui6wqfm .kinstacdn.com/wp-content/uploads/2021/05/MRM-Results_and-Data_2021.pdf. That trend has wavered little from year to year. Victoria Knight, "American Medical Students Less Likely to Choose to Become Primary Care Doctors," Kaiser Health News, last updated July 3, 2019, https://khn.org/news/american-medical-students -less-likely-to-choose-to-become-primary-care-doctors/.

56. Leslie Kane et al., "International Physician Compensation Report 2019: Do US Physicians Have It Best?," Medscape, September 16, 2019, https://www.medscape .com/slideshow/2019-international-compensation-report-6011814#6.

57. Mark J. Prashker and Robert F. Meenan, "Subspecialty Training: Is It Financially Worthwhile?," *Annals of Internal Medicine* 115, no. 9 (November 1, 1991): 715–19, https://doi.org/10.7326/0003-4819-115-9-715.

58. Roger A. Rosenblatt and C. Holly A. Andrilla, "The Impact of U.S. Medical Students' Debt on Their Choice of Primary Care Careers: An Analysis of Data from the 2002 Medical School Graduation Questionnaire," *Academic Medicine* 80, no. 9 (September 2005): 815–19, https://doi.org/10.1097/00001888-200509000-00006.

59. David W. Chen, "Surprise Gift: Free Tuition for All N.Y.U Medical Students," *New York Times*, August 16, 2018, https://www.nytimes.com/2018/08/16/nyregion /nyu-free-tuition-medical-school.html; Mark S. Lachs and Augustine M. K. Choi, "Eliminating Medical Student Debt: A Dean and a Geriatrician's View from Opposite Ends of the Training Pipeline," *Annals of Internal Medicine* 172, no. 4 (February 18, 2020): 279–80, https://doi.org/10.7326/M19-2897.

60. Erin Barry, "Why NYU's Tuition-Free Medical School Offer May Not Live Up to Its Hype," CNBC On the Money, September 9, 2018, https://www.cnbc.com/2018/09/08/why-nyus-tuition-free-medical-school-may-not-live-up-to-its-hype.html.

61. Ryne Lane, "8 Medical School Loan Forgiveness Programs for Doctors," Nerdwallet, July 1, 2020, https://www.nerdwallet.com/article/loans/student-loans/medical-school-loan-forgiveness-programs.

62. Andrew Abbott, *The System of Professions: An Essay on the Division of Expert Labor* (Chicago: University of Chicago Press, 1988), 59–85.

63. Mark D. Schwartz et al., "Medical Student Interest in Internal Medicine: Initial Report of the Society of General Internal Medicine Interest Group Survey on Factors Influencing Career Choice in Internal Medicine," *Annals of Internal Medicine* 114, no.1 (January 1, 1991): 6–15, https://doi.org/10.7326/0003-4819-114-1-6.

64. Eliot Freidson, *Profession of Medicine, a Study of the Sociology of Applied Knowledge* (New York: Dodd Mead, 1973), 345; Ezekiel J. Emanuel and Linda L. Emanuel, "Four Models of the Physician-Patient Relationship," JAMA 267, no. 16 (April 22–29, 1992): 2221–26, https://doi.org/10.1001/jama.1992.03480160079038.

65. Marie-Anne Durand et al., "Shared Decision Making Embedded in the Undergraduate Medical Curriculum: A Scoping Review," *PLOS One* 13, no. 11 (November 14, 2018): e0207012, https://doi.org/10.1371/journal.pone.0207012.

66. B. Hodges et al., "Evaluating Communication Skills in the OSCE Format: Reliability and Generalizability," *Medical Education* 30, no. 1 (January 1996): 38–43, https://doi.org/10.1111/j.1365-2973.1996.tb00715.x.

67. N. Pattni et al., "Challenging Authority and Speaking Up in the Operating Room Environment: A Narrative Synthesis," *British Journal of Anaesthesia* 122, no. 2 (February 2019): 233–44, https://doi.org/10.1016/j.bja.2018.10.056.

68. Huug Obertop, "How Surgeons Make Decisions: Authority and Evidence," *Annals of Surgery* 242, no. 6 (December 2005): 753–56, https://doi.org/10.1097/01.sla.0000189110.37637.6b; Julian Barling, Amy Akers, and Darren Beiko, "The Impact of Positive and Negative Intraoperative Surgeons' Leadership Behaviors on Surgical Team Performance," *American Journal of Surgery* 215, no. 1 (January 2018): 14–18, https://doi.org/10.1016/j.amjsurg.2017.07.006; Nancy L. Keating et al., "Treatment Decision Making in Early-Stage Breast Cancer: Should Surgeons Match Patients' Desired Level of Involvement?," *Journal of Clinical Oncology* 20, no. 6 (March 2002): 1473–79, https://doi.org/10.1200/JCO.2002.20.6.1473.

69. Erich Fromm, *Escape from Freedom* (New York: Farrar & Rinehart, 1941).

70. Martin Shapiro, *Getting Doctored: Critical Reflections on Becoming a Physician* (Toronto: Between the Lines, 1978), 196–205.

71. Dominick L. Frosch et al., "Authoritarian Physicians and Patients' Fear of Being Labeled 'Difficult' among Key Obstacles to Shared Decision Making," *Health Affairs* (Millwood) 31, no. 5 (May 2012): 1030–38, https://doi.org/10.1377/hlthaff.2011.0576.

72. Thomas S. Szasz and Marc N. Hollander, "A Contribution to the Philosophy of Medicine: The Basic Models of the Doctor-Patient Relationship," *Archives of*

Internal Medicine 97, no. 5 (May 1956): 585–92, https://doi.org/10.1001/archinte.1956
.00250230079008. In "Four Models," Emanuel and Emanuel build on this work by
identifying four models of the doctor-patient relationship: paternalistic (closest to
activity-passivity); informative (providing information so that a patient can make a
decision); interpretive (elucidating a patient's values); and deliberative (delineating
the clinical situation and the values inherent in a patient's options and suggesting
why some values are more worthy of aspiring to).

73. Albert Camus, L'Étranger (Paris: Gallimard, 1942).

74. Martin F. Shapiro, "The Last Breath—Enriching End-of-Life Moments,"
JAMA Internal Medicine 179, no. 7 (July 1, 2019): 865–66, https://doi.org/10.1001
/jamaimternmed.2019.1451.

75. Rita Charon, "The Patient-Physician Relationship. Narrative Medicine: A
Model for Empathy, Reflection, Profession, and Trust," JAMA 286, no. 15 (Octo-
ber 2001): 1897–902, https://doi.org/10.1001/jama.286.15.1897; Danielle Ofri,
"Medical Humanities: The Rx for Uncertainty?," Academic Medicine 92, no. 12
(December 2017): 1657–58, https://doi.org/10.1097/ACM.0000000000001983.

Errors of (com)Mission

Misdirected Priorities in Education, Practice, and Research

Selflessness is a rare virtue because it doesn't pay for itself.
—Bertolt Brecht, *Mother Courage and Her Children*

The Tripartite Mission

In addition to the instruction of medical students, schools of medicine are engaged in a number of other activities, including the further training of medical school graduates (postgraduate education), research, and clinical practice by members of their faculty and their trainees. This is often referred to as their tripartite mission. The mission statements of many American medical schools mention compassion, professionalism, critical thinking, community, and, most recently, diversity and inclusion. At their core, however, they profess to be most devoted to education, research, and practice.[1] We will examine each component of the tripartite mission in some detail in this chapter and in chapters 7 and 8. This chapter is largely concerned with the education of residents and fellows. In so doing, it considers the impact of the clinical and research programs of the schools upon the trainees.

Postgraduate Medical Education
The Growth of Specialization and the Complicity of Medical Schools

Postgraduate medical education entails training residents and fellows in their specialties and subspecialties. It is a major business of academic medical centers and of the medical schools with which many of them are affiliated. Medical school faculties train the doctors who enter highly specialized fields. It is worth considering just how specialized American medicine has become, as well as the role that medical schools have played in the evolution toward the current configuration of medical practice.

Historical Trends

In the colonies and the early years of the republic, the great majority of physicians were generalists. There always had been physicians with particular skills, but they did not tend to identify themselves formally as part of any specialties. That began to change in the 1860s, when some started to advertise as specialists.[2] A torrent of specialization followed. The emergence of anesthesia and antisepsis made surgeries much less lethal. From the 1890s through the 1920s, surgical fields proliferated to include abdominal surgery, gynecology, neurosurgery, urology, and ear, nose, and throat surgery. Beginning in 1910, annual national congresses of surgeons were held in the United States. In 1912, the American College of Surgeons was founded. Internal medicine was not too far behind. Internists were anxious to distinguish themselves, in terms of prestige, from general practitioners. In 1915, they founded the American College of Physicians.[3]

After World War II, the subspecialization and sub-subspecialization of medicine began to explode in earnest, a process that continues to this day. In cardiology, there are now cardiologists who do catheterizations and others who specialize in placement of pacemakers, insertion of valves into the heart through arterial catheters, echocardiography, electrophysiology (rhythm disturbances), congenital heart disease, congestive heart failure, geriatric cardiology, and so on. The American Board of Internal Medicine now issues sub-subspecialty certification (through examination) in four of these areas: interventional cardiology, clinical cardiac electrophysiology, advanced heart failure and transplant cardiology, and adult congenital heart disease.[4]

In urology, there are subspecialists in kidney transplantation, cancer of the bladder and prostate, benign prostatic disease, kidney and bladder stones, sexual dysfunction, gender reassignment surgery, female pelvic medicine and reconstructive surgery, and pediatric urology. (There are subspecialty certificates available in the last two fields.)[5] In ophthalmology, specialization has emerged in cataract, cornea, glaucoma, low vision, neuro-ophthalmology, plastic surgery, retina, strabismus, and refractive surgery.[6]

Proliferation, the Lack of Regulation, and Their Consequences

There is little regulation at the societal level in the United States of the number of people entering a given subspecialty or sub-subspecialty. If a training program is approved by the Residency Review Committee and specialties are sanctioned by a component of the American Board of Medical Specialties, that position is available. In some other countries, the government specifies how many people can train in a particular field and how many can practice in that field in a particular community.

When my friends Dana and Benoît, both nephrologists, moved to Montreal from Paris, there was only one nephrologist slot available at McGill University where they were hired. That was because the responsible agency for the province of Quebec specifies the number of positions in each specialty to which each university and regional hospital in the province is entitled. Dana filled that position, while Benoît, who also was certified in critical care, took an available position as an intensive care specialist. The point here is that the sanctioning of training in a specialty predictably generates costs in that area for the health care system. Society has a fiduciary interest in the number of people practicing a specialty and should be able to specify appropriate limits on their numbers. There also should be a means to ensure that specialists' geographic distribution is consistent with society's needs.

In the United States, no government authority takes responsibility or exercises authority to ensure that specialist numbers meet, but do not exceed, society's need in this way. Consequently, the market (mediated by individuals in that specialty) makes these determinations for society, but not necessarily in the interest of society. At the same time, there is considerable concern that there are insufficient numbers of practitioners who don't do procedures, particularly in primary care.

The Association of American Medical Colleges, which represents broadly the interests of medical schools and their many specialties, recently projected a shortfall of 46,900 to 121,900 physicians by 2032, among whom nearly half would be primary care physicians (PCPs).[7] Their projection reflected an estimated need for a total of 283,400 PCPs out of 915,100 total physicians (about 31%).[8] Even that relative increase would result in a smaller proportion of PCPs than in other advanced, industrialized countries. In Canada, 51% of doctors were general practitioners in 2020.[9] Most advanced economies have ratios comparable to that in Canada.[10] In one analysis, increasing the numbers of PCPs in US counties with shortages would increase life expectancy substantially.[11]

Specialty Training and Practice in Medical Schools

How did academic medical centers respond to these developments? Those seeking to enter the proliferating subspecialties needed training in them, much of which occurred in medical schools. Many of the schools came to strongly emphasize subspecialty medicine. One consequence was that there were few generalist physicians working within most medical schools in the 1950s and 1960s. In the 1970s, this imbalance began to get some notice, and some schools started to recruit more generalists to their faculty.[12] This trend accelerated when clinical leaders decided that they needed to build primary care networks to feed their specialties.

Accordingly, some medical schools began to hire more general internists and assigned some of their residency positions in internal medicine to tracks for students specifically interested in primary care. These tracks typically comprise only a small proportion of the training positions in a hospital's internal medicine residency program. At Cornell's New York-Presbyterian Hospital, for example, they accept 4 internal medicine residents each year into a primary care track, out of 45 new interns. At UCLA, there are 12 such slots each year among 60 in internal medicine. While the trainees in the regular slots do have the option of not doing a subspecialty, those in primary care tracks are more likely to make that choice.

The Scramble for Slots in Lucrative Fields

Within internal medicine training programs, residents are well aware of income differences between subspecialties. There is a clear hierarchy of desirable subspecialty fields that reflect their relative incomes. At the top of the heap are the major procedural fields of cardiology, gastroenterology, oncology, and pulmonary/critical care. Nephrology (kidney disease) is an intermediate-income field owing to the care of dialysis patients. Rheumatology (which involves some joint injections and aspirations) and endocrinology (with occasional thyroid biopsies) are largely evaluation and management fields and are much closer in prestige (and income) to the lowly infectious disease specialists and the general internists, who rarely do procedures.[13]

Some of the physicians within these subspecialties are able to earn even more. Examples of this include so-called invasive cardiologists who do catheterizations, electrophysiology procedures, and pacemaker insertion (as opposed to those whose practices emphasize fields like geriatric cardiology and congestive heart failure), and gastroenterologists who specialize in inserting tubes and doing procedures through them, including colonoscopists, upper endoscopists, and those who put scopes into the pancreatic and hepatic (liver) ducts to do procedures in them, as opposed to those gastroenterologists who manage liver failure and chronic inflammatory bowel diseases. Incomes for generalist physicians are not at all bad, but the differences are stark. Many internal medicine trainees want to get into a high-paying subspecialty, and the competition is fiercest for cardiology and gastroenterology. I recall one typical year in which at least 10 of the 30 residents in our internal medicine residency program were applying for fellowships in cardiology. In contrast, the chief of infectious diseases lamented to me how difficult it was to attract talented individuals into academic training as clinician investigators in that field.

Shouldn't medical schools that claim a mission of population health want to make sure that health care resources are allocated in relation to what society needs and can afford? The numbers and distribution of physicians across specialties are some of the most important variables in any calculus relating to constraining health care costs. More people trained in procedures means that more of them get done. A person who passes tubes will pass tubes, and one who puts in pacemakers will put in pacemakers. Excessive numbers of procedural specialists drive use of technologies, hospitals, and associated resources. They thereby ratchet up costs in ways that affect affordability of health insurance and access to medical care. Certainly, lots of organizations have been interested in developing strategies to lower the cost of specialty services, but they rarely talk about the obvious step of limiting the number of people who are trained to do them.[14]

A More Rational Approach

Is there an appropriate number of practitioners of a particular specialty in a community? If we allow the market to decide, there will be overuse so long as insurance permits it, because doctors will find patients on whom to do the procedures. If it is done by regulation, there is a danger of shortages, and mechanisms are needed to monitor the decision-making process with that in mind. Conversely, clinicians who do more than a minimum number of procedures often have better outcomes. This would suggest that there should be some objective approach to determining the level of societal need for a procedure, and that we then limit the numbers of individuals doing these procedures, such that all who need them can get them done by someone who is experienced. Doctors should welcome the opportunity to share data on their level of experience with procedures as well as on their complication rates, but they rarely offer such information, even to sophisticated consumers.

Ed Park, an economist colleague and friend of mine, developed colon cancer. The surgeon whom he consulted planned to remove part of the colon through a small incision, using a laparoscope. Ed inquired as to how often he performed this procedure.

"Often," he responded.

"Could you quantify that?" asked Ed.

The surgeon then told him that he did that procedure up to 100 times per year. Ed was satisfied and went forward with the operation. Ed told me that the surgeon would not have shared those data if he had not pushed for it. As an economist, Ed spent his time analyzing quantitative data, expected specificity about numbers, and didn't hesitate to request that information when it was not forthcoming. Most patients are not quantitative scientists and may not feel entitled to ask probing questions about their doctor's experience or anticipated outcomes. It shouldn't take someone with the background of an economist to successfully elicit such basic information when it is not readily available![15]

Why don't the leaders of medical schools sit down with health authorities to determine whether they need to train more cardiologists and gastroenterologists, and if so, how many are needed to perform the procedures that are supported by the evidence and that are required for their population? They don't do that, in part, because having trainees for the specialty faculty makes their work much more efficient. They can see more patients in less time, and either generate more revenue or have additional time for other pursuits such as research, without having to sacrifice income. It is also financially beneficial to medical schools and their hospitals to be highly specialized. As discussed in chapter 7, they talk about population health, but they don't mean it. To paraphrase Claudius in *Hamlet*, "their words fly up, but their thoughts remain below." In this respect, they are failing society.[16]

The specialties themselves do not seem to be trying very hard to limit the numbers entering the fields. Indeed, much of the recent literature talks about shortfalls in the number of specialists in some fields relative to the need or demand in America's unregulated medical market.[17]

Residents' Experiences in Providing Longitudinal Care

Another aspect of postgraduate medical training aligns with failings in undergraduate training. Residency programs find it difficult to provide meaningful experiences in clinics, where trainees should have the opportunity to learn that outpatient visits are so much more than "cognitive services." They can introduce the young physician to the joy of building relationships with patients, the opportunity to empathize with their difficulties, the exhilaration (and frustration) of working with them to address their life challenges and crises, and the importance of taking the time to collaborate with their patients on decision-making about their medical care. As if it were not enough that specialty procedures seem more glamorous and exciting to residents, and are more lucrative, one of the problems in attracting physicians into lower-paying fields is that trainees' experiences of providing such care in clinic settings are generally awful.[18]

Difficult Patients and Discontinuity

The patients whom residents get to see often are the ones the faculty don't want to take care of, either because they are difficult, demanding patients, or because they are poor and have many health problems. Patients who have chronic pain with substantial need for analgesia, who have other conditions like sickle cell disease that are difficult to treat, or who have many social problems, often predominate. It is challenging for residents to meet their needs in the time available, and most have not yet had sufficient experience to be able to prioritize problems well in outpatient care. Some residents and students love the work and the relationships, but many are resentful and would prefer to get back to inpatient medicine, where the problems are urgent, the priorities clear, the expectations reasonable, and the support more extensive.

Recently, residents at many medical schools have been moved to outpatient blocks of a week or two every four to eight weeks, but this approach means that the possibility of continuity, a component of which is accessibility and which is a key intended benefit to the trainee of providing ongoing outpatient care, is not prioritized.[19] A problem with the block approach is that patients often need to return sooner than the time when the residents can see them. Trainees may have partners who cover their patients when they are away, but if they are away most of the time, it is hard to conceive of this as the same kind of ongoing relationship that practicing physicians have with their patients. In one analysis, residents considered the patients whom they actually saw with the block model to be their own patients a little more often than in the old model, but that was only about half of patients they saw. Clearly, neither approach is achieving a high degree of continuity.[20]

If one of the joys of being a doctor is getting to know your patients as you take responsibility for them, that is being lost. That would require a program structure, for example, in which the resident would be relieved of inpatient responsibilities for the rest of the day when they have a weekly clinic, so that outpatient care is not regarded as a distraction from the resident's main job.[21] The demands of inpatient care are intense, and solving this problem is not a simple one and may require multiple interventions.[22]

Discontented Doctors

Residents sometimes comment that primary care doctors in their health systems seem unhappy, while proceduralists seem less stressed and much happier.[23] Small wonder! Academic primary care physicians are under pressure to see more and more patients. The specialists, who are being paid up to two or three times as much, may face similar pressures but with less consequence for their personal financial situations. Resident clinics may be understaffed, with both mentors who can focus on the resident experience and other support staff and resources.[24] In academic institutions, the administrative burden on primary care physicians may be greater than that in the specialties (where, for example, there may be scribes to write the notes). Higher administrative burden, in turn, is associated with career dissatisfaction.[25]

Medical students and residents notice these challenges and make their choices accordingly. The time line for deciding about a subspecialty in internal medicine is short. In a typical program of three years, applications need to be submitted by the beginning of the third year for most programs. At that point, the trainee will not have experienced many subspecialties, and their total exposure to outpatient care in their continuity clinic will be perhaps 80 or 90 half days. If even a few of those experiences are unpleasant, that may be decisive.

So unsatisfactory are the ambulatory experiences that even many of the physicians who choose not to do a subspecialty opt for jobs as "hospitalists," doctors who limit their practices to the care of the hospitalized patient. Hospital medicine can be an interesting and fulfilling career, but when I asked one resident who was choosing to be a hospitalist what else he had considered, he told me, "Well, I don't want to do a specialty, and I don't want to do clinic." He regarded his experience as a student, in the clinic where residents saw patients (often the ones that faculty members chose not to follow), as being comparable to what it would be like to have his own practice and follow a diverse group of patients over time.

American medical schools have been icons of innovation: in vaccines to prevent feared diseases, machines to enhance diagnosis, and treatments that prolong life. Can't they come up with a sensible approach and sufficient resources that would give residents more positive experiences in ambulatory care? Such models exist in some programs, but many medical schools do not implement them because it is inconvenient. Apart from the scheduling issues, faculty members would need to care for patients who are more socioeconomically diverse (patients like the ones not troubled by seeing residents) and work side by side with their trainees in their care. In so doing, they could model approaches to the challenges that the patients pose and show how fulfilling such care can be. Reimbursement likely would be less, given that many would have public insurance or none at all. Investing societal resources in multiple studies of strategies for improving ambulatory experiences in training would pay substantial dividends if they resulted in fewer future physicians devoting their careers to doing procedures.

The hospitalist model has been shown to shorten length of stay slightly, but it can produce discontinuity in care, particularly when the outpatient doctor is not fully informed about the hospital course. That can have adverse effects on health as well as raise costs. It is well recognized that patients with complex health problems are at greater risk of hospitalization and that they might well benefit from better coordination of care.[26] A group at the University of Chicago is conducting a multihospital study of the impact of "comprehensive care physicians" who provide both inpatient and outpatient care (as had been common in the prehospitalist era) for particularly complex patients. They have found that patients receiving comprehensive care from one physician report more satisfaction and fewer hospitalizations than those seeing different doctors inside and outside of the hospital.[27] The fact that comprehensive (inpatient and outpatient) care has been identified as a needed innovation indicates how far we have strayed from the notion that one's doctor will be around for the major health-related moments in an individual's life.

The Conflict between Teaching and Clinical Work

With the massive expansion of the clinical programs associated with medical schools, at multiple clinic sites, and often at multiple hospitals, most of the faculty are clinicians, and most of the revenue to support their salaries comes from clinical work. To account for this activity, medical school departments tend to assign targets of productivity, which as we saw in chapter 3 are defined by relative value units (RVUs) of care. While there is some ability to adjust visits and other medical acts for complexity, there is an incentive to move through visits expeditiously. Primary care and specialty visits in the US average about 20 minutes and 21 minutes, respectively.[28] Medical schools reward faculty physicians who churn through more RVUs and generate more revenue to support their salaries. Sometimes they do this through brevity. As noted previously, some physicians bill at the highest allowable rate for complex visits when they have had far more limited interactions with patients.

I was referred to an orthopedic surgeon on the faculty because of back pain that had persisted for several months. When I called, his receptionist said that I needed to have a magnetic resonance imaging (MRI) study before I could be seen. I got it done, then showed up for the appointment. When I was placed in the examining room, a resident came in for a couple of minutes, asked me half a dozen questions, and tapped on my knees, but did no other parts of a physical examination. I assumed that he was waiting for the orthopedic surgeon to do the rest of the examination with him.

When the latter showed up, he poked his head in the door, and said that the MRI told the whole story, and that I should come to another room to see it. I did. While standing in front of the images, he told me that surgery was an option, but I might want to wait until things got worse. He didn't ask any questions. He didn't examine me. He billed my insurance for a new patient complex history and physical examination. This was an instance of so-called upcoding, in the extreme. Disgusted, I went to another back surgeon in the community. He actually examined me and came to a different conclusion about my problem that led to a nonsurgical cure.

This culture of "efficiency" means not spending as much time as is needed with the patient to take a meticulous history, not doing a thorough physical examination, not carefully explaining what is going on, and not making sure that the patient truly understands it. It does not embrace the inevitable "inefficiency" of shared decision-making, nor give the patient full rein to express what is on his or her mind. Most residents and students have opportunities to watch clinicians interview and examine patients. They learn to reproduce the modeled behavior. They may also notice that this style of drive-by care is reinforced not infrequently by clinic staff who complain about physicians who take "too much time" with each patient and "fall behind."

In this context, the busy work of the faculty member in generating revenue often leads to giving much less priority to taking time with a resident (or student) to discuss the details of a case and their implications. When the resident has seen the patient first, the faculty supervisor might spend little time with the patient (shaking hands or asking a cursory question or two), or even none at all. There are numerous clinicians who buck this trend, often paying a price in revenue generation. Students see for themselves.

One such exception, my friend Dana, the nephrologist mentioned previously, is utterly devoted to her patients. Unlike the kidney specialist who treated my father as little more than a series of laboratory test values, she spends enormous amounts of time attending to the full range of her patients' clinical and social needs. That is not the example that most students get to see. When patients come in with complex needs, how consistently do they get addressed? Wealthy patients in the concierge practices certainly get that attention. For those who are poor, it is another matter entirely.

Socioeconomic Triage: Where the Poor Get Seen

Teaching hospitals are core institutions for clinical education and clinical research. I discuss them in more detail in chapter 7. Here, we are concerned with the implications of the academic clinician's practice style for the education of medical students and postgraduate trainees. These academic centers receive substantial government funding for research and some adjustment of Medicare rates to account for the additional costs of care that are associated with their teaching roles.[29]

While some are public hospitals, such as Bellevue in New York City and Cook County in Chicago, and some are private, for-profit hospitals, most are so-called voluntary hospitals, which are technically nonprofit institutions. In general, hospitals are not allowed to turn away patients in an emergency. Thus there are Medicaid and uninsured patients on inpatient services. In the case of the uninsured, many of these hospitals recognize no obligation to continue to provide care once patients are discharged. They may refer them to public hospitals and free clinics for follow-up. As for Medicaid patients, some do receive care at university hospitals, but it varies a lot.

When I was working at the University of California, Los Angeles, which is a state institution, I noticed that there had been a decrease in the number of MediCal (California Medicaid) patients in the general medicine clinic where I worked. I collected data on the trend over time in our proportion of MediCal patients: it had fallen from more than 30% to

10% to 15% over the previous few years. I presented the data at a faculty meeting. Many of my colleagues were sympathetic but we were not in a position to get our hospital and health system leadership to do anything about their contracting, their policies regarding visits for patients being discharged from the hospital, or their willingness to allow new patient visits for MediCal beneficiaries.

In the ensuing years, those numbers continued to decline to the point where, by 2015, 5% or fewer of patients being seen had MediCal. Some of the decline related to not offering clinic appointments to MediCal patients who were being discharged from the hospital. Some was related to not contracting with MediCal managed care. Some other specialties at UCLA, such as orthopedics and ear, nose, and throat, would not see any MediCal patients for elective surgeries; many others relegated them to trainee clinics, if they could get in at all. This trend, which has characterized other University of California hospitals as well, shows no signs of abating.[30]

In New York City, medical schools such as Cornell's provide a follow-up visit for Medicaid patients who have been hospitalized, but typically not at the office of a faculty member. They only provide continuity of care for them in some primary care clinics: those in which residents and a minority of the generalist faculty see their patients. Many more generalist physicians who are affiliated with the medical school do not take Medicaid insurance at all. In the case of specialty care, residents or fellows are first-line providers for the patients, with few exceptions.

Faculty members do supervise in the clinics, but it is the residents who are expected to provide continuity for the patients whom they see. Continuity of care is considered to be a key component of quality. Studies consistently have found that continuity is far from optimal in many resident and fellow clinics, and inferior to that provided by practicing physicians because these trainees have intensive inpatient rotations that limit availability, and in most cases, they will leave the institution or move onto subspecialties.[31] These discriminatory patterns of care aroused anger in the wake of the Black Lives Matter movement at both UCLA and Cornell in 2020.

Many practicing doctors do not take Medicaid patients because the reimbursement is substantially lower than it is with other forms of insurance. Bureaucratic challenges in getting reimbursed can lead to additional lost revenue in the care of those with Medicaid coverage.[32] Even those who graduate with sufficiently intact moral compasses to want to provide care to that population find that many corporate provider systems that offer them employment do not give them the option of taking care of the poor. Getting specialist care, especially for complex problems, can be challenging for Medicaid patients, and the wait times can be long.[33]

This pattern of providing "steerage" care to the poor in academic institutions is ethically and pedagogically problematic. First, it is inferior care for the patients in terms of continuity. Second, in at least some cases, the faculty physicians do not go into the room to see the patients seen by trainees whom they supervise, even though they are billing for the visits. Many of these patients are complex, and trainees might well benefit from more active participation by the professor. Third, the trainees "see for themselves" and learn from the behavior of supervising physicians who do not take on the care of such patients. Understandably, they interpret what they observe as permission similarly to refuse to care for patients whose insurance does not pay well when they enter practice. They are being educated profoundly in their ambulatory experiences, in the acceptability of morally reprehensible behavior.

The "Free Clinic" as a Teaching Venue

When I came to the United States from Canada, I was surprised to learn that many of the more idealistic doctors were going to "free clinics" a couple of times a month to provide care for the poor. In Canada, there were no free clinics to speak of, because virtually everyone had insurance for health care and did not have to pay deductibles or a proportion of the cost of care.

These free clinics are now an institutionalized component of care in the US. Many become Federally Qualified Health Centers, or FQHCs, which meet certain regulatory requirements. Some idealistic doctors who are employed at these facilities earn far less than their colleagues in academic or private practice. Care is clearly inferior in FQHCs to that in other practice settings, in continuity, resources, convenience, availability of referrals, and some measures of quality of care.[34]

When I worked in such a free clinic, supervising residents who rotated through it, the patients saw a different resident at almost every visit. We tried to come up with a way to improve continuity of care with the residents (who were there for a half-day session only one or two weeks out of every five or six) by scheduling patients whom they saw to come back on a half day when their resident was scheduled to be there. This initiative failed. Some patients needed to come back sooner. Others had interceding events needing care. Still others came back but were scheduled on the wrong day or half day. Some were unable to make it on the day the resident was there.

Was this a worthwhile experience for the residents? Yes, insofar as they occasionally gained some insight into what life was like for the disadvantaged. But some learned the wrong lesson: that volunteering to work without pay in such a clinic once in a while is sufficient, even if you spend the rest of your time only caring for those with "good" insurance.

Not My Responsibility

When I came to Los Angeles, I had a colleague in my research fellowship training program who had been a resident at a local public hospital. He was a smart young man, liberal in disposition, so I was shocked when we got around to talking about undocumented persons who needed care. He told me that some Mexican immigrants with kidney failure showed up at his hospital for dialysis treatment. He added that, as a chief resident, he collaborated in turning them away. He told me, "We can't be taking on all of these people from Mexico who need dialysis and can't get it there." I understood that his public hospital had a policy about that. I was more bothered by his lack of outrage. It was a death sentence for the patients, and he did not seem particularly distressed by that realization.

He was one of many young doctors who had learned socially regressive lessons, even when working in public hospitals and taking care of the poor. He went on to have several prominent jobs in American medicine. I always wondered if his perspective changed as his responsibilities grew, or if that indifference poisoned his decision-making and values in all of his career stops.

Clinical Practice in Medical Schools: "No Margin, No Mission" or "Margin Is the Mission"?

Medical schools derive revenue from a limited number of sources. Student tuition can be a burden for the student, but its contribution to the cost of running a medical school is trivial. Medical schools in public universities often receive direct financial support from the state government. That funding, however, has declined in many places as state budgets have been strained, and it has contributed a progressively smaller share of the coverage of medical school costs. Gifts and bequests are another source of support. The medical schools best known for their research programs are most effective in garnering such funding. Research and educational grants are still another channel for revenue. Educational grants tend not be substantial. Research grants are invaluable, but the level of such funding varies a great deal. Other than these sources, there is only clinical revenue. Virtually all medical schools and/or their affiliated hospitals are centrally concerned with the generation of clinical business.[35]

The Pursuit of Clinical Revenue

Jess Unruh, a renowned California secretary of state who once ran for governor against Ronald Reagan, famously said that money is the mother's milk of politics. Well, money also is the mother's milk of academic medicine. Clinical revenues are crucial, and schools go to great lengths to capture market share, improve case mix (meaning get rid of the patients with poor insurance or no insurance, including Medicaid beneficiaries), and improve productivity (meaning get doctors to produce more widgets per day, and to do lots of the kinds of procedures that reimburse well).

Academic "health systems" of hospitals and clinics are laser-focused on profitable product lines. How does that relate to the mission of medical schools? All medical schools consider the education of medical students, residents, and fellows to be a core component of their mission. It is worth considering, then, what education is supposed to be. The word "educate" has two Latin sources: *educare*, to rear, and *educere*, to lead forth. Since the time of the Flexner report, clinical programs have been essential to undergraduate and postgraduate education. Given that much of the educational activity now is centered in "clinical enterprises," it is fair to consider where those experiences are leading the students. Do academic health systems behave differently from those not affiliated with medical schools? Not really.

There is little doubt that medical schools lead their students toward the styles of practice and values that their trainees participate in every day in their health systems, and what they see is doctors, departments, and whole institutions centrally focused upon revenue generation. In a survey of more than 12,000 internal medicine residents and of the directors of their programs in teaching hospitals, only 47.8% of the residents and 54% of their program directors reported that a majority of the faculty who work with residents consistently role modeled cost-conscious care.[36] In 2018, 91% of teaching hospitals received $832 million in biomedical industry payments for royalties, education programs, compensation for services, gifts, or charitable contributions.[37] Academic practitioners and other physicians were equally likely to believe that physicians over-order tests when they have a financial incentive to do so.[38] One joke poses the question, "What is the difference between academic medicine and private practice?" The answer is, "In the private sector, it's dog eat dog; in academic medicine, it's the other way around!"

The Need for Clinicians and Patients

Educationally, medical schools need clinicians to teach patient care. The clinicians need "clinical material" (patients) to demonstrate clinical findings, model styles of practice, teach clinical therapeutics, and the like. Although government support, tuition, and educational grants might provide funding for didactic courses, these sources cannot begin to cover the cost of clinical teaching. Accordingly, medical schools hire clinicians, and the clinicians expect to be paid competitive salaries. Furthermore, the schools need to have clinicians qualified to teach in all of the major clinical areas. Toward this end, they cannot count on busy outside practicing clinicians to come in as an avocation and do the bulk of the clinical instruction and supervision.

To support these clinicians, medical schools need dependable supplies of patients, clinics for outpatient visits, and hospital beds for inpatient care. These require investments. The clinicians also want to be able to provide full service to their patients: the cardiologist wants colleagues who catheterize, replace valves, put in pacemakers, obliterate sources of arrhythmias, manage chronic heart failure, and so on. They are even happier if there is a cardiac transplant program with which they can affiliate. This is completely consistent with the academic hospital's interest in having many state-of-the-art product lines that they can advertise ("where miracles happen") and that generate lots of revenue. Complicating all of this is health sector consolidation and the dominance of private insurance. Each academic clinical enterprise needs to effectively negotiate the rates of reimbursement with the various insurers that allow them to extract surplus revenue from their clinical activity. To accomplish that, it is essential to have a sufficiently large population of patients who want to receive care from them, and whom the insurance companies want to keep (or acquire) as policyholders.

Thus academic systems actively compete with other clinical systems (academic and nonacademic) in their communities for business and have greatly expanded their numbers of practitioners, particularly in the area of primary care, in order to be able to maintain a pipeline of patients being sent to their specialists and to their hospitals for consultations and procedures. This trend has accelerated greatly since about 2000.

At UCLA, I became chief of the Division of General Internal Medicine and Health Services Research in 1991. For the first few years, we had only a few doctors whose principal professional activity was primary care. But our department's chair, Alan Fogelman, understood the need for patients to feed specialty practices and to fill beds in the hospital, so he invested in clinical growth. By the time I left in 2016, we had well over 100 outpatient general internists as well as a comparable number of generalists providing inpatient "hospitalist" care.

Where did we install these physicians? Certainly not all could practice in our limited academic space in or near the hospital. Some of the outpatient physicians admitted patients to our main teaching hospital. Others admitted to a community hospital that UCLA acquired in Santa Monica. Still others worked in practices located in other parts of greater Los Angeles where most patients had private insurance. They admitted to other hospitals that were not owned by our system but that were happy to have our patients fill their beds. The hospitalists were deployed to all the sites where our patients were admitted. Where did these clinicians come from? Some came directly from training programs such as ours (which began to promote generalist careers more aggressively). Others came from private practices that became less viable as standalone activities as consolidation proceeded apace.

The appetite for clinical revenue is not delimited. Physician faculty want to earn more. Some academicians do even better than private practitioners because of the free labor of trainees to handle some of their tasks. In addition, clinical revenue can offset some of the costs of teaching that are not supported from other sources.

Subsidizing the Costs of Research

Further, most medical schools report that they lose money on research. How can that be? The grants that the federal government funds pay directly for the salaries, benefits, and supplies for those engaged in the research and include some additional support for research-related infrastructure. There are, however, many things that this funding does not cover, such as the cost of constructing buildings to house the research, the costs associated with writing and submitting research grants, most of which do not get funded, and the cost of conducting further analyses and preparing research papers for publication after the funding runs out. Finally, the National Institutes of Health (NIH) provides little such infrastructure support on training grants, and many other funders pay only a fraction of what the NIH covers toward these costs.

For all of these reasons, robust collection of clinical revenue can underwrite some of the costs of research and the costs of supporting faculty who are not fully funded for their research programs. To make matters worse, in 2012, Congress reduced the maximum salary payable to a research faculty member (even a Nobel laureate) from $199,700 to $179,700. This limit has crept back up slowly, but as of 2021, it still had not reached the prior level.[39] In many cities, that is less than the starting salary of a practicing physician.

Academicians, Entrepreneurs, or Corporate Employees?

The salary of the clinical investigator must be underwritten by other revenues if it is to be competitive. Some faculty members do some consulting with industry (conflicts of interest emerge), and some are lucky enough to get endowed chairs. The others have to find a way to survive. In procedural fields, doing procedures such as echocardiograms and colonoscopies, say 20% of the time, can cover a large chunk of salary. For those (like me) who do not do procedures, net clinical revenue does not even cover the cost of the time spent doing the clinical work. So, the mission of the dean, department chair, or division chief is to raise money. They can do this by begging for support from their hospital system; by building big, revenue-generating clinical programs with expectations for high productivity; and by providing incentives to the clinicians to accomplish these goals themselves. As one department chair put it, "I want my faculty, at the margin, to consider it preferable to see another patient than to spend more quality time at home with their family." Another patient seen is another aliquot of income.

With so much on the line, academic health systems do not behave like other components of universities, where the notion of academic freedom is supposed to be sacrosanct. Some physicians publicly criticize their health systems, but doing so is relatively uncommon. Health system leadership may even seek to control other kinds of speech. One physician I know was removed from an institutional role by a hospital administrator who did not like the tenor of some public comments he made about a general health issue. In this context, "academic freedom" is far from absolute.

Every year, most medical school faculty have the opportunity to renegotiate their salaries and need to show how their salary is going to be covered. The negotiation may well involve review of teaching evaluations, research productivity, and participation in committees and other institutional roles. Inevitably, however, these negotiations are largely driven by the issue of how the institution will cover the individual's salary for the coming year. Yet even those faculty members who draw an institutional base salary for a hospital or departmental role, who have ongoing salary support from a government contract or grant, or who have an endowed chair or other such enduring source of funding almost always have more salary to cover.

At UCLA, there were thousands of medical school faculty. Something like 335 of them received a university salary. I was fortunate enough to receive one of the 65 or 70 such slots assigned to my department. The university paid me exactly as much as they did to a professor of history, chemistry, or drama at my level. That was not nearly what doctors made in the community and was far less than the total compensation that the medical school negotiated for me and other faculty members, the rest of which had to be generated by the professor. As my department chair once commented, "every faculty member runs a business." They must cover their salary, and they must cover their staff.

Spending time mentoring and nurturing students often loses out to clinical demands. To be sure, there are many altruistic, generative faculty members who devote their hearts and souls to education tirelessly, but there really is an incentive for faculty members not to compromise their ability to generate more revenue and support higher salaries. In some specialties, having residents and fellows working long hours and doing much of the clinical work (admitting and following up patients) can free up the faculty member to do more procedures or otherwise generate revenue more efficiently.[40]

Academic clinicians can bring in the big bucks, sometimes not for doing anything wondrous. Like many other academic institutions, UCLA has an executive health program.[41] The chief executive officer (CEO) of the health system pitches it as "a world class program for annual executive health care, with a level of individualized service and attention second to none . . . in a manner respectful of the needs of this important part of our community." Its physicians are "experts in prevention—as well as detection of diseases in their earliest stages."[42]

As this message implies, this is not cost-effective, evidence-based care. Lots of stuff gets done that cannot be justified on the basis of published studies. One clear consequence is that the doctors who work in the program do very well. The program director earned more than $2 million in 2019, and other faculty members made as much as $815,000. Not bad pay for doing things not found in clinical guidelines.[43]

On one occasion, several years before this program was established, a medical student of mine referred his father-in-law, the CEO of an important company in Los Angeles, to my medical clinic. That man came and saw me for a few years, but he regularly asked why he was not getting all the tests and procedures that his other executives received. I told him that I followed the evidence. He eventually found another doctor.

Evaluating the Clinical Performance of Trainees

The system for assessment of residents as they progress through residency and of the programs themselves offers interesting insights into what educational leaders believe that they should be conveying to their trainees. The programs are designed to comply with the requirements of the Accreditation Council for Graduate Medical Education (ACGME), which has Residency Review Committees (RRCs) in each specialty that meet twice yearly to accredit (or not) training programs in their respective clinical areas.

There currently are 28 such committees, each of which includes 6 to 20 physician volunteers and one resident.[44] Members are appointed by the American Medical Association's Council on Medical Education, the specialty board in that field, and the professional college or organization of that specialty. The RRC reviews every program at least every five years. The process includes a site visit, survey of residents, analysis of scores of the trainees on specialty board examinations, and details of the program content at participating institutions (hospitals).[45] In conjunction with specialty boards, ACGME has established a program to characterize each trainee's performance on a scale ranging from "novice" through "graduation goal" up to "expert resident/greater than the expectation."

The internal medicine committee implemented an updated list of twenty-one milestones in July 2021 in six areas: patient care, medical knowledge, system-based practice, practice-based learning improvement, professionalism, and interpersonal communication skills.[46] Most would agree that these categories are important. Physicians need to be knowledgeable, technically competent, ethical, responsible, conscientious, and open to learning how to improve in any number of ways.

A few of the milestones relate to understanding and engaging meaningfully with patients and their experience. One concerns patient- and family-centered communication, and encouragingly refers to using effective communication behaviors, engaging in shared decision-making, identifying barriers to effective communication, including personal bias, and mitigating communication barriers. There are several problems with these admirable metrics.

Faculty evaluators observe residents' interactions with patients only occasionally and generally quite briefly. They are rarely present for in-depth conversations, even in clinic. Second, the faculty themselves often are poor communicators. Studies described in chapter 4 showed that many physicians do not allow patients to complete their opening statements about why they are there. Are the faculty competent to judge adequately residents' communication skills and ability to mitigate communication barriers? It is unclear what is being done to address "communication disorders" in the faculty, particularly in disciplines such as surgery, in which interactions on the part of the faculty with patients are most problematic.

Several of the competencies allude to the importance of social and cultural factors in care. An earlier version of the milestones called for assessing whether residents respond to and consistently models respect for "each patient's unique characteristic and needs." The new version is vague and may not capture issues relevant to the patient's experience. For example, the competencies of history-taking and inpatient and outpatient patient management mention "incorporating psychosocial and other determinants of health," and one on therapeutic knowledge mentions formulating treatment plans "within the clinical and psychosocial context of the patient."

Unfortunately, even though the social history is part of the traditional medical history, all that many residents document as social history is any tobacco and alcohol use. It is unusual for them to document financial challenges, ability to pay for medications, relationship problems, issues pertaining to housing environment and safety, social network, religious beliefs, literacy, work history, legal or immigration issues, health or social problems being encountered by family members, caregiving demands that are sources of stress or that interfere with the ability to receive medical care, problems accessing social and medical services, and many more, all of which are potentially of great relevance to the encounter.[47]

Again, many evaluators may be poorly-equipped to provide meaningful assessments in these domains. Learning about a patient's "psychosocial context" or "unique characteristics and needs," is a crucial dimension of medical care. Eliciting such information is a complex task. Trainees need experienced instructors who model the skills involved, the empathy required, and humility needed when there is a cultural gap or chasm, and something more than a translator on a video hookup to close that gap. They also need to be observed and critiqued in this process.

Finally, in the area of system-based practice, the milestones call for assessing whether residents use local resources to meet the needs of patients and communities and advocate "for populations and communities with health care inequities." Of course, many of them are trained in institutions that contribute to these inequities. Meeting this milestone by publicly criticizing institutional practices might well earn the approbation of their professors!

While milestones might prove useful to educators and learners in certain substantive clinical areas, much research is needed regarding the validity of the assessments. Objective Structured Clinical Examinations can be used to evaluate and provide feedback to trainees about communication competency[48] and could be used to evaluate attention to patients' social circumstances, but they rarely are used to assess residents, and it is unclear whether clinician teachers who evaluate trainees are in a position to judge such domains. That is particularly the case in areas in which evaluators may not have observed the relevant activities and in some cases may lack competence themselves.[49]

If the ability to relate to patients were not deficient, would transplant doctors be sending their patients to another service to be informed that they would not be getting a transplant? Would physicians assign to their 26-year-old interns the job of discussing with patients and their families the reasons why aggressive treatment should not continue near the end of life? Would oncologists be pouring poisons into cancer patients in the last two weeks of life? Would doctors who earn $400,000 to $600,000 or more per year be unwilling to provide personalized care (or even any care) for persons whose insurance coverage (Medicaid) reimburses a lot less than that of other carriers? What should we think about the judgments such individuals render about the qualifications and characteristics of physicians-in-training?

There has been some discussion in medical education about hidden curricula.[50] The formal, didactic education may send one message, but the observed behavior of faculty physicians and residents may send a different message to trainees. Thus showing respect for patients and communicating effectively with them may be important, but if the trainee sees practitioners being inconsiderate of the patient's perspective or needs, that undermines what was taught in the classroom. Similarly, the explicit lesson may be to make your services available to all who need them, but the "hidden" lesson may be to be more attentive to the wealthy patient, to be unwilling to see patients with Medicaid insurance, or to be anxious to push the uninsured patient out of the hospital with considerable uncertainty about follow-up. When that is seen as "the way it is," the student or resident learns that lesson very well.[51] As discussed in chapter 5, "doctoring"-type courses that may address this problem often are undermined by the failure to continue the course throughout all four years of medical school. It is no less important to provide such ongoing education throughout residency training, during which the clinical experiences that send different messages are profuse.[52]

The American College of Physicians committee considering this issue suggested that the best approach to the hidden curriculum is to "uncover it, integrate its positive aspects into the formal curriculum, and lead to development of approaches to understand and mitigate its negative aspects by educators and practicing clinicians." They suggest that doing so could "reshape not only education but also the culture of medicine."[53]

Those are admirable notions, but when negative features are pervasive, limiting such efforts to the first two years of medical school is like trying to drain an ocean with a teaspoon. A group of Dutch educators described a program that showed promise, but it involved reflecting upon these issues in the clinical workplace and involving both faculty and trainees.[54] Even if such approaches prove effective, they may never neutralize many negative (and not-always-so-hidden) aspects of the curricula.

How do you reshape policies and practice in an orthopedic hospital that rarely takes any patients with Medicaid insurance? How do you come to terms with the ubiquitous socioeconomic class discrimination when a hospital's leadership does not tolerate any criticism of their discrimination against the poor, while rushing to the bedside of the rich and famous? If a clinician has an occasional slip into inappropriate behavior, that may be remediable with opportunities to reflect and "coaches" (as some medical schools have instituted). In contrast, how can trainees not be profoundly and permanently shaped by the widespread patterns of behavior by members of a specialty that is inhospitable to women and minorities,[55] a hospital that caters primarily to the well-to-do (while claiming to care about population health), or a training program in a subspecialty in which the clinical bar or threshold for performing money-generating procedures is so low as to be almost nonexistent?

Even outstanding courses on ethics and professional responsibility fade into an ether of inconsequence, as trainees adopt the norms that permeate their environments in the intense years of clinical training. Young doctors like my former colleague may still do no more than shrug as they accept the inevitability of turning away uninsured immigrants with renal failure. Internists like my friend Henry may continue to lament only vaguely ordering the pulmonary function tests that are not needed clinically but are ordered nonetheless to cover the rent.

Some residents completing training may opt for careers caring for the disadvantaged, but many others are likely to feel that they have no choice but to join a group that will pay well while not caring for those with Medicaid. Young subspecialists entering practice may be determined to do procedures only when the evidence warrants it, but soon many never doubt the value of their procedures for every patient, while generating incomes of several hundred thousand dollars a year. When the environment is sick, where can the student look for a vaccine or a cure?

The practitioners in academic health care systems are not wicked, but few of them have the inclination to resist what they experience daily. Instead, they accept a way of practicing medicine that provides them with substantial rewards. When the system offers that choice, the outcome is predictable. Meaningful change is unlikely to come from within, and they teach their disciples well.

Research in the Medical School: Its Impact upon Education
Lack of Intellectual Diversity in the Medical School Faculty

Even with robust clinical programs, and notwithstanding protestations that they lose money on research, research revenues remain attractive to medical schools. There are a number of reasons for this. Medical schools see the generation of new knowledge as one of their core missions. Many faculty members want to be able to conduct research. Medical students and postgraduate trainees also often have an interest in engaging in research or at least in studying in a research-rich environment. Yet research is expensive whether it is basic science, clinical studies, or other forms of translational research. Funding from outside sources is needed, and schools direct their hiring of investigators toward those individuals whom they believe will be able to pull in large grants in the areas that are well funded.

In chapter 8, we will examine the influence of the National Institutes of Health and of recent legislation that allows medical schools and their faculty members to participate in patents and royalty revenue. Here, we consider the impact of current research patterns and practices on life in the academic institutions.

The contrast between the culture of medical school research and that undertaken by faculty in such departments as history, sociology, and anthropology is instructive. There is little funding for scholars in these latter disciplines, relative to what is available to medical school researchers. The Social Sciences Research Council gives out some grants, as do the National Endowment for the Humanities and some foundations. But these grants tend, for the most part, to be small. They pay for a faculty member to spend a year or two abroad doing research, for the cost of conducting a survey, or for a few research assistants. Grants typically are in the tens of thousands of dollars.[56] Even in institutions with sterling reputations in the social sciences and humanities, it is common for most faculty in these departments to have little or no funding for research, other than coverage of their salaries. Accordingly, almost all of the faculty get most of their support directly from the university.

Universities assign faculty slots to departments in relation to their teaching loads (which in turn reflect the numbers of students selecting majors in their fields). In general, college students seek majors that lead to lucrative careers, or at least more certainty of a job, and social sciences have increasing difficulty attracting students in the face of competition from computer sciences and preprofessional school programs.[57]

Thus the number of faculty positions in these disciplines has dwindled in recent decades. Sociology has a lot to tell us about many aspects of society and about health and health care. Yet this discipline retains few positions. In 2020, there were between 22 and 39 full-time sociologists at each of eight prestigious universities, all of which ranked in the top ten nationally in the field.[58]

What about medical schools? In departments of internal medicine, the magnitude of the grants and the numbers of faculty are vastly greater. At UCLA, there were nearly 1,000 members in that department when I was there. Numbers are comparable in other schools. Ponder what it means to the nature of the university when one department has hundreds or thousands of faculty in gleaming new buildings, while many other have 10, 20, or occasionally 30 who are tucked away in aging rabbit warrens. Years ago, a colleague who had come from Europe complained that American campuses are cluttered with the uniforms of football players. Social scientists might well view the proliferation of faculty in medical school departments in a similar way.

Many of these medical school faculty members are largely, or entirely, engaged in clinical work, but quite a few are researchers as well. There were close to 70 positions funded by the university in my department (nearly twice the number in sociology), but many more faculty members than that were engaged in research. These additional faculty had to fund their entire salaries without university support. Some (the clinicians) did clinical work. Others had clinical or educational administrative roles (running a unit or a program). But for those engaged exclusively in research, if they had no university support, all or most of their funding had to come from so-called soft money (grants and donations).

For PhD social scientists, full salary coverage without some university funding is hard to come by.[59] Clinician-investigators interested in the social sciences can fund some of their salaries with clinical revenue, but unless they do procedures, substantial funding at the level of what physicians earn is a stretch. It is hard for clinician scientists in basic or clinical science fields to cover themselves fully, but if they bring in a major grant, the medical school will be more inclined to pay for some of their research time beyond that covered by the grant.

Following Sutton's Law, medical school researchers go where the money is. If funding is available to study a particular problem, grants get written. So, there is considerable institutional pressure for academic physicians to follow the money, not because they don't have intellectual curiosity, but because they can't survive academically without the grants.

Lack of Priority or Rewards for Teaching

Social scientists may do the same, but those in tenure track positions in such departments as sociology may be in a position to do research with relatively little grant support (or even none at all). Toward this end, teaching is a low priority relative to obtaining grants for many medical school researchers. Some have nonteaching appointments (with titles such as "research scientist"). Social scientists in most medical schools are expected to cover much of their salaries if they are to be involved in research.

Whatever the discipline, however, even those appointed as professors, who have students, and who are expected to teach are rewarded for their scholarship, not their teaching. Faculty promotion criteria at the University of California require excellence in creative activity, teaching, and community service. But it is unusual for researchers to be punished for inadequacy of their teaching performance. I spent several years on the promotions committee of my department at UCLA. I recall one dossier for which the primary reviewer judged research productivity to be marginal for promotion and said of the teaching, "I guess these are the worst teaching evaluations we have seen." Nonetheless, he recommended promotion, and the majority of the committee went along.

There were other instances in which a dossier was held up because of poor teaching evaluations, but I do not recall any in which they were ultimately decisive. When I served on a similar committee at Cornell's medical college, I once asked why we did not receive copies of teaching evaluations when considering candidates for promotion. I was told that those can be included, but it is at the discretion of the division chief or candidate whether to provide them. Cornell's medical school does not seem to care, at least in the promotions process, about the quality of the instruction that their faculty provide.

Even at institutions like UCLA, where teaching evaluations are a required part of the dossier for academic researchers, perhaps 2% of the decision rests on them. Scholarship is the whole ball game, and without funding, faculty members don't even get to stay around to be considered for promotion.

In this context, attentiveness to pedagogical needs of students and residents is a lower priority for many faculty than meeting expectations for research productivity. While some researchers are wonderful teachers, others are often distracted when in clinic or on the hospital wards and don't devote the time and attention to teaching that they might. Really connecting with trainees matters in any effort to instill good values and ethics, and to help trainees prioritize caring over revenue generation; many research faculty fall short. William Osler once said that "the most important thing a professor of medicine can give to his student is the key to his front door." Academic researchers, struggling to survive, may not even give student directions to their office.

Arguably, medical schools are society's representatives in identifying people who should practice medicine and in equipping them with abilities and values that will best serve to promote the health and well-being of the population. In these respects, medical schools fail decisively. As I have attempted to illustrate in these last two chapters, for the most part, medical schools admit students with values, attitudes, and traits that make many problems worse. They do not do a very good job of nurturing desired characteristics, nor of giving students the opportunities to flourish in an environment that reinforces, rather than undermines, concern for societal well-being. They also clutter the profession with so many specialists doing procedures of marginal value that drive up the cost of care, and with practitioners who are far too often indifferent to the needs of the population.

Their eloquent mission statements are monuments to insincerity: educational programs fail to promote the values or produce the providers that society needs, clinical programs prioritize revenue over morality, and research ignores disciplines that could advance health and knowledge and enrich education. Nor are they always contrite about these shortcomings. A distinguished physician who lectured at Harvard some years ago about his research on an impending oversupply of physicians relative to society's needs told me that a senior faculty member in attendance said, "There never can be too many Harvard Medical School graduates."[60]

In the coming chapters, we will examine some of the problems relating to medical practice in large clinical corporations (including those affiliated with medical schools), as well as broader issues concerning academic scientists, their disciplines, and their organizations.

Notes

1. See, e.g., "Mission Statement," Johns Hopkins School of Medicine, accessed July 17, 2021, https://www.hopkinsmedicine.org/som/about-us/mission.html; "Mission, Vision and Core Values," Indiana University School of Medicine, accessed July 17, 2021, https://medicine.iu.edu/about/mission-vision-values; "About Us," David Geffen School of Medicine at UCLA, accessed July 17, 2021, https://medschool.ucla.edu/about; "Mission Statement and Community Values," Harvard Medical School, accessed July 17, 2021, https://hms.harvard.edu/about-hms/campus-culture/mission-statement-community-values; "School's Core Values," Duke University School of Medicine, accessed July 17, 2021, https://medschool.duke.edu/about-us; "MD Program Mission Statement," Stanford Medicine MD Program, accessed July 17, 2021, https://med.stanford.edu/md.html.

2. Rosemary Stevens, *American Medicine and the Public Interest* (Berkeley: University of California Press, 1998), 101.

3. Stevens, *American Medicine*, 77–97.

4. "Exam Administration History," American Board of Internal Medicine, accessed June 17, 2020, https://www.abim.org/about/exam-information/exam-administration-history.aspx.

5. "Subspecialties," American Board of Urology, accessed June 18, 2020, https://www.abu.org/subspecialty/.

6. Paul P. Lee, Daniel A. Relles, and Catherin A. Jackson, "Subspecialty Distributions of Ophthalmologists in the Workforce," *Archives of Ophthalmology* 116, no. 7 (July 1998): 917–20, https://doi.org/10.1001/archopht.116.7.917.

7. "New Findings Confirm Predictions of Physician Shortage," Association of American Medical Colleges, April 23, 2019, https://www.aamc.org/news-insights/press-releases/new-findings-confirm-predictions-physician-shortage.

8. IHS Markit Ltd., *The Complexities of Physician Supply and Demand: Projections from 2017 to 2032* (Washington, DC: Association of American Medical Colleges, April 2019), http://aamc-black.global.ssl.fastly.net/production/media/filer_public/31/13/3113ee5c-a038-4c16-89af-294a69826650/2019_update_-_the_complexities_of_physician_supply_and_demand_-_projections_from_2017-2032.pdf.

9. "Number of Family Medicine and General Practice Physicians in Canada as of 2020, by Province," Statista, accessed August 19, 2022, https://www.statista.com/statistics/831118/canada-family-general-practitioners-by-province/; "Number of Medical Specialists in Canada as of 2022 by Province," Statista, accessed August 19, 2022, https://www.statista.com/statistics/831147/canada-medical-specialists-by-province/. There were 46,665 general practitioners and 45,346 specialists in Canada, according to those analyses.

10. Sherine E. Gabriel, "Primary Care: Specialists or Generalists," *Mayo Clinic Proceedings* 71, no. 4 (April 1996): 415–19, https://doi.org/10.4065/71.4.415.

11. Sanjay Basu et al., "Estimated Effect on Life Expectancy of Alleviating Primary Care Shortages in the United States," *Annals of Internal Medicine* 174, no. 7 (July 2021): 920–35, https://doi.org/10.7326/M20-7381.

12. Michael Karpf and Gerald S. Levey, "Divisions of General Internal Medicine: Accomplishments and Needs," *Annals of Internal Medicine* 103, no. 3 (September 1, 1985): 456–58, https://doi.org/10.7326/0003-4819-103-3-456.

13. Leslie Kane, "Medscape Physician Compensation Report 2019," Medscape, April 10, 2019, https://www.medscape.com/slideshow/2019-compensation-overview-6011286#3.

14. N. Baker et al., *Reducing Costs through the Appropriate Use of Specialty Services*, IHI Innovation Series White Paper (Cambridge, MA: Institute for Healthcare Improvement, 2010), http://www.ihi.org/resources/Pages/IHIWhitePapers/ReducingCostsAppropriateUseSpecialtyServicesWhitePaper.aspx.

15. R. E. Park, personal communication, February 15, 2010.

16. S. Claiborne Johnson, "Academic Medical Centers: Too Large for Their Own Health?," *JAMA* 322, no. 3 (July 2019): 203–4, https://doi.org/10.1001/jama.2019.6834.

17. Ryan Dornbier and Christopher M. Gonzalez, "Workforce Issues in Urology," *Urologic Clinics of North America* 48, no. 2 (May 2021): 161–71, https://doi.org/10.1016/j.ucl.2021.01.001; Jin Suk C. Kim, Richard A. Cooper, and David W. Kennedy,

"Otolaryngology—Head and Neck Surgery Physician Work Force Issues: An Analysis for Future Specialty Planning," *Otolaryngology—Head and Neck Surgery* 146, no. 2 (February 2012): 196–202, https://doi.org/10.1177/0194599811433977; Michael R. Go et al., "An Updated Physician Workforce Model Predicts Shortage of Vascular Surgeons for the Next 20 Years," *Annals of Vascular Surgery* 66 (July 1, 2020): 282–88, https://doi.org/10.1016/j.avsg.2020.01.097.

18. Joanna Veazey Brooks et al., "Feeling Inadequate: Residents' Stress and Learning at Primary Care Clinics in the United States," *Medical Teacher* 40, no. 9 (September 2018): 920–27, https://doi.org/10.1080/0142159X.2017.1413216; Carla C. Keirns and Charles C. Bosk, "Perspective: The Unintended Consequences of Training Residents in Dysfunctional Outpatient Settings," *Academic Medicine* 83, no. 5 (May 2008): 498–502, https://doi.org/10.1097/ACM.0b013e31816be3ab.

19. Craig Noronha et al., "X+Y Scheduling Models in Internal Medicine Residency Programs: A National Survey of Program Directors' Perspectives," *American Journal of Medicine* 131, no. 1 (January 2018): 107–14, https://doi.org/10.1016/j.amjmed.2017.09.012.

20. Kathleen Heist et al., "Impact of 4 + 1 Block Scheduling on Patient Care Continuity in Resident Clinic," *Journal of General Internal Medicine* 29, no. 8 (August 2014): 1195–99, https://doi.org/10.1007/s11606-013-2750-4.

21. J. Stepczynski et al., "Factors Affecting Resident Satisfaction in Continuity Clinic—A Systematic Review," *Journal of General Internal Medicine* 33, no. 8 (August 2018): 1386–93, https://doi.org/10.1007/s11606-018-4469-8.

22. Jeremy Walker et al., "Continuity of Care in Resident Outpatient Clinics: A Scoping Review of the Literature," *Journal of Graduate Medical Education* 10, no. 1 (February 2018): 16–25, https://doi.org/10.4300/JGME-D-17-00256.1.

23. Mark D. Schwartz et al., "Medical Student Interest in Internal Medicine: Initial Report of the Society of General Internal Medicine Interest Group Survey on Factors Influencing Career Choice in Internal Medicine," *Annals of Internal Medicine* 114, no. 1 (January 1, 1991): 6–15, https://doi.org/10.7326/0003-4819-114-1-6.

24. Carla C. Keirns and Charles L. Bosk, "Perspective: The Unintended Consequences of Training Residents in Dysfunctional Outpatient Settings," *Academic Medicine* 83, no. 5 (May 2008): 498–502, https://doi.org/10.1097/ACM.0b013e31816be3ab; L. A. Peccoralo et al., "Resident Satisfaction with Continuity Clinic and Career Choice in General Internal Medicine," *Journal of General Internal Medicine* 28, no. 8 (August 2013): 1020–27, https://doi.org/10.1007/s11606-012-2280-5.

25. Sandhya K. Rao et al., "The Impact of Administrative Burden on Academic Physicians: Results of a Hospital-Wide Physician Survey," *Academic Medicine* 92, no. 2 (February 2017): 237–43, https://doi.org/10.1097/ACM.0000000000001461.

26. David Blumenthal and Melinda K. Abrams, "Tailoring Complex Care Management for High-Need, High-Cost Patients," *JAMA* 316, no. 16 (October 25, 2016): 1657–58, https://doi.org/10.1001/jama.2016.12388; Douglas W. Roblin et al., "Comparative Effectiveness of a Complex Care Program for High-Cost/High-Need Patients: A Retrospective Cohort Study," *Journal of General Internal Medicine* 36, no. 7 (July 2021): 2021–29, https://doi.org/10.1007/s11606-021-06676-x; R. Gupta et al., "A

System-Wide Population Health Value Approach to Reduce Hospitalization among Chronic Kidney Patients: An Observational Study," *Journal of General Internal Medicine* 36, no. 6 (June 2020): 1613–21, https://doi.org/10.1007/s11606-020-06272-5.

27. They estimate that it is economically viable and logistically possible for them to follow about 200 outpatients while caring for about 5 inpatients on a given day. David O. Meltzer and Gregory W. Ruhnke, "Redesigning Care for Patients at Increased Hospitalization Risk: The Comprehensive Care Model," *Health Affairs* (Millwood) 33, no. 5 (May 2014): 779–87, https://doi.org/10.1377/hlthaff.2014.0072; "Comprehensive Care Physician: Integrated Inpatient and Outpatient Care for Patients at High Risk of Hospitalization (CCP)," ClinicalTrials.gov, accessed September 22, 2021, clinicaltrials.gov/ct2/show/NCT01929005; David O. Meltzer, "Effects of Comprehensive Care Physicians on Patient Experience, Outcomes and Hospitalization: Preliminary Results of a Randomized Controlled Trial," paper presented at Hospital Medicine 2019, March 24–27, 2019, National Harbor, MD, https://shmabstracts.org/abstract/effects-of-comprehensive-care-physicians-on-patient-experience-outcomes-and-hospitalization-preliminary-results-of-a-randomized-controlled-trial/.

28. Matthew K. Shaw et al., "The Duration of Office Visits in the United States, 1993 to 2010," *American Journal of Managed Care* 20, no. 10 (October 2014): 820–26, PMID 25365685.

29. "Indirect Medical Education (IME)," Center for Medicare and Medicaid Services, last modified August 4, 2014, https://www.cms.gov/Medicare/Medicare-Fee-for-Service-Payment/AcuteInpatientPPS/Indirect-Medical-Education-IME.

30. Michael Wilkes and David Schriger, "Op-Ed: Why Won't UC Clinics Serve Patients with State-Funded Health Insurance?," *Los Angeles Times*, April 4, 2022, https://www.latimes.com/opinion/story/2022-04-04/university-of-california-uc-medi-cal-healthcare-insurance.

31. Walker, "Continuity of Care"; Rahul Vanjani, Andrea Pitts, and Pranav Aurora, "Dismantling Structural Racism in the Academic Residency Clinic," *New England Journal of Medicine* 368, no. 21 (May 26, 2022): 2054–58, https://doi.org/10.1056/NEJMms2117023.

32. Abe Dunn et al., "A Denial a Day Keeps the Doctor Away," National Bureau of Economic Research, July 1, 2021, https://www.nber.org/system/files/working_papers/w29010/w29010.pdf.

33. Anthony Hollenberg, the chair of the Department of Medicine at Cornell has expressed his intention to end this pattern of segregation. It will be interesting to see how far good intentions can go in getting clinicians to accept the lower payments and associated bureaucratic challenges of caring for Medicaid patients. There are many ways for them to avoid doing so.

34. See, e.g., Steven B. Zeliadt et al., "Challenges Implementing Lung Cancer Screening in Federally Qualified Health Centers," *American Journal of Preventive Medicine* 54, no. 4 (April 2018): 568–75, https://doi.org/10.1016/j.amepre.2018.01.001; Susan Wood et al., "Scope of Family Planning Services Available in Federally Qualified Health Centers," *Contraception* 89, no. 2 (February 2014): 85–90,

https://doi.org/10.1016/j.contraception.2013.09.015; Balambal Bharti et al., "Diagnostic Colonoscopy Completion after Abnormal Fecal Immunochemical Testing and Quality of Tests Used at 8 Federally Qualified Health Centers in Southern California: Opportunities for Improving Screening Outcomes," *Cancer* 125, no. 23 (December 1, 2019): 4203–9, https://doi.org/10.1002/cncr.32440; Sara J. Rosenbaum et al., "Community Health Centers: Challenges of Health Reform," Kaiser Commission on Medicaid and the Uninsured, accessed July 12, 2020, https://hsrc.himmelfarb.gwu.edu/cgi /viewcontent.cgi?article=1195&context=sphhs_policy_facpubs.

35. Richard A. Culbertson, Leslie D. Goode, and Robert M. Dickler, "Organizational Models of Medical School Relationships to the Clinical Enterprise," *Academic Medicine* 71, no. 11 (November 1996): 1258–74, https://doi.org/10.1097 /00001888-199611000-00026; Jacqueline LaPointe, "Academic Medical Centers Adapting with New Business Models," Recycle Intelligence, Practice Management News, May 6, 2019, https://revcycleintelligence.com/news/academic-medical -centers-adapting-with-new-business-models.

36. Mitesh S. Patel et al., "Role-Modeling Cost-Conscious Care—A National Evaluation of Perceptions of Faculty at Teaching Hospitals in the United States," *Journal of General Internal Medicine* 30 (September 2015): 1294–98, https://doi.org/10 .1007/s11606-015-3242-5.

37. Timothy S. Anderson, Walid F. Gellad, and Chester B. Good, "Characteristics of Biomedical Industry Payments to Teaching Hospitals," *Health Affairs* (Millwood) 39, no. 9 (September 2020): 1583–91, https://doi.org/10.1377/hlthaff.2020.00385.

38. Heather Lyu et al., "Overtreatment in the United States," *PLOS One* 12, no. 9 (September 6, 2017): e0181970, https://doi.org/10.1371/journal.pone.0181970.

39. "Salary Limitation on Grants, Cooperative Agreements, and Contracts," National Institutes of Health, accessed April 20, 2020, https://grants.nih.gov/grants /guide/notice-files/not-od-11-073.html; "Notice of Salary Limitation on Grants, Cooperative Agreements, and Contracts," National Institutes of Health, accessed April 20, 2020, https://grants.nih.gov/grants/guide/notice-files/not-od-12-035.html; "Guidance on Salary Limitation for Grants and Cooperative Agreements FY 2021," National Institutes of Health, accessed May 27, 2021, https://grants.nih.gov/grants /guide/notice-files/NOT-OD-21-057.html.

40. Ryan Park, "Why So Many Young Doctors Work Such Awful Hours," *The Atlantic*, February 21, 2017, https://www.theatlantic.com/business/archive/2017/02 /doctors-long-hours-schedules/516639/.

41. "About Us," UCLA Health, accessed April 14, 2020, https://www.uclahealth .org/executivehealth/about-us.

42. "Message from Our CEO, UCLA Health System," UCLA Health, accessed April 14, 2020, https://www.uclahealth.org/executivehealth/message-from-ceo.

43. "2019 Salaries for University of California," Transparent California, accessed May 27, 2021, https://transparentcalifornia.com/salaries/2019/university-of -california/.

44. There also is a committee concerned with transitional year programs and another concerned with overall institutional review.

45. "Committees and Members Selection Process," Accreditation Council for Graduate Medical Education, accessed April 16, 2020, https://www.acgme.org/About-Us/Committees-and-Members-Selection-Process.

46. "Internal Medicine Milestones," Accreditation Council for Graduate Medical Education, accessed April 15, 2022, https://www.acgme.org/globalassets/pdfs/milestones/internalmedicinemilestones.pdf.

47. Heidi L. Behforouz, Paul K. Drain, and Joseph J. Rhatigan, "Rethinking the Social History," *New England Journal of Medicine* 371, no. 14 (October 2, 2014): 1277–79, https://doi.org/10.1056/NEJMp1404846.

48. Elizabeth A. Rider, Margaret M. Hinrichs, and Beth A. Lown, "A Model for Communication Skills Assessment across the Undergraduate Curriculum," *Medical Teacher* 28, no. 5 (August 2006): e127–e134, https://doi.org/10.1080/01421590600726540; B. Hodges et al., "Evaluating Communication Skills in the OSCE Format: Reliability and Generalizability," *Medical Education* 30, no. 1 (January 1996): 38–43, https://doi.org/10.1111/j.1365-2923.1996.tb00715.x.

49. Su-Ting T. Li, "The Promise of Milestones: Are They Living Up to Our Expectations?," *Journal of Graduate Medical Education* 9, no. 1 (February 2017): 54–57, https://doi.org/10.4300/JGME-D-16-00694.1.

50. Nandini Nittur and Jonathan Kibble, "Current Practices in Assessing Professionalism in United States and Canadian Allopathic Medical Students and Residents," *Cureus* 9, no. 5 (May 2017): e1267, https://doi.org/10.7759/cureus.1267; Carlton Lawrence et al., "The Hidden Curriculum in Medical Education: A Scoping Review," *Academic Medicine* 93, no. 4 (April 2018): 648–56, https://doi.org/10.1097/ACM.0000000000002004.

51. Lisa Soleymani Lehmann et al., "Hidden Curricula, Ethics and Professionalism: Optimizing Clinical Learning Environments and Being a Physician: A Position Paper of the American College of Physicians," *Annals of Internal Medicine* 168, no. 7 (April 2018): 506–8, https://doi.org/10.7326/M17-2058.

52. Frederic W. Hafferty, Elizabeth H. Gaufberg, and Joseph F. O'Donnell, "The Role of the Hidden Curriculum in 'On Doctoring' Courses," *AMA Journal of Ethics* 17, no. 2 (February 1, 2015): 130–39, https://doi.org/10.1001/virtualmentor.2015.17.02.medu1-1502.

53. Suleymani Lehmann, "Hidden Curricula."

54. Hanneke Mulder et al., "Addressing the Hidden Curriculum in the Clinical Workplace: A Practical Tool for Trainees and Faculty," *Medical Teacher* 41, no. 1 (January 2019): 36–43, https://doi.org/10.1080/0142159X.2018.1436760.

55. K. Lauren Barnes et al., "Gender Bias Experiences of Female Surgical Trainees," *Journal of Surgical Education* 76, no. 6 (November–December 2019): e1–e14, https://doi.org/10.1016/j.jsurg.2019.07.024.

56. There are some major survey research centers, such as that of University of Michigan and one affiliated with the University of Chicago, that do get much more substantial funding.

57. In this context, it is less and less common for students to pay much attention to the relevance of a discipline like history in today's world. As George Santayana

might have said ironically, today's ethos may be that those who fail to learn from the mistakes of prior software engineers and programmers are destined to repeat them.

58. Here are numbers of faculty with their primary professorial appointments in some sociology departments that ranked among the top 10, according to *U.S. News and World Report* (excluding lecturers and emeritus faculty; I have not counted those who appear to have primary appointments in other departments): UCLA and the University of Michigan, 39 each; the University of Wisconsin, 29; Princeton, 31; the University of Chicago, 24; Harvard, 26; University of North Carolina, Chapel Hill, 24; and Stanford, 22. Thus these eight departments had 234 professors of sociology among them. "Ladder Faculty," UCLA Sociology, accessed April 15, 2022, https://soc.ucla.edu/faculty; "Faculty," Harvard University Department of Sociology, accessed April 15, 2022, https://sociology.fas.harvard.edu/people/sociology-faculty?page=1; "Faculty," Sociology University of Michigan, accessed April 15, 2022, https://lsa.umich.edu/soc/people/faculty.html; "Faculty Directory," Princeton University Department of Sociology, accessed April 15, 2022, https://sociology.princeton.edu/people/faculty; "Faculty," Stanford Sociology, accessed April 15, 2022, https://sociology.stanford.edu/people/faculty; "Sociology Faculty," Department of Sociology, University of Chicago, accessed April 15, 2020, https://sociology.uchicago.edu/directories/full/sociology-faculty; "Sociology Faculty," Department of Sociology, University of Wisconsin–Madison, accessed April 15, 2022, https://sociology.wisc.edu/faculty/; "Faculty," Department of Sociology, University of North Carolina College of Arts and Sciences, accessed April 15, 2022, https://sociology.unc.edu/people/faculty/.

59. Some do get substantial funding from the NIH, as social scientists on the "community core" of large center grants, but those opportunities are relatively uncommon in most medical schools.

60. Alvin Tarlov, personal communication, 1985.

Dialogue #5

Professor (reading the document): Good work.

Student: This was pretty depressing. There are so many things that the medical schools should be doing differently. Who they admit. What they teach. The influence of the clinicians and other trainees on the students. The kind of practice they model. Where do you begin?

Professor: Good question. It does seem that the issues are related, and the impact is cumulative.

Student: Professor, we have identified a lot of problems in the health care system. I'd like to get on to thinking about solutions.

Professor: Which parts of the system do you propose to fix? And how do you know if your alterations will get the job done? Believe me, I share your frustration. But before we prescribe any solutions, we need to be clear about the scope of the disorder. I think that we may still be missing some important elements beyond the medical schools and the behavior of physicians and patients that may need to be addressed. Can you think of any?

Student: Well, we haven't talked about hospitals and other corporations that deliver care. They seem to be developing big networks, and they sure advertise a lot on television these days. Are they up to anything nefarious?

Professor: That is a great point. How did they get to be so big? What external factors are driving their behavior? What are the motivations of the individuals who run these organizations? How is it that some hospitals just take care of the poor while others rarely do so? How does this affect the patients who go there?

Student: Let's take a look at this stuff. I would have thought they mostly just respond to what their patients need. We don't want to get distracted from the big issues of cost, access, and outcomes.

Professor: We'll keep them in focus, but we won't know how relevant these clinical corporations are to what we are getting at unless we look "under the hood" at what they are up to.

7

Making a Killing

Corporate Providers of Medical Care

Earth provides enough to satisfy every man's needs, but not every man's greed.
—Mohandas Gandhi

One year, the faculty members of my department of internal medicine at the University of California, Los Angeles, held a retreat to talk about our clinical programs. We had a guest speaker who was a senior executive at Henry Ford Hospital and Health System in Michigan. He spoke about the strategy that they had employed to expand their clinical practices, describing the impact as an increase in "sales." He paused and said, "That is what you call admissions and visits." It was shocking to hear clinical activity characterized in that way. Are we selling things, or are we taking care of patients?

In fact, his comments were clarifying. The distinction between taking care of patients and promoting revenue through sales has been obliterated in recent decades. During that time, more and more of the practice of medicine in the United States has come to be controlled by large clinical corporations, some for-profit, but many nominally not-for-profit or "voluntary." Notwithstanding their often-noble mission statements, these corporations are primarily focused upon extracting surplus revenue from their clinical operations in order to expand their enterprises, reward their investors financially, or both. How did it come to this? A step back in time to look at the evolution of hospitals in the

United States will show that although the development of the current state of affairs was not inevitable, it is far from surprising.

Emergence of Hospitals in the United States

In 1800, there were no real health systems in the United States and few hospitals. Historian Charles Rosenberg writes, "if we define 'hospital' as an institution devoted exclusively to the inpatient care of the sick, then there were only two hospitals in America: Philadelphia's Pennsylvania Hospital and the New York Hospital."[1] Nonpoor individuals avoided such establishments. Workers too sick for care at home would often go to almshouses, which housed orphans and persons who were destitute or permanently incapacitated. These establishments also had accommodations for those who were physically or mentally ill. Some later evolved into the municipal hospitals that we know today. For example, New York's first almshouse, founded in 1736, eventually begat Bellevue Hospital in 1824. These hospitals also provided outpatient care to those who could not afford the services of doctors in private practice.

Even by the time of the Civil War, there were fewer than 200 hospitals in the United States, including mental hospitals, and few with relationships to medical schools.[2] Some private hospitals had begun to emerge, but most hospitalized patients were poor people going to the municipal hospitals. In the ensuing decades, there was a revolution in care and a vast expansion in the role of hospitals, with the emergence of procedures that required hospital care, notably most surgeries.[3] By the first decade of the twentieth century, there were more than 4,300 hospitals in the US (not counting mental hospitals and chronic hospitals for conditions such as tuberculosis). The number of beds increased from about 50,000 in 1873 to more than 420,000 in 1909.

Hospitals for the Deserving and Undeserving

While some of the earliest hospitals were established as benevolent institutions, they were never able to depend entirely upon donations. A few hospitals had large endowments and could take care of many poor individuals without charge (Massachusetts General Hospital in Boston, Pennsylvania Hospital in Philadelphia, New York and Roosevelt Hospitals in New York were examples). Others were strongly dependent on patient-related revenues: either out-of-pocket payments from patients, support from charities for the provision of care, or appropriations by the local government. Accordingly, there was always at least some effort to collect fees from patients. As the numbers of such hospitals grew, many had much smaller endowments, and patient fees became an increasingly important source of revenue. Early in the twentieth century, private hospitals began to compete aggressively for the paying patients.[4] The municipal almshouse hospitals had always been regarded as the place for the poor. Other hospitals sought to admit the more "deserving" clientele. Some even required references, attesting to the good standing of prospective patients seeking admission. Thus the system of bifurcated care in America came to define where many people would go when sick.

Hospitals and Their Clinical Networks

For much of the twentieth century, hospitals were standalone institutions. The practitioners who admitted patients to them operated practices that were independent of the hospitals. Even though clinical teaching had become integral to medical education in France by 1800,[5] medical schools were not closely tied operationally either to networks of practitioners or to hospitals in the United States a century after that. Many had outpatient clinics and some full-time staff who saw some outpatients, but many of their patients came from independent practices outside of the hospital. There were few networks of hospitals.

The first real efforts to build systems of care that included hospitals and outpatient practices were created by health maintenance organizations such as Kaiser Permanente, which catered mostly to workers who were insured through large companies for which they worked. Starting in California, in the 1930s, Kaiser built a series of hospitals and outpatient practices, with a group of physicians who were formally affiliated with them providing care for the contracted population as full-time members of the Permanente Medical Group.[6] With the exception of organizations such as Kaiser, and the municipal hospitals and their affiliated clinics, the health systems that emerged in America in the past century developed patterns of practice that have relentlessly driven up the cost of care.

The Emergence and Impact of Health Insurance

As health insurance became more widespread, hospitals needed to contract with the insurers for rates of reimbursement for services. It became clear that larger networks were in a better position to obtain favorable rates from the insurers, since the insurers' prospective enrollees would want to have a wide set of options as to where they would obtain care. A crucial moment was the introduction of Medicare and Medicaid in the 1960s. Medicare gave hospitals an assured source of revenue for the care of the elderly without giving them any associated responsibility for the care of the disadvantaged. Medicare payments to providers and hospitals inflated rapidly because of their approach to reimbursement. This led to considerable revenue for hospitals, which began to make major capital investments to support services that would maximize Medicare income.[7]

A key feature of Medicare was enormously beneficial to the hospitals and the ways in which they financed growth. They could include the cost of borrowing money in the calculation of their costs for the purpose of determining their Medicare reimbursement rates. They did this by entering depreciation costs of buildings and other assets into their balance sheets. Crucially, they were able to use the "current replacement costs" of the assets as the basis for calculating the amount of depreciation instead of original costs. Thus they were able to use their federal funds partly as a source of revenue for construction. This led to massive capital expansion by the hospitals and to assumption of substantial long-term debt to accomplish that. Whereas 21% of voluntary hospital funding of new construction came from long-term debt financing in 1965, the proportion reached 69% by 1981. This trend also propelled them toward clinical programs, sites of activity, and marketing strategies that would generate surpluses, in order to build up their capital reserves.[8]

Consolidation of Health Care Markets

When managed care began to be more widespread in the 1980s, it placed pressure on other health care systems, including academic and private practices, whose prices were not particularly competitive with those of the managed care organizations. One of the responses to this situation was the beginning of consolidation in the health care delivery market, which has been substantial and breathtakingly rapid. One goal of this consolidation in recent decades has been to give hospital systems more leverage in their negotiation of rates with insurers. Individual practitioners were in no position to bargain in this way and often had to join larger health systems. The requirement to use electronic medical records also has been a financial burden for individual practitioners and small groups, given the cost of adopting these technologies.[9]

Accordingly, three to five large consolidated health care systems have emerged in many urban areas, often centered around academic health centers but including many smaller, regional hospitals. At the same time, these systems have pursued aggressively the building of networks of practitioners (many generalists, but also specialists) to provide the full range of services to their "covered lives" and to make sure that they can fill the beds in their hospitals.

The insurance industry has had a decisive impact on consolidation. Unlike countries in which the entire population have more or less the same insurance coverage (such as in Western Europe and Canada), in the United States there have been many insurers, public and private, with different standard or negotiated rates that they pay for services. A doctor in the US can get paid directly by the government for care of individuals with Medicare coverage or Medicaid (unless the patient is enrolled in a managed care Medicaid program), but for patients with private insurance, doctors are only compensated directly for care if contracted with that individual's insurance company. The US also lacks a systematic program for financing hospital care such as Canada's, in which the government-sponsored insurance program makes global payments to all hospitals for all the care that they provide. Hospital care in the US is fee-for-service or fee-for-a-package-of-services.[10]

Practically speaking, it is hard for a small group of doctors or even a small hospital to negotiate fair compensation. It is far easier for insurers to negotiate with large entities. For systems to be in a strong position to negotiate prices, they need to demonstrate that they take care of a large group of people who are desirable to the insurers. Not surprisingly, the degree of hospital and health system consolidation within health care markets has been found to correlate with increases in health care prices (and hence costs to recipients of care and to society as a whole), as well as with less satisfaction with care. Paradoxically, reduction in the number of insurers in a market has correlated with lower prices of care.[11]

As these clinical corporations have seen their negotiating positions improve with increased market share, it is hardly surprising that they seek to grow and corner ever larger shares of the market. Hence, in recent decades, hospitals have scrambled to build larger and larger networks of clinicians. The systems advertise for business, often highlighting their miraculous cures or scientific advances. They also aggressively hire young physicians, both in primary care and the specialties, and buy up, or contract with, existing groups of physicians working in areas with favorable insurance profiles. The goal of this activity is to have so many covered lives in their systems that they will be able to dominate their negotiations with the insurers. It is these covered lives for whose health care they want to be responsible.

Covered Lives

We should pause for a moment and reflect upon that term, *covered lives*. Words matter. When leaders of health systems talk about covered lives, they are not committing themselves to "helping the sick in whatever houses they enter," as the Hippocratic Oath would have it. They are discounting the lives of real people whom they assemble on the altar of the coveted coverage-that-means-revenue. Why not talk about people for whom we are responsible? Why not speak urgently about communities who need us? "Covered" implies that the "uncovered" are the other people, about whom we do not care, for whom we do not feel responsible. Covered in this usage does not even include the 75 million or so individuals who had Medicaid coverage and another 7 million who were enrolled in the Children's Health Insurance Program (CHIP) as of April 2021.[12] It only envelops those with desirable insurance. Indeed, terms like covered and uncovered harkens back to the early days of hospitals that distinguished between the "deserving" and "undeserving." "Lives" is not an empathic category—it is a dehumanized accounting denomination in this context. This notion of the "undeserving poor" is embedded deeply in the consciousnesses of a large slice of American society.[13]

Because executives of health systems recognize that they can improve their leverage by maximizing their market share, the pressure to keep expanding is enormous. The promotion aimed at accomplishing this is sophisticated and ubiquitous. Like sharks, they seem to feel that if they do not continuously move forward and expand, they will perish.

The structure and organization of these health systems reflect an unswerving commitment to health—their own fiscal health. The specialization of medicine led to the creation of groups that coordinated related components of care but mostly did not include primary care practitioners. The newer systems are all about building primary care networks to feed the hospitals and the specialists, whose procedures generate much of the hospitals' revenue. All of these systems are interested in generating as much revenue as they can. Toward this end, they mostly are inclined to place their practices and, when possible, their hospitals in locations that will attract patients with good insurance.

Los Angeles is a case in point. In chapter 6, I talked about the growth of UCLA's network in recent years. Cedars-Sinai Health System, centered in Beverly Hills, competes vigorously with UCLA for the business of the well insured. Technically part of the same medical school, there is no love lost between them. They both strive continuously and vigorously for greater shares of the same market of well-insured patients. Their relationship reminds me of the conversation between the president and the alien in the film *Independence Day*. When asked by the president, "What do you want us to do?" the alien replied, "Die."

UCLA has built a network of hospitals and clinics in west Los Angeles, Santa Monica, Pacific Palisades, the beach communities, the San Fernando Valley, and the Simi Valley. They have noticeably avoided placing their practices in south Los Angeles, east Los Angeles, Watts, Compton, and other communities with heavily minority populations, who are either uninsured or covered by the California version of Medicaid. Cedars-Sinai's practices follow a similar demographic strategy to that of UCLA.

When I was an assistant professor at UCLA, I had the opportunity to deliver a lecture for Medical Grand Rounds. I chose the topic "The Social Responsibilities of the Physician," which is related to my area of research. My plan was to discuss the historical context of physicians caring for the poor back to the time of the ancient Greeks, then review some contemporary data on disparities in health, life expectancy, and medical care between whites and nonwhites, and between the poor and nonpoor. Finally, I planned to conclude with some criticism of our hospital's failure to take care of more people who were poor or ethnically diverse, including those who were Medicaid beneficiaries.

As I began my talk, I noticed a senior administrator of our medical center was sitting in the middle of the third row. I wondered what he would think of my comments, but I thought it was good that he would hear what I had to say. Because of where he was sitting, I could see him throughout my talk. As it went on, he became more and more uncomfortable. His face was red and he appeared to be angry. I girded myself for his expected attack during question period.

He raised his hand immediately when I finished. Ken Shine, the chair of the department at the time, was fielding questions. Happily, he recognized the situation, saw what was coming, and did not recognize the hospital director for a question. He spared me from a rather unpleasant confrontation. The administrator never did speak to me about my talk. I don't think that he found it enlightening. In the corporate suites of health systems, concerns such as the ones that I raised rarely are heard and certainly are not welcomed. Health systems that work hard to capture the population that is demographically desirable do not like to hear criticism of their discriminatory practices.

Another academic health system in the Los Angeles area belongs to the University of Southern California, whose major teaching hospital had been a public one (Los Angeles County-USC Medical Center). In recent years, however, they have moved aggressively to build their privately insured business and have a private hospital now next to the county facility. One major health maintenance organization (Kaiser Permanente), which has a large number of enrollees in Southern California, recently opened a medical school. Kaiser is not in direct competition with these other systems for patients (theirs come largely from major corporate employer contracts), but UCLA has had to match their salary structure for primary care physicians in order to attract practitioners.

USC, whose main hospitals are in a less affluent part of town, has placed many of its practices in more advantaged areas, including Pasadena, Beverly Hills, and Newport Beach.[14] Kaiser, with a different mission, has clinics throughout more diverse communities, although not in the poorest areas. Kaiser's medical school also seems to be much more genuinely committed to the health of a broader population.[15] These are not the only systems in the second-largest city in the United States, but they are influential, and other than Kaiser (which is self-insured), they have been really good at negotiating with insurers. None of them do much business in the poor parts of town. That is left to the public system and some free clinics, with their paucity of specialist care services.

In some other metropolitan areas, consolidation by academic systems has been even more aggressive. In Boston, two leading general hospitals (Massachusetts General Hospital and Brigham and Women's Hospital) merged. Their system now includes hospitals in Belmont, Jamaica Plain, Martha's Vineyard, Nantucket, Newton, Northampton, and Salem in Massachusetts as well as in Dover, New Hampshire, a network of rehabilitation hospitals, and multiple practice sites.[16]

In New York, Cornell's Medical School faculty worked in the independent New York Hospital, while Columbia University's faculty worked in Presbyterian Hospital. The two hospitals merged to form New York Presbyterian Hospital, which now has about eight other hospital components to their system in Brooklyn, Manhattan, and Queens in New York City and nearby.[17] Northwell, a new medical school system, has twenty-three hospitals, including twenty-two in New York (New York City, Long Island, Westchester County, and various other locations in New York State) and affiliates in Syracuse and in Boca Raton, Florida.[18] Mount Sinai Health System in New York has about eight hospitals, including the former Roosevelt and St. Luke's Hospitals, now rebranded as Mount Sinai West and Mount Sinai Morningside.[19] New York University (NYU) and Albert Einstein Medical College have also built hospital and clinical systems aggressively in New York City and environs.

All of these health systems are zealous in seeking customers. Years ago, I was on the board of directors of the West Los Angeles Little League, which sponsored baseball and softball programs in my neighborhood close to where I worked. The league was always interested in raising more money to improve the facilities and support the programs. At one meeting, we were asked to think about whom we knew that might be willing to buy advertising space on our fields. It occurred to me that I worked for the largest employer in the area, so I contacted someone at hospital administration.

She was able to come up with $10,000 annually, in exchange for a large sign that appropriately advertised their pediatrics programs. I was surprised at their generosity but should not have been. The families who frequented the field were the kind of people whom they hoped to attract: well-insured and well-off. Not long after that, such promotions for our health system and others in the area became a nearly constant presence in advertising on radio and television, on buses and in sports stadiums. It is now not possible to watch a Los Angeles Dodgers home game in person or on television without seeing one of the banners for UCLA's health care system. I am pretty sure they are paying more for that prime locale than they did for their spot on the fence of our Little League field.

In New York, it is hard to watch television for more than a few minutes without seeing an advertisement for one or another academic health system. The promotions are not, shall we say, evidence based. One analysis estimated that health care providers spent at least $10 billion in 2017 and $11.8 billion in 2019 on advertising on radio and television spots, newspaper advertisements, direct mailers, and on digital advertising, which now consumes a large proportion of their media budgets.[20] Many of these advertisements are aimed at local audiences, but some systems, such as the University of Pittsburgh, Sidney Farber Cancer Center in Boston, and New York's Hospital for Special Surgery, have run national television advertising campaigns.[21] The marketers leave no well-insured groups unsolicited in their campaigns to capture more covered lives.

All of the New York City health systems seek to spread their tentacles into most or all of the boroughs of the city, although their efforts vary geographically. They vie for populations in Manhattan and the more affluent areas of Brooklyn and Queens, but (with the exception of Albert Einstein) pay far less attention to the Bronx, Harlem, and other areas that will not bring surplus revenue to their organizations. Competition for business is fierce. New York Presbyterian proclaims, "amazing things are happening here." Mount Sinai warns, "Which hospital you choose can make all the difference." NYU's health system is "made for New York."

As is consistent with the national data, while the expanded health care delivery systems in Los Angeles, New York, and elsewhere have consolidated, they have not achieved greater financial efficiency. In fact, in many communities, the prices of care covered by insurers other than federal Medicare and state Medicaid programs have increased because the insurers are hard-pressed to negotiate effectively with organizations that control one-fifth or one-third of the local market. Nor is it clear that there is any improvement in quality of care, notwithstanding the expectation that such systems would compete on quality. Market clout is everything.

Cash Is King: The Accumulation of Capital by Health Systems

Most health care delivery systems and the hospitals that comprise them are supposed to be not-for-profit, "voluntary" organizations. In reality, they have always been interested in maintaining positive streams of revenue. In the past 20 to 30 years, the appetite for surplus has been limitless. As health care systems have evolved and the revenue for highly technical care for well-insured patients has grown, these institutions have found themselves in a position to expand enormously their surplus-at-the-end-of-the-year-that-we-cannot-call-profit. The ability continually to extract revenue from their systems is not surprising.

The organizations argue that they need the revenue to expand services, reach more people, modernize, and so on, and they regularly sound the alarm that their financial positions are threatened. The reality is that while small organizations such as rural hospitals often lose money, and some go out of business, the large systems are doing fine.

In 2018, the Mayo Clinic's operating revenue yielded a surplus of $799 million ($706 million net from all activities).[22] The five hospitals owned by the University of California reported net cash from their operating activities of over $1.407 billion and cash on hand (even after some prepayment of existing debts, including mortgages on buildings and the like) of just over $3 billion for fiscal year 2017–18.[23]

New York Presbyterian Hospital showed net revenue of more than $412 million in 2017 (an increase of about $25 million from the previous year) and net assets of $6.884 billion, a $900 million increase from 2016.[24] NYP's pattern of net revenue continued, at least through the first six months of 2018.[25]

Similar patterns of robust surplus revenue accumulation were seen for Partners Health Care in Boston (now Mass General Brigham), Barnes-Jewish in St. Louis, and the University of Chicago.[26] Many of the most profitable hospitals in the United States are so-called nonprofits.[27]

In order to achieve their surpluses, hospitals invest in strategic planning that can optimize such factors as the impact of the location of their practices and hospitals on who uses their services and what kind of insurance they have.[28] Like other corporate interests, health systems do not always have good radar for realizing when their lust for revenue morphs into morally reprehensible behavior. Health systems such as the University of Virginia routinely sue patients for unpaid medical bills, seizing their paychecks, often putting liens on patients' homes, and placing them at risk of bankruptcy. According to one analysis, the University of Virginia sued 36,000 patients and former patients over a six-year period. That works out to about 120 suits per week.[29]

The centrality of surplus revenue to these enterprises is reinforced by the broader system, in which they compete with other enterprises and feel compelled to improve their physical plants, get better equipment, expand networks, and try to position themselves to get the most favorable contracts. Accordingly, the administrations of these organizations, which have expanded remarkably in recent decades,[30] now include top executives who frequently make several million dollars annually, and whose compensation is tied to revenue. In 2018, US hospital chief executive officer (CEO) bonuses averaged 33.2% of their base salaries, and bonuses for five other key hospital executive positions averaged 19.2% to 30.6%, according to the *Hospital Executive Compensation Report*.[31] In 2019, the CEOs of 82 of the largest voluntary hospital systems were paid an average of $3.629 million.[32]

In one analysis, when including return on investments of accumulated surplus, the 84 largest nonprofit health care systems accrued total profit of $35.6 billion in 2017, an average of over $400 million each.[33] The pursuit of surplus revenue is limitless for many of these health systems. Some profitable ones sought and obtained COVID-19 bailout funds from the US government even though they had plenty of cash on hand and were investing some of their accumulated billions in venture capital.[34] Still others, including Cedars-Sinai in Los Angeles and NYU Langone in New York City, clearly were not nearly as financially distressed as they claimed. They used COVID-19 relief funds to pursue mergers with other hospitals in their regions, thereby diminishing competition and improving even further the prospects for more surplus revenue extraction.[35]

Cathedrals for the Deserving

What kinds of people do modern health systems consider to be deserving or undeserving of their care? Are there clues in their histories, as well as in their policies and practices?

Even after the Jim Crow era ended with the passage of civil rights legislation in the 1960s, structural evidence of that racist history remained. When I was a medical student, I did an elective at Charity Hospital in New Orleans in 1973. I learned that until a few years earlier, one of the hospital's wings had been limited to white patients, while the other wing was for Black patients. Seeing that concrete embodiment of very recent segregation in a hospital was chilling.

When I was an intern, I again visited the South, this time to see a community health research program in a small town in Georgia. An immigrant doctor who worked in the program told me that it was hard being there, given the persistent racism. In the clinic where his program was situated, he indicated that there were two waiting rooms for the non-research patients, one for the Blacks and one for the whites. Learning about that in a small town, where desegregation presumably was occurring with "deliberate speed," was even more bothersome to me. Happily, those were vestiges of a fading era. Or were they?

Among the most important stops during a tour of Europe are the magnificent cathedrals and churches in every city and town. In the smaller towns, they often dominate the skyline. Many were built over decades or centuries at enormous cost. Today, in the United States, the hospitals are like secular cathedrals. As they accumulate large surpluses, these corporations invest some of their profits in magnificent new structures, sometimes designed by famous architects. When UCLA built a new hospital, it was designed by I. M. Pei and associates, famous, among other things, for their spectacular work at the Louvre.[36]

Hospital buildings can be architectural icons. They also are monuments to the values embodied, and the choices made, by the organizations working therein, just as Charity Hospital's very structure evoked memories of segregated care. It is not surprising that health systems develop policies to leverage these investments to continue to attract the kinds of patients that will allow their surpluses to keep on accumulating. Consider the lengths to which health systems go today to cater to patients with "good insurance," the great majority of whom are white and nonpoor.

I saw my patients and supervised residents in UCLA's main clinic building, which is right next to the hospital. I always enjoyed walking through the lobby, which featured a piano and some seats nearby. An older volunteer sat at the piano most afternoons, banging on the ivories and playing old popular songs. One day, to my dismay, the pianist was gone, and so was the piano. When I asked what had happened, I was told that it had been removed because the quality of the playing was not up the standard appropriate for the patients who were coming in. Clearly, the desired clientele came from a slice of society whose cultural tastes were more refined than my own!

At Cornell, a beautiful new outpatient and procedure building recently was erected across from the hospital, bearing the name of a billionaire-philanthropist. When I went there for a procedure not too long after it opened, I was struck by the vastness and emptiness of the elegant lobby. When I commented on that to one of the nurses, who was African American, she told me that staff had to use a service entrance and were not allowed to enter through the lobby. The staff included many nurses and others who were people of color. They weren't meant to mingle with the customers.

How successful are these efforts to refine their population, to make sure that the customers whom they value are never made to feel uncomfortable by mingling with the rabble in "steerage class"? In racially diverse New York City, where 23.8% of the population is African American, African Americans are three times as likely as whites to go to public hospitals. The proportion of patients who are African American at two renowned specialty hospitals are 5% at Hospital for Special Surgery

(HSS) and 9% at Memorial Sloan Kettering Cancer Center. As for being Black and poor, only 0.3% of HSS's patients are Blacks with Medicaid insurance.[37]

Robert Downey Sr.'s classic 1969 cult film *Putney Swope* is a satiric send-up of racism in America. In it, a Black man is appointed as the only minority member on the board of directors of a Madison Avenue advertising firm. Because he is Black, he is not allowed to use the main elevator to get to the board meetings, only the service elevator. Of course, that was satire. (He eventually became the company's CEO, telling the other board members that his philosophy is "Don't rock the boat; sink it.") The film was making an exaggerated point about racism.

Today, a similar point could be made about the racial and socioeconomic sorting (or should we say segregation) achieved by health care systems' relentless pursuit of patients who are well insured. In the case of hospital care in major American cities, the structural racism could be conveyed equally well in a documentary, with no need for any exaggeration at all.

Medical Schools and the Hospital Corporations

Since the time of Bichat in revolutionary France, bedside teaching has been an important component of medical education, and much of it has been focused in the hospital.[38] The associations between hospitals and medical schools in the United States became increasingly important to the medical schools throughout the twentieth century. While public hospitals were important and had many teaching cases, so too did the private, voluntary hospitals with paying patients. Eventually, these became sources of important revenue for the medical schools to cover faculty salaries and some other expenses.

As health systems seek to improve their financial leverage, they need more doctors to care for their ever-expanding numbers of "covered lives." Insofar as medical schools have the clinicians that the hospitals need, the relationships can be mutually beneficial. When medical schools don't own the hospitals, the latter hold the purse strings and the power. For example, New York Presbyterian Hospital does share some of its revenue with the Columbia and Cornell University medical schools, but often it is stingy with the resources that it passes on. As one observer of this trend, an academic cardiologist, has observed, this change in the role of the medical school has been fundamental:

> With health systems in charge, medical schools have become financially starved and have lost control of their faculty. The vestiges of the academic structures are still in place, meaning that there are still deans, departmental and divisional leaders, people with educational titles, and students. But unless they also have authority over the health system or service lines, the men and women in leadership positions are often only figureheads. . . . [with] no funding and little decision-making capacity . . . If academic leaders pursue a parallel "academic mission," they do so at their own peril. As a result, deans at modern medical schools serve a ceremonial function.[39]

The prose is rather hyperbolic, and schools in which hospitals are administratively subordinate to leaders of the medical schools are somewhat different, but the point is sobering nonetheless.

Even if they are not satisfied financially with the proceeds that they have been able to extract from their relationships with their hospitals, medical schools such as these have taken what amounts to a blood oath. They are bound to their health systems and the values inherent in the business practices of those systems. Those values infect them and crowd out any contrary notions of what their values and ideals as institutions should be.

Their care becomes increasingly expensive because they have an incentive to do the most expensive, technical procedures on every patient. Their clinical programs become more racially and socioeconomically exclusive when the practices operate in that way. This infection not only obliterates any independent priorities that they may have as institutions. It also becomes established in their students, who see how their professors and resident teachers operationalize their own ethical postures.

Cherry-Picking Populations

Finally, these hospitals, whether academic or nonacademic, for-profit or voluntary, work hard to "improve" patient mix to maximize the revenue they accrue for the care they provide. While they cannot turn away persons who show up at the emergency department, we have seen that their faculty grow comfortable with the provision of little or no ongoing service to Medicaid beneficiaries or to those with other kinds of coverage that do not pay well, and their students and other trainees only occasionally complain.

Many teaching hospitals and medical schools prominently profess their commitment to population health. On the face of it, one might think that they are committed to the well-being of the broader populations of the communities that they serve. In reality, the only populations about whom they care (in the practical sense of being prepared to do something about their well-being) are the covered lives of the well-insured individuals who can fill the beds and coffers of their hospitals and pay the fees of their doctors. They are not interested in the health of the population as a whole. At best, they want to achieve some efficiencies and to have some "outcomes" that they can advertise to the people for whom they have contracted responsibility.

The power of teaching hospitals can overwhelm all educational priorities, greatly diminishing the influence of academic leaders such as deans and department chairs. Clinicians are strongly discouraged from saying anything publicly that might threaten market share.[40] The masters of the universe in medicine these days are the hospital directors. Often, they are physicians who have MBA degrees. Their primary responsibilities are revenue accrual and surplus generation.

As part of their efforts to promote their hospitals and health systems in their refined catchment areas, they often provide a modicum of community service, in the form of health screenings for those lacking insurance and the like. That is a distraction from their primary goals. They are most attentive to prominent members of the community and to potential donors. When such individuals are in the hospital, the hospital director often goes to see them and pressures the staff to provide better service. Not so for Medicaid patients, who rarely receive follow-up care, and, if they do, certainly not with the faculty physicians, in most instances.

Any doubt in my mind about the slice of society who are the target population for these systems was extinguished when I was interviewing for a position in New York City. I was scheduled to meet with a senior administrator in a prominent teaching hospital. Early in our meeting, he stated that his hospital took care of people like a distinguished former federal official, whom he named. Shortly thereafter, he received a phone call, and told me that he had to terminate our meeting because a well-known former New York politician, whom he also named, was in the emergency department. Quite apart from the inappropriateness of disclosing these names to me, it was clear that these were the cherished customers to whom they catered.

Providing Value

In recent years, the catastrophe of the high cost of medical care in the United States has led to more discussion in health policy circles about "value" and cost-effectiveness. These discussions have trickled down to the level of provider systems, in part stimulated by the threat to hold them responsible for all the costs of care of the patients whom they see in "accountable care organizations." These incentive schemes have had some impact, but not as much as some hoped.[41] They do remain a threat to the perpetual lavish revenue streams to which health systems believe they are entitled. Many of the systems talk value but continue to promote profligacy.

Thus they want lots of referrals to their specialists who do procedures. They rarely do much to discourage unnecessary interventions, and they continue to reward the high producers (of revenue) with more income. They have the fantasy that they can veer sharply toward financial responsibility on the day that they no longer can squeeze the system for every penny. That is about as likely as turning an aircraft carrier on a dime.

In pursuit of ever greater market share, they develop and market "product lines" intended to attract well-insured patients, touting the wonders wrought within their systems with advertising that is potentially as misleading as that of the pharmaceutic industry. While ambulatory practices suffered considerable losses during the COVID-19 pandemic, hospitals were not lacking for patients to fill their beds. Their claims of lost revenue and successful pleas for bailout funds largely had to do with the loss of the elective procedures and operations that comprise these product lines and from which they generate their surplus.[42]

Medical schools and their universities also make deals with manufacturers, at times getting kickbacks and acquiring financial interests in products. Rather than something to be avoided, conflicts of interests, which are legal, are consummations devoutly to be wished. Some of these deals, as I discuss in chapter 8, defy any reasonable sense of what is decent or ethical. The problem is not merely disclosure, about which patients are unlikely to learn in any event, but the actual conflicts of interest themselves.[43] Systems built on series of product lines will not see value the way that patients do.

Doing It All

Some other countries are making earnest efforts to regionalize and specialize facilities. Patients can be sent to the best place for care, where the treatment is most likely to produce the best results. That occurs for some services in the US, but it is more difficult to implement broadly when health systems are battling one another to the death.

The struggle for market share creates an upward spiral of high-technology medicine. If one system has a doctor who can do an exotic procedure, they will advertise that, particularly if the competition lacks that capacity. From the patient's perspective, why not go to the place with the heart transplantation program if you have a heart problem? Or to the place that does robotic prostate removal? Or some innovative approach to chemotherapy (regardless of whether or not it produces better outcomes)? Once the high-technology physician is on board, he or she must perform tasks that will generate coverage for a high salary, so more procedures get done using the fancy technology, and costs escalate.

Other Corporate Providers

Specialty services providers—such as nursing homes, dialysis providers, and home care companies—are another important corporate element in health care. They tend to comply with requests for their services, rarely declining to provide care that might be clinically inappropriate, such as kidney dialysis for people who are soon to die from another health problem, or promoting expensive rehabilitation services in the last month of life.[44] They, too, are focused upon maintaining revenue streams, even when there are questions about their quality of care. They spend lavishly to protect their interests, as occurred in 2018, when a California initiative to limit costs of dialysis was defeated with more than $110 million in opposition funding, 90% from two corporate providers of 80% of all dialysis in the US.[45]

Investors

Private equity corporations and hedge funds are particularly avaricious participants in the health care market. After all, why would they stay away from this 18% slice of the economy? Their business model is straightforward: buy a company, intervene to maximize extractable revenue (hence its value), then sell it. In health care, they target lucrative areas of medical practice that can be modified to enable rapid valuation and revenue extraction. After a failed expansion of physician management companies in the 1990s,[46] the 2010s saw exponential growth of private equity investment in health care, notably buying up medical practices. Some of the incentive to do this was the inherent inefficiency of small provider groups in billing and ineffective negotiation of rates with insurers. But these firms also have identified other opportunities through these investments, which totaled more than $42 billion in 2017 alone.[47]

They can augment revenue by increasing the numbers of procedures being done and incorporating charges for ancillary services, such as pathology and radiology. Consequently, they have been interested in acquiring practices with many discretionary services, such as dermatology, in which there are skin biopsies, injections, pathology costs, and Mohs surgery procedures. There is some evidence that dermatology practices acquired by private equity do inordinately large numbers of such procedures.[48]

Other areas of practice that have been attractive to private equity include otolaryngology,[49] gastroenterology, ophthalmology,[50] urology, and allergy.[51] There has also been some movement of private equity into behavioral health care, in which they have identified opportunities to increase revenue (by attracting more clients with eating disorders, for example) or decrease costs (such as in the "autism sector") by providing less care.[52]

The goal of these firms clearly is to extract profit. The investors expect an annual return of at least 20%. Prices are based on EBITDA (earnings before interest, taxes, depreciation, and amortization). The firms will pay up to 10 to 12 times this number to acquire an initial prominent practice in a community, and then they will pay less than that for additional practices that they absorb. They then set about increasing revenue and decreasing costs, generally with the goal of selling it off in several years.[53]

As noted above, revenue increases come from increasing the volume of high-paying procedures, as well as from negotiating higher reimbursement from insurers. Costs can be reduced by decreasing administrative inefficiencies, but also by trimming aspects of service (e.g., by using physician assistants in place of physicians, by hiring untrained technicians in place of those with training, and by moving some inpatient care to the outpatient setting).[54] The firms typically keep some clinicians as minority owners of the practices to show their commitment to the success of the business. Inevitably, clinicians are expected to respond to the new norms of the practice.

Private equity managers can be ambitious, even buying hospitals. If their investments don't produce the kinds of returns that they anticipate, they are not shy about shutting these facilities down, whatever the im-plications for the communities that they serve.[55]

There has been almost no research done on the impact of the private equity firms on the costs, quality, outcomes, and patient perceptions of the care provided in these acquired practice settings.[56] The role of private equity in health care will continue to grow. Given that health care in the US is financially inefficient compared to other countries, with enormous administrative costs,[57] it is hard to see how this activity will decrease that level of inefficiency, given the expectation of revenue extraction by the investors. Meeting societal needs, constraining health care costs, and optimizing population health are not what their investors are looking for.

Collateral Damage

Is it such a bad thing that hospital corporations and those who invest in them are devoted to the generation of surplus revenue and the accumu-lation of capital? Isn't that the American way? Well, that style of doing business can have profound consequences for real people.

William, a man in his late sixties, was admitted to the hospital with congestive heart failure and was assigned to my care. In this condition, one's heart is too weak to keep up with the flow of blood through the circulation. Each time the heart contracts, it needs to pump out most of the blood that has entered it through the veins. If it does not, the fluid backs up behind the heart and can flood the lungs.

A normally functioning heart has an ejection fraction of 50% or greater, meaning that it removes half of the blood in the left ventricle with each heartbeat. William had an ejection fraction of 11%. That is really bad heart failure. The risk of dying is great. We treated him with medications that were designed to remove fluid and to relax blood vessels, so that more fluid would flow into the arteries and stay out of the lungs. His condition began to improve.

The morning after his admission, I received a call from a member of the hospital administrative staff. "Your patient does not have insurance, but he is a veteran, so we can transfer him to the VA [Veterans Affairs] hospital today," he said.

"I'm sorry, but he is not stable for transfer."

"Yes, he is. You've been treating him since yesterday."

"He still is unstable. His ejection fraction is only 11%. He could easily develop pulmonary edema again or have an arrhythmia."

"That's very unlikely. The risk is extremely low," said the administrator, who was not a clinician.

"I disagree with you and refuse to discharge him.," I responded.

In this case, the hospital was all too willing to chalk up William to collateral damage, if necessary, when business considerations are paramount. On this occasion, I managed to carry the day, but that is not always the case. Too often, the first inclination of administrators is to protect the interests of their business, not the best interest of the patients. Too often, the pressure that they apply to the clinical staff pays dividends. As in the case in chapter 1 of Luis, who needed a new liver, the people who ran our teaching hospital, a state-owned institution with an annual surplus of hundreds of millions of dollars, could have seen things differently.

Notes

1. Charles E. Rosenberg, *The Care of Strangers: The Rise of America's Hospital System* (New York: Basic Books, 1987), 4.

2. Rosenberg, *Care of Strangers*, 5.

3. Rosenberg, *Care of Strangers*, 5.

4. Rosenberg, *Care of Strangers*, 237–61.

5. Michel Foucault, *The Birth of the Clinic: An Archaeology of Medical Perception* (New York: Pantheon, 1973), 64–87.

6. Cecil C. Cutting and Morris Frank Collen, "A Historical Review of the Kaiser Permanente Medical Care Program," *Journal of the Society for Health Systems* 3, no. 4 (1992): 25–30, PMID 1288670.

7. Rosemary Stevens, *In Sickness and in Wealth: American Hospitals in the Twentieth Century* (Baltimore: Johns Hopkins University Press, 1999), 284–320.

8. Stevens, *In Sickness and in Wealth*, 293–97.

9. Erik W. J. Kokkonan et al., "Use of Electronic Records by Different Specialty and Office Settings," *Journal of the American Medical Informatics Association* 20, e1 (June 2013): e33–e38, https://doi.org/10.1136/amiajnl-2012-001609.

10. There have been isolated experiments in the area of financing hospital care, such as one successful initiative for hospitals in Maryland. That has not been

translated into broader policy up to now. J. M. Sharfstein et al., "An Emerging Approach to Payment Reform: All-Payer Global Budgets for Large Safety-Net Hospital Systems," Commonwealth Fund, August 16, 2017, https://www.common wealthfund.org/publications/fund-reports/2017/aug/emerging-approach-payment -reform-all-payer-global-budgets-large.

11. Asako S. Moriya, William B. Vogt, and Martin Gaynor, "Hospital Prices and Market Structure in the Hospital and Insurance Industries," *Health Economics, Policy, and Law* 5, no. 4 (October 2010): 458–79, https://doi.org/10.1017/S1744133110000083; Seidu Dauda, "Hospital and Health Insurance Markets Concentration and Inpatient Transaction Prices in the U.S. Health Care Market," *Health Services Research* 53, no. 2 (April 2018): 1203–26, https://doi.org/10.1111/1475-6773.12706; David Cutler and Fiona Scott Morton, "Hospitals, Market Share, and Consolidation," JAMA 310, no. 18 (November 13, 2013): 1964–70, https://doi.org/10.1001/jama.2013.281675; Richard M. Scheffler, Daniel R. Arnold, and Christopher M. Whaley, "Consolidation Trends in California's Health Care System: Impacts on ACA Premiums and Outpatient Visit Prices," *Health Affairs* (Millwood) 37, no. 9 (September 2018): 1409–16, https://doi.org /10.1377/hlthaff.2018.0472; Andrew S. Boozary et al., "The Association between Hospital Concentration and Insurance Premiums in ACA Marketplaces," *Health Affairs* (Millwood) 38, no. 4 (April 2019): 668–74, https://doi.org/10.1377/hlthaff.2018 .05491; Emily Gee and Ethan Gurwitz, "Provider Consolidation Drives Up Health Care Costs: Policy Recommendations to Curb Abuses of Market Power and Protect Patients," Center for American Progress, December 5, 2018, https://www .americanprogress.org/issues/health care/reports/2018/12/05/461780/provider-consolidation-drives-health-care-costs/; Caroline Hanson, Bradley Herring, and Erin Trish, "Do Health Insurance and Hospital Market Concentration Influence Hospital Patients' Experience of Care?," *Health Services Research* 54, no. 4 (August 2019): 805–15, https://doi.org/10.1111/1475-6773.13168.

12. "April 2021 Medicaid and CHIP Enrollment Data Highlights," Medicaid.gov, accessed October 24, 2021, https://www.medicaid.gov/medicaid/program -information/medicaid-and-chip-enrollment-data/report-highlights/index.html.

13. Michael B. Katz, *The Undeserving Poor: America's Enduring Confrontation with Poverty* (Oxford: Oxford University Press, 2013).

14. "Our Hospitals and Clinic Locations," Keck Medicine of USC, accessed July 13, 2021, https://www.keckmedicine.org/locations/.

15. "The Medical School for the Doctor You Want to Be," Kaiser Permanente Bernard J. Tyson School of Medicine, accessed September 12, 2020, https:// medschool.kp.org/homepage?kp_shortcut_referrer=kp.org/schoolofmedicine.

16. Major facilities are Faulkner (a community hospital in Jamaica Plain); Mass Eye and Ear in Boston; Newton-Wellesley Hospital in suburban Boston; McLean (a psychiatric hospital in Belmont); Cooley Dickinson (a community hospital in Northampton, in western Massachusetts); North Shore Medical Center in Salem; Nantucket Cottage Hospital and Martha's Vineyard Hospital (on islands off the coast); the Spaulding Rehabilitation facilities throughout eastern Massachusetts; and, just for good measure, Wentworth-Douglas Hospital in Dover, New Hampshire.

"Members and Affiliates," Mass General Brigham, accessed July 13, 2021, https://www.massgeneralbrigham.org/who-we-are/members-affiliations.

17. "Our Locations," New York-Presbyterian, accessed April 14, 2020, https://www.nyp.org/locations.

18. "Locations: Hospitals," Northwell Health, accessed April 14, 2020, https://www.northwell.edu/doctors-and-care/locations?type=hospitals&user_filtered=true&page=2.

19. "Mount Sinai Locations," Mount Sinai, accessed April 14, 2020, https://www.mountsinai.org/locations.

20. Paige Minemyer, "Hospitals Spend Big Bucks on Advertising. Here's a Look at the Cost of 8 Ad Campaigns," Fierce Healthcare, August 27, 2018, https://www.fiercehealth care.com/hospitals-health-systems/hospitals-spending-big-bucks-advertising-a-look-cost-8-ad-campaigns; "Advertising Spending in the Hospital Industry in the United States from 2018 to 2019," Statista, accessed June 11, 2021, https://www.statista.com/statistics/470699/hospitals-industry-ad-spend-usa/#statisticContainer.

21. Shefali Luthra, "Playing on Fear and Fun, Hospitals Follow Pharma in Direct-To-Consumer Advertising," Kaiser Health News, November 19, 2018, https://khn.org/news/hospitals-direct-to-consumer-health-care-advertising-marketing/.

22. "Mayo Clinic Consolidated Financial Report December 31, 2018," Mayo Clinic, accessed January 28, 2020, https://cdn.prod-carehubs.net/n1/802899ec472ea3d8/uploads/2019/02/Mayo-Clinic-Year-End-2018-Consolidated-Short-Form.pdf; Dusta Anastasijevic, "Strong Performance Bolsters Mayo Clinic's Humanitarian Mission, Resilience for Future Growth," Mayo Clinic News Network, accessed September 4, 2020, https://newsnetwork.mayoclinic.org/discusson/strong-performance-in-2018-bolsters-mayo-clinics-humanitarian-mission-resilience-for-future-growth/.

23. "University of California Medical Centers Report 17/18," University of California, accessed September 4, 2020, https://regents.universityofcalifornia.edu/regmeet/nov18/c3attach5.pdf.

24. "New York and Presbyterian Hospital Full Text of 'Form 990' for Fiscal Year Ending Dec. 2017," ProPublica Nonprofit Explorer, accessed January 28, 2020, https://projects.propublica.org/nonprofits/organizations/133957095/201843199349304239/IRS990.

25. "Unaudited Consolidated Financial Statements and Supplementary Information: The New York Presbyterian Hospital, As of and for the Six Months Ended June 30, 2018," Electronic Municipal Market Access, Municipal Services Rulemaking Board, accessed January 28, 2020, https://emma.msrb.org/ES1194379-ES933433-.pdf; Kelly Gooch, "New York-Presbyterian's Net Income Climbs 364.5%," Becker's Hospital CFO Report, June 4, 2019, https://www.beckershospitalreview.com/finance/newyork-presbyterian-s-net-income-climbs-364-5.html.

26. "Partners Health Care Reports Fourth Quarter 2018 Financial Results," Electronic Municipal Market Access, Municipal Services Rulemaking Board, accessed April 15, 2020, https://emma.msrb.org/ES1221774-ES953956-.pdf; "Consolidated Financial Statements BJC HealthCare, Years Ended December 31, 2018 and 2017,

with Report of Independent Auditors," Electronic Municipal Market Access, Municipal Services Rulemaking Board, accessed April 15, 2020, https://emma.msrb.org/ER1201479 -ER940449-.pdf; KMPG, "The University of Chicago Medical Center Consolidated Statements June 30, 2018 and 2017," accessed September 4, 2020, https://www .uchicagomedicine.org/-/media/pdfs/adult-pdfs/about-us/financial-information/2018 audited.pdf?la=en&hash=9D7F9E9150B53819292385E06555AB9EE0F9A566.

27. Lena H. Sun, "These Hospitals Make the Most Money off Patients—and They're Mostly Nonprofits," *Washington Post*, May 3, 2016, https://www.washingtonpost .com/news/to-your-health/wp/2016/05/02/these-hospitals-make-the-most-money -off-patients-and-theyre-mostly-nonprofits/.

28. Ge Bai and Gerald F. Anderson, "A More Detailed Understanding of Factors Associated with Hospital Profitability," *Health Affairs* (Millwood) 35, no. 5 (May 2016): 889–97, https://doi.org/10.1377/hlthaff.2015.1193.

29. Jay Hancock and Elizabeth Lucas, "'UVA Has Ruined Us': Health System Sues Thousands of Patients, Seizing Paychecks and Putting Liens on Homes," *Washington Post*, September 9, 2019, https://www.washingtonpost.com/health/uva-has-ruined -us-health-system-sues-thousands-of-patients-seizing-paychecks-and-putting-liens -on-homes/2019/09/09/5eb23306-c807-11e9-be05-f76ac4ec618c_story.html.

30. Stevens, *In Sickness and in Wealth*, 332–44.

31. "Average Bonus for a Hospital CEO is 33.2% of Base Salary," Cision PRWeb News Center, April 10, 2018, http://www.prweb.com/releases/2018/04 /prweb15398416.htm.

32. Adam Andrzejewski, "Top U.S. 'Non-profit' Hospitals and CEOs Are Racking Up Huge Profits," *Forbes*, June 26, 2019, https://www.forbes.com/sites /adamandrzejewski/2019/06/26/top-u-s-non-profit-hospitals-ceos-are-racking-up -huge-profits/#131c3ad19dfb.

33. Meg Bryant, "CEO Salaries at Nonprofit Hospitals Up 93% Since 2005," Healthcaredive, August 17, 2018, https://www.healthcaredive.com/news/ceo -salaries-at-nonprofit-hospitals-up-93-since-2005/530353/.

34. Jesse Drucker, Jessica Silver-Greenberg, and Sarah Kliff, "Wealthiest Hospitals Got Billions in Bailout for Struggling Health Providers," *New York Times*, May 25, 2020, https://www.nytimes.com/2020/05/25/business/coronavirus -hospitals-bailout.html.

35. Reed Abelson, "Buoyed by Federal Covid Aid, Big Hospital Chains Buy Up Competitors," *New York Times*, May 22, 2021, https://www.nytimes.com/2021/05/21 /health/covid-bailout-hospital-merger.html?searchResultPosition=1.

36. Martha Groves, "New UCLA Hospital Is Dedicated," *Los Angeles Times*, June 5, 2007, https://www.latimes.com/archives/la-xpm-2007-jun-05-me-ucla5-story.html.

37. Barbara Caress, "Hospital Care in Black and White: How Systemic Racism Persists," New School Center for New York City Affairs, September 16, 2020, http://www.centernyc.org/urban-matters-2/2020/9/15/hospital-care-in-black-and -white-how-systemic-racism-persists-saved; "New York City, New York, Population Estimates, July 1, 2021," US Census Quick Facts, accessed August 21, 2022, https:// www.census.gov/quickfacts/newyorkcitynewyork.

38. Foucault, *Birth of the Clinic*, 64–87.

39. Milton Packer, "Med Schools' Business Model Is Officially Dead," Medpage Today, November 28, 2018, www.medpagetoday.com/blogs/revolutionandrevelation /76553.

40. Conor Friedersdorf, "Hospitals Must Let Doctors and Nurses Speak Out," *The Atlantic*, April 10, 2020, https://www.theatlantic.com/ideas/archive/2020/04/why -are-hospitals-censoring-doctors-and-nurses/609766/.

41. Shashank S. Sinha et al., "The Effect of Medicare Accountable Care Organizations on Early and Late Payments for Cardiovascular Disease Episodes," *Circulation: Cardiovascular Quality and Outcomes* 11, no. 8 (August 2018): e004495, https://doi .org/10.1161/CIRCOUTCOMES.117.004495.

42. Sourav K. Bose et al., "The Cost of Quarantine: Projecting the Financial Impact of Canceled Elective Surgery on the Nation's Hospitals," *Annals of Surgery* 273, no. 5 (May 2021): 844–49, https://doi.org/10.1097/SLA.0000000000004766.

43. Marcia Angell, "Transparency Hasn't Stopped Drug Companies from Corrupting Medical Research," *New York Times*, September 14, 2018, https://www .nytimes.com/2018/09/14/opinion/jose-baselga-research-disclosure-bias.html.

44. Helena Temkin-Greener et al., "Rehabilitation Therapy for Nursing Home Residents at the End-of-Life," *Journal of the American Medical Directors Association* 20, no. 4 (April 2019): 476–80.e1, https://doi.org/10.1016/j.jamda.2018.07.024.

45. "California Proposition 8, Limits on Dialysis Clinics' Revenue and Required Refunds Initiative (2018)," Ballotpedia, accessed July 1, 2019, https://ballotpedia.org /California_Proposition_8,_Limits_on_Dialysis_Clinics%27_Revenue_and_Required _Refunds_Initiative_(2018).

46. Uwe E. Reinhardt, "The Rise and Fall of the Physician Practice Management Industry," *Health Affairs (Millwood)* 19, no. 1 (January–February 2000): 42–55, https://doi.org/10.1377/hlthaff.19.1.42.

47. Suhas Gondi and Zirui Song, "Potential Implications of Private Equity Investments in Health Care Delivery," JAMA 321, no. 11 (March 19, 2019): 1047–48, https://doi.org/10.1001/jama.2019.1077.

48. Sally Tan Set al., "Trends in Private Equity Acquisition of Dermatology Practices in the United States," *JAMA Dermatology* 155, no. 9 (September 2019): 1013–21, https://doi.org/10.1001/jamadermatol.2019.1634; Sailesh Konda et al., "Private Equity Acquisition of Physician Practices," *Annals of Internal Medicine* 171, no. 1 (July 2, 2019): 77–78, https://doi.org/10.7326/L19-0255; Jack S. Resneck Jr., "Dermatology Practice Consolidation Fueled by Private Equity Investment: Potential Consequences for the Specialty and Patients," *JAMA Dermatology* 154, no. 1 (January 2018): 13–14, https://doi.org/10.1001/jamadermatol.2017.5558.

49. Lauren E. Miller, Vinay K. Rathi, and Matthew R. Naunheim, "Implications of Private Equity Acquisition of Otolaryngology Physician Practices," *JAMA Otolaryngology* 146, no. 2 (February 2020): 97–98, https://doi.org/10.1001/jamaoto.2019.3738.

50. Shriji N. Patel, Sylvia Groth, and Paul Sternberg Jr., "The Emergence of Private Equity in Ophthalmology," *JAMA Ophthalmology* 137, no. 6 (June 2019): 601–2, https://doi.org/10.1001/jamaophthalmol.2019.0964.

51. Gondi and Song, "Potential Implications."

52. Benjamin Brown, Eloise O'Donnell, and Lawrence P. Casalino, "Private Equity Investment in Behavioral Health Treatment Centers," *JAMA Psychiatry* 77, no. 3 (March 2019): 229–30, https://doi.org/10.1001/jamapsychiatry.2019.3880.

53. Lawrence P. Casalino et al., "Private Equity Acquisition of Physician Practices," *Annals of Internal Medicine* 170, no. 2 (January 15, 2019): 114–15, https://doi.org/10.7326/M18-2363.

54. Brown et al., "Private Equity Investment."

55. Chris Pomorski, "The Death of Hahnemann Hospital," *New Yorker*, May 31, 2021, https://www.newyorker.com/magazine/2021/06/07/the-death-of-hahnemann-hospital.

56. Ryan Crowley et al., "Financial Profit in Medicine: A Position Paper from the American College of Physicians," *Annals of Internal Medicine* 174, no. 10 (October 2021): 1447–49, https://doi.org/10.7326/M21-1178.

57. David U. Himmelstein, Terry Campbell, and Steffie Woolhandler, "Health Care Administrative Costs in the United States and Canada, 2017," *Annals of Internal Medicine* 172, no. 2 (January 21, 2020): 134–42, https://doi.org/10.7326/M19-2818.

Dialogue #6

Student: That was revealing. These health corporations are powerful and don't seem to be prepared to do much to solve any of the problems.

Professor: I agree. Most troubling to me is their indifference to the well-being of so many people in their communities who are dying and suffering needlessly. Emma Lazarus would have characterized their position as "Give me your huddled masses, but only if they have good insurance."

Student: Yes. They love to have their doctors do procedures, and the wallet biopsy seems to be their favorite one! But do they really have a choice? Given the way the overall health care system is financed, they have to find ways to remain solvent.

Professor: They are more than solvent. They could choose to be a little less obsessed with their bottom lines. The level of vertical and horizontal consolidation—acquiring practices and creating networks of hospitals— also is stunning. It's at a greed-is-good level, apparently without much concern for its implications.

Student: Well, some hospitals lost hundreds of millions of dollars when the COVID-19 pandemic hit.

Professor: And some invested their bailouts in new acquisitions. There are other ways to protect against possible catastrophic losses than with their current business practices. Remember the point about global budgets for hospitals being an option. As the quality improvement folks observe, every system is perfectly designed to get the results it gets.[1]

Student: So, in one respect, the health care system is perfect.

Professor: Slim pickings for $3 trillion a year. What else are we missing?

Student: Well, as I said, we need to look at the insurance and pharmaceutical industries, but I suspect that you again are going to send me down a different path.

Professor: They will not escape our scrutiny, but there is more to do, and some of it is highly relevant to understanding corporate behavior in health care. We have not yet looked at biomedical scientists and the organizations and institutions that support their work.

Student: There are corporate interests at play, but American science has made wonderful contributions to scientific knowledge and medical therapy. Surely you aren't a science denier.

Professor: No, but don't prejudge how scintillatingly wonderful the scientists' contributions are. We need to look at them objectively. Are their priorities motivated by financial considerations? By career-related needs? Are there issues in their backgrounds, their training, their characteristics, and their interests that affect their motivations, choices, and behavior? What is the role of institutions and funders in shaping the priorities of biomedical science? What kind of evidence would convince you that this topic is pertinent?

Student: We would need to look at the kinds of clinical care problems that do and don't get studied, and see if there is insufficient funding in areas that may be important to health.

Professor: I like that. Perhaps we can figure out whether there is a distinction between science as a discipline or set of disciplines and the ways in which the practitioners and sponsors of scientific work enact and prioritize scientific work.

Student: We also need to figure out if the priorities of science and the consequences of discoveries can adversely affect costs, access, and outcomes of care along with the good they may do.

Professor: Let's do that.

Note

1. These words are sometimes attributed to W. Edwards Deming but likely originated with Paul Batalden. Doug McInnis, "What System?," *Dartmouth Medicine* 30, no. 4 (Summer 2006): https://dartmed.dartmouth.edu/summer06/html/what _system.php.

8

Biomedical Scientists and Their Truths

Disinterested Investigation or Prioritized Self-Interest?

Science is but an image of the truth.
—Francis Bacon

I was invited to Washington University in St. Louis some years ago to advise the leadership of the Department of Internal Medicine and the medical school on developing a research program in general internal medicine that would focus upon health care delivery. In my research on health care delivery, I look at such problems as access to care, disparities in who gets treated, cost and cost-effectiveness of treatments, quality of medical care, and the impact of treatment on health outcomes that patients care about. Washington University School of Medicine is a great institution with numerous scientists who have won Nobel Prizes. But the school was known at that time to have little interest in the kinds of research that examined whether people were getting the care that they needed.

I was encouraged that the leadership seemed to want to move in that direction, but the medical school lacked some of the intellectual infrastructure that they would need. When I met with the dean at the end of my visit, I told him that to have a successful program, they would need to provide institutional support for at least six clinician scientists and for a comparable number of social scientists focused upon health care, as well as clinical epidemiologists to build the program.

"That would take an endowment of $25 million," he said.

"I suppose it might," I responded.

"But that is what I am spending on a new animal house!" responded the dean.

Seemingly irritated by my comment, he terminated our meeting at that point, earlier than scheduled. An animal house is a facility to house animals that are being used in research. This senior, distinguished academic leader, who was in the midst of a lengthy tenure as both dean and executive vice chancellor for medical affairs, could not imagine investing as much money in building a program to study and improve medical care for the population as he was spending on better accommodations for their research animals. To understand how that came to be a common point of view of the leadership and practitioners of American biomedical science, let's take a look at how we got there.

America is justifiably proud of its medical science, which is preeminent in the world and has contributed greatly to our understanding and treatment of disease. As one measure of those contributions, the Nobel Prize in Physiology or Medicine was not awarded to an American the first 26 times that it was given. From 1930 to 2021, however, one or more scientists who were Americans or who worked in the United States won or shared the prize 61 of 89 times. The contributions have included the discovery of human blood groups (Karl Landsteiner, 1930); characterization of the chemical nature of vitamin K (Edward Doisy, 1943); the structure and function of adrenal hormones (Philip Hench and Edward Kendall, 1950); the discovery of streptomycin, which treated tuberculosis (Selman Waksman, 1952); genetic regulation and recombination (George Beadle, Joshua Lederberg, and Edward Tatum, 1958); the causes and treatments of certain cancers (Charles Huggins and Peyton Rous, 1966); description of the interaction between tumor viruses and genetic material in cells (David Baltimore, Renato Dulbecco, and Howard Temin, 1975); discoveries leading to a treatment of elevated cholesterol (Michael Brown and Joseph Goldstein, 1985); cancer-causing genes (Michael Bishop and Harold Varmus, 1989); kidney and bone marrow transplantation (Joseph Murray and Donnall Thomas, 1990); and the roles of telomeres and telomerase in health (Elizabeth Blackburn, Carol Greider, and Jack Szostak, 2009).[1]

There is much to be proud of in this record. Medical science has become a major, complex enterprise in the United States, with numerous centers of excellence in scientific research. Building it has required a system for prioritizing possible areas of inquiry and for soliciting and evaluating proposals for research studies. There also has been enormous growth in research funding, in the training of the scientific workforce, and in organizations to produce and disseminate the products and inventions that emanate from the work.

This story seems noncontroversial, but it is important to understand whether all of this investment and effort is directed toward doing the most good possible for the health of the population. In a number of respects, it is not. To understand why, let us first briefly consider the norms of science and their implications.

The Values and Worldview of the Scientist

A useful framework for thinking about these questions is one developed by sociologist Robert Merton. He points out that, in response to attacks on scientific integrity, the field of science had assumed an ethos, or culture, characterized by norms of what is appropriate behavior.[2] Merton describes the ethos of science as having four sets of "institutional imperatives":

- *Universalism*, which implies that scientific assertions are subject to verification by preestablished criteria that are independent of those making the assertions. It also implies that anyone is eligible to make scientific contributions.
- *Communalism*, in the sense that "the substantive findings of science are products of social collaboration and are assigned to the community." He notes that part of this imperative is communication of the findings: "Secrecy is the antithesis of this norm; full and open communication is its enactment." Further, "the communalism of the scientific ethos is

incompatible with definition of technology as 'private property.'" In this spirit, some renowned scientists took out patents to *ensure* availability for public use.[3]

- *Disinterestedness* means being objective about the outcome. Merton does not think that this norm reflects any moral superiority of the scientist (greater altruism) or less propensity for moral failings (greed or dishonesty), but rather the fact that so much of science is subject to rigorous verification. He notes that there is competition for "priority" or credit for discovery (witness the double helix competition) but suggests that this is a reason why there is so little falsification in science.[4]

- *Organized skepticism* is suspension of judgment and detached scrutiny of beliefs. This skepticism may bring participants in science into conflict with other elements of society with more fixed beliefs. Notably, the ethos applies not just to the individual scientists, but also to the institutions that are involved in the scientific enterprise as a whole (presumably including funding agencies, universities, and independent research organizations).

American medical science often fails to live up to these norms in a number of respects. This chapter explores how this has come to be the case, starting with the mother ship, the National Institutes of Health (NIH).

The Emergence and Growth of the National Institutes of Health

The NIH has been the engine of growth of the medical scientific enterprise in the United States. It traces its origins to a system of marine hospitals and coastal and inland waterways, created in 1798 through passage of an Act for the Relief of Sick and Disabled Seamen, and initially funded through a tax on the seamen's wages. An 1870 law centralized the administration of these hospitals under a Washington-based Marine Hospital Service directed by a former army surgeon who bore the title "Supervising Surgeon General." The service was responsible for running quarantine stations.

In 1887, the quarantine station in New York (which had just moved to Staten Island from nearby Bedloe Island to make way for installation of the Statue of Liberty) provided space to establish a bacteriological laboratory under the directorship of Dr. Joseph Kinyoun, a 26-year-old physician who had acquired an interest in bacteriology while training at Bellevue Hospital in New York. The new laboratory was organized primarily to identify dangerous infectious diseases, such as cholera (which was an active threat that year) and yellow fever, in people arriving from abroad. This "Hygienic Laboratory" soon moved to Washington, DC, and the director established a training program in bacteriology. It received a federal appropriation in 1901 of $35,000 for a new building to study "infectious and contagious diseases and matters pertaining to public health." The laboratory expanded, adding divisions of chemistry, pharmacology, and zoology to the existing division of pathology and bacteriology, and it began to hire PhD scientists. It assumed responsibility for regulating vaccines, antitoxins, and blood under the Biologics Control Act of 1902, following an episode of contamination of diphtheria antitoxin with multiple fatalities. In 1912, the organization in which the laboratory resided became the Public Health Service.[5]

At that time, the laboratory received authorization also to study noncontagious diseases and water pollution. During World War I, it mostly focused on sanitation in the area of military bases. In 1930, the Ramsdell Act gave the laboratory a new name: the National Institute of Health. The National Institute of Health was authorized to award research fellowships. There was no categorical budget for the institute at first, but in 1937, congressional concern about cancer led to the creation of a National Cancer Institute (NCI). The NCI was able to give grant awards to researchers outside of the government. By 1944, the NCI was formally made a part of the NIH. Even then, the research budget was small.[6]

Prior to World War II, there was not much of a medical science establishment in the United States because there was not much of a government budget for medical research. With the creation of the NCI, the first budget appropriation to the linked organization came in 1938, in the amount of $464,000 (all but $64,000 for the NCI). By 1945, the budget had increased modestly to about $2.8 million, but by 1949, it had jumped tenfold to $28.5 million, then rose to $1.1 billion in 1969, $7.4 billion in 1989, $27.2 billion in 2003, and $42.9 billion in 2021. The president's budget for 2022 called for a further one-year increase of $9 billion.[7]

During World War II, much of the NIH's activity focused upon matters related to the war effort. In 1944, the Public Health Service Act authorized expansion of the NCI grants program to the rest of the NIH, created a two-step peer-review system for grants and contracts, and authorized clinical research within the NIH. This led to the creation of centers for reviewing grants and for conducting research at the NIH, as well as eight new institutes between 1946 and 1956. Nine more institutes and centers were added between 1962 and 1974, four more in the late 1980s, and another four between 1999 and 2011, to reach the current complement of twenty-one institutes and six centers. A Division of Research Grants administered the proliferating program of "extramural" grants to outside organizations, and the internal research program, centered on a Clinical Center, was conducted though the various institutes.[8]

The NIH does not present itself to the world as an arcane, academic organization, concerned with esoteric questions with few proximate implications for the health of the public. If it did, it would have much more difficulty extracting appropriations from the US government. The NIH's mission statement unambiguously promises to deliver the goods: "NIH's mission is to seek fundamental knowledge about the nature and behavior of living systems *and the application of that knowledge to enhance health, lengthen life, and reduce illness and disability*" (emphasis added). Thus the NIH is interested in the fundamental (the basic sciences), but also in the application of that knowledge to improve health.[9] The mission statement also says that its programs are "designed to improve the health of the nation by conducting and supporting research . . . in the causes, diagnosis, prevention, and cure of human diseases."[10] This mandate includes research to understand the causes and mechanisms of disease, but improving health always has been the core of the mission.

That the intention of Congress has been to address the health of populations is reflected in the names of the twenty-one institutes.

- Fifteen of them are focused upon specific diseases or patient populations: National Cancer Institute (established 1937), National Eye Institute (1968), National Heart, Lung, and Blood Institute (1948), National Institute on Aging (1974), National Institute on Alcohol Abuse and Alcoholism (1970), National Institute of Allergy and Infectious Diseases (1948), National Institute of Arthritis and Musculoskeletal and Skin Diseases (1986), National Institute of Child Health and Human Development (1962), National Institute on Deafness and Other Communication Disorders (1988), National Institute of Dental and Craniofacial Research (1948), National Institute of Diabetes and Digestive and Kidney Diseases (1950), National Institute on Drug Abuse (1974), National Institute of Mental Health (1949), National Institute on Minority Health and Disparities (2010), and National Institute of Neurological Disorders and Stroke (1950).
- Two others are highly relevant to patient care: National Institute of Nursing Research (1948) and the National Library of Medicine (1956).
- The other four can be clinically relevant but also reflect central interests of basic sciences: National Human Genome Research Institute (1989), National Institute of Biomedical Imaging and Biomedical Engineering (2000), National Institute of General Medical Sciences (1962), and National Institute of Environmental Health Sciences (1969).
- The six centers also have clinical relevance: NIH Clinical Center (1953), Center for Information Technology (1964), Center for Scientific Review (review of grant proposals, 1964), Fogarty International Center (international programs, 1968), National Center for Advancing Translational Sciences (translation to patients and populations, 2011), and National Center for Complementary and Integrative Health (1999).[11]

The Scientific Workforce: Institutions and Constituency

The NIH conducts some research internally within its institutes, but the great majority of its funding goes to investigators elsewhere. These grants are awarded through "peer review," a process that tends to be conservative. The reviewers are biased in favor of the kinds of work that they do. Scientists who participate in the reviews are most enthusiastic about the problems that they study themselves and the methods that they use. It is not surprising that their reviews tend to look favorably upon the potential impact of work in areas to which they devote their own efforts. Thus bias, which may be unconscious (or not), affects the review process. Beyond their participation in peer review, as discussed below, scientists are unrestrained in advocating for funding of their work. They want more resources because they believe in what they do, but also because it builds their programs and advances their careers, regardless of whether that is society's greatest need.

An important component of the NIH's program is the training of the scientific workforce. The vast expansion of the NIH's intramural and extramural programs has made possible rapid growth in the scientific workforce. Of all PhD graduates in the United States in 2018, 15.9% were in the biological and biomedical sciences, 4.6% were in other health sciences, and 2.1% were in bioengineering and biomedical engineering. These percentages do not include psychologists and some social scientists who also may compete for NIH grants.[12]

The numbers in these disciplines have increased far more rapidly than the overall growth in the numbers of PhDs in the country. From 1988 to 2018, PhDs in the biological/biomedical disciplines in the US increased by 149%, compared to 50% in all other fields.[13] Some of those who train in these bioscientific fields head to careers in industry, but many others populate universities, either in professorships or pure research positions. Even if they do not ultimately pursue academic careers, a large proportion of these newly minted PhDs do postdoctoral training in academic institutions. Between the predocs, postdocs, research scholars, and professors, the universities have built up a large and formidable scientific workforce.

Research Dollars: Direct and Indirect

Grants and contracts funding from NIH pay for the research costs and contribute to infrastructure to support the research, including institutional facilities and administration. Not surprisingly, many of these expenditures (called F&A, for facilities and administration, popularly known as indirect costs) are concentrated in elite research universities. For example, in Fiscal Year 2020, Johns Hopkins University School of Medicine received nearly $534 million in grants from NIH (excluding research and development contracts). Of that amount, $138 million was to support indirect costs. The rest was for direct expenditures on grants that included the salaries and benefits of faculty and other researcher staff. A public institution, University of California San Francisco Medical School, received $602 million that year, of which $161 million was for indirect costs.[14] These institutions depend upon the continuing flow of NIH funds to maintain their programs and facilities, and to support their personnel. They also publicize their NIH rankings to add prestige to their institutions.[15]

The Perils of the Scientific Career

The interests of scientists and their academic institutions coincide in these respects. Medical schools are frequently strapped for resources and worry about covering their bottom-line expenses. Academic scientists must overcome a number of hurdles. Most of them need to cover their research time with grant funding. It often is not enough for a researcher to have one or even two grants if he or she wants to devote substantial time to research. Scientists in medical schools generally earn less than they would in private corporations.

In order to be at least somewhat competitive with the private sector, medical schools often offer established investigators salaries that exceed the NIH salary cap (the maximum salary allowed) and must underwrite the portion of the scientists' time that is devoted to the grant beyond the amount of salary that the NIH will cover. Thus a senior scientist whose salary is $260,000, and who has grants that pay for 100% of their time, needs $260,000 plus the cost of benefits to be fully funded. If the NIH cap is about $200,000, they only will get coverage from NIH for the percentage of salary covered by the grant, up to a maximum of $200,000.[16] This leaves $60,000 of salary, plus the benefits on that proportion of the salary (perhaps $20,000) uncovered by the grant in our example. The medical school needs to cover the difference ($80,000 in this instance).

In that context, any unfunded research time would require substantial additional subsidization of the scientist's salary and benefits, so it is a luxury that relatively few institutions can afford. Furthermore, it is unusual for a grant to cover more than 30% to 40% of a senior investigator's time (often less than that, even when they are the principal investigator). Thus funding on multiple projects is needed to get close to full coverage of time for research. Accordingly, scientists need to pursue grants aggressively.

As one colleague of mine, then at Harvard but later dean of public health at Yale, put it, "we write grants to cover 300% of our time, and hope to get funded for 150%."[17] In pursuing such grants, the scientists have to be strategic: only about 10% to 20% of such grants currently get funded, so those who receive the grants are the most productive, with many good results and publications. The review committees often want to see substantial preliminary data, which curbs innovation and often leads to overstatement of the quality and implications of the work, particularly by male scientists.[18]

Within the institutes of the NIH, certain disciplines or targets have their advocates. For example, longtime director of the NIH, Francis Collins, was formerly the leader of the Human Genome Project. This close association with that field led to some criticism of his appointment as NIH director.[19] Similarly, the National Institute of Allergy and Infectious Disease (NIAID) invested heavily in HIV vaccine development (a particular interest of that institute's director) for many years even though there was little progress and lots of reasons to think that it would be difficult to develop a vaccine that would prevent infection.[20]

Lobbying

The importance of the NIH to the scientific workforce is reflected in the organized efforts of scientists to lobby for continued growth of the NIH budget, as well as for funding within that budget of their own lines of work. Part of the project of selling your work is to tout how promising the findings are not just in your grant proposals, but also to potential funders of the work, especially the government. A scientist invested in a particular line of inquiry is reluctant to give it up. Consistent with their interest in maximizing their take of NIH dollars, medical schools encourage their faculty to participate in these lobbying efforts.

Scientific groups lobby, in collaboration with the Association of American Medical Colleges, with great vigor and considerable success to maintain the flow of revenue from NIH.[21] Thus there is close collaboration between the scientific research establishment (represented by NIH leadership and national organizations in the sciences), medical schools, and the scientists in the field, to get more money for what they do. They accomplish this by lobbying Congress and by promoting their work to the public.

In so doing, they almost never advise legislators or the administration to rethink the priorities of those budgets. Scientists lobby for more funding in their areas of specialization. Is such lobbying consistent with the social responsibilities of scientists? Stephanie Bird notes, "Scientists are often rightly perceived as largely indiscriminate advocates for science funding over other possible public expenditures. Yet, when mindful of the limitations, uncertainties, risks, and hazards of the science, scientists have the capacity to reflect on what kinds of science meet the needs of society."[22] Notwithstanding such a capacity, it would be a reportable event for a scientist to say that higher priority should be given to figuring out how to help people control their hypertension than to pouring more funding into their own scientific niche.

Often, the extramural research that NIH funds is not particularly creative, representing only marginal advances in directions that already have the funder's imprimatur as being valuable lines of inquiry. The "high risk, high reward" project that proposes something truly original has much more difficulty getting funded.[23]

Although the NIH now does have specific high-risk, high-reward funding opportunities, and funded 93 such projects in 2020 with $267 million over five years, it is a small part of their budget.[24] While these projects do represent something distinct from other funded work, few of them deviate from the main streams of inquiry that have been supported by the NIH. A recent analysis concluded that despite such efforts, the extent to which funding builds on the most recent advances has declined over time and has become more conservative.[25]

While there have been strenuous efforts in Congress to reduce discretionary domestic spending over the years, the scientific research budgets of the NIH and the National Science Foundation have been able to avoid budget cuts by drawing support from both political parties in Congress. Lobbying by their constituents for grants in their districts and states is one approach. To stoke congressional support for generous funding of medical research, the NIH can create good feeling in a member of Congress by providing medical care to them or a family member. For example, Orrin Hatch, a cost-cutting former Republican senator who chaired the Senate's Health, Education, Labor and Pensions Committee, detected a lump under his arm and called the NIH director. The director had him come to their campus, where they quickly reassured him that it was benign. He has acknowledged that ever since that episode, he has been a strong supporter of the NIH.[26]

Disease-specific interest groups play a key role in aiding the efforts of the scientific organizations, medical schools, and universities in their extraction efforts in Washington. There is evidence that the disease-specific lobbies are effective in shaping NIH funding priorities: the more they spend on lobbying, the more funding that their disease gets. They tend to achieve this mostly through congressional earmarks, which specify that some amount of funding to the NIH will be used for research on their disease. In one study of more than 50 conditions over a 19-year period, each $1,000 spent on lobbying was found to correlate with an increase of subsequent funding of about $25,000.[27]

Does the NIH Do All It Can to Advance the Nation's Health? What It Mostly Ignores

It would seem self-evident that NIH's commitment in their mission statement to supporting research on "causes, diagnosis, and prevention" should include societal factors such as poverty, prejudice, stress, diet, and the like, and that "application of that knowledge to improve health" would include making sure that people get seen and treated in accordance with what the evidence shows improves health. The ability to cure or ameliorate diseases depends on people receiving treatment. If that is the goal, then surely part of the effort to cure disease and improve human health necessarily involves addressing the important roles played by social causes of disease and by societal factors that impede treatment. But the NIH has been inconsistent in looking at the care that people receive.

Some institutes have shown a lot of interest in such problems at times, but other institutes have not. The National Institute of Mental Health (NIMH) has supported research on mental health services over the years, but it has moved away from that recently, with the proportion of the budget devoted to all applied (non-basic) research falling from nearly 50% to less than 30% between 2008 and 2016.[28] The National Cancer Institute (NCI) has a small component of its program targeting implementation science in cancer care, and the National Institute of Drug Abuse (NIDA) does likewise in its area.

One analysis looked at the number of projects funded each year between 2005 and 2016 by NIH institutes that were devoted to the study of the delivery of medical care. During that period, numbers of projects declined dramatically at some institutes, rose in a few, and fluctuated wildly in still others, while another group rarely funded any.[29]

Basic science and applied research, related to drug development and the like, have undergone some relatively modest variations in the funding of new grants, depending on the trend in the overall NIH budget, but they have never been subjected to these kinds of wild swings in support seen for health services research and other work that extends beyond the laboratory bench or the clinic. It is difficult to build a robust research program if it is unclear what, if any, funding will be available, even on a competitive basis, from year to year. Notwithstanding NIH's assertions that "translation" of scientific advances to the health of populations is an area of interest to them, the evidence of such commitment in their pattern of investments is scant.[30]

Why is there so much variability in the extent to which the NIH's institutes look at the full range of factors that affect health in the population in their areas of emphasis, at the medical care that people do or do not receive, and at how effective that care is?[31] Some scientists and scientific administrators have broad visions of the world and of the role of science within it. Others are narrowly focused upon their work and do not think much about the context in which it occurs. The precipitous drop in NIMH support for services research was not due to a decline in quality of the proposals, but rather to the appointment of a new director who wanted to prioritize basic research.

The scientists who are in positions to influence the priorities of science, including those who lead the NIH's institutes and the overall director of the NIH, rarely threaten the status quo of which areas of investigation get the overwhelming majority of government (and nongovernment) funding. When one does challenge the status quo, the institutional inertia is likely to bring that institute back in line with the overall organizational ethos when the next director of that institute comes along. To be fair, the National Institute on Minority Health and Disparities and the National Institute of Nursing Research do have more consistent interest in these areas, but their budgets are small ($392 million and $175 million, respectively, in Fiscal Year 2021 out of the NIH's budget of $42.9 billion).

NIAID has the second-largest budget at the NIH. They are responsible for research relating to HIV; new and emerging infectious diseases such as SARS-CoV-2; the virus responsible for the COVID-19 pandemic; immune disorders; and many aspects of international health. They are interested in development of vaccines and other preventive treatments, as well as medicines to treat these disorders. Their priority always has been scientific discovery, development of drugs, and the like. These are important needs that deserve much attention, but NIAID (along with several other institutes) gives little emphasis and few grants to the downstream aspects of improving health (sometimes called types three and four translational research). In the case of NIAID, these would include assessing the care that people with HIV and hepatitis C are receiving, studying behavioral interventions to reduce the spread of the disease, and measuring the impact of factors that might deter receipt of treatment, such as stigmatization, structural and financial barriers to care, discrimination, and misinformation. NIAID does not prioritize these areas, presumably regarding those important problems as someone else's responsibility.

Likewise, even though the NIMH does provide some diminishing support to mental health services research, remarkably, it is not the major thrust of the organization. People with chronic mental illness often live in the streets and die prematurely of a range of diseases, in part because there is not an effective system for ensuring that they get the treatment that they need. Similarly, depression is such an important and common disease, debilitating for many, leading to suicide for others. While it is appropriate to try to develop even better treatments, how about making sure that the patients who clearly need some treatment get what is currently available? Doesn't that have something to do with "improving the health of the nation"? The NIH does not give that much priority.

Can Other Agencies and Institutes Fill the Gap?

The Agency for Healthcare Research and Quality (AHRQ) is another federal agency with the mission of evaluating medical care. Their ability to fulfill that mission is limited by having a budget that is only about onehundredth the size of that of NIH. The agency was created in 1974 as the National Center for Health Services Research. Its budget was spotty: there were years when they had no funds to award new grants. In 1984, the Center had "and Health Care Technology Assessment" added to its name. In 1989, it was transformed into a full-fledged agency, the Agency for Health Care Policy and Research (AHCPR), within the Department of Health and Human Services. It was reauthorized in 1999 with its current name, AHRQ.

In theory, this organization could do a great deal of the research needed to make health care more responsive to the needs of the population, more equitable, and more efficient. In practice, it has been suffocated by grossly inadequate funding and a great deal of political interference.

There have been multiple efforts to eliminate the agency because some of the research it supports has offended powerful interests. Notably, a series of studies about the failure of spinal fusion therapy to improve health outcomes in many situations aroused the ire of the North American Spine Society (NASS). NASS was highly critical of guidelines that came out of that work in the early 1990s, which led to the creation of a lobbying group that launched a campaign attacking what was then AHCPR. Their campaign culminated in the House of Representatives passing a budget for 1996 that zeroed out the agency. Only strenuous efforts in the Senate eventually saved it, but with substantial reduction in its budget.[32]

The agency foreswore guidelines development thereafter. It did maintain a National Guideline Clearinghouse of evidence-based guidelines developed by others, but the Trump administration ended funding for that in 2018 (as well as for their National Quality Measures Clearinghouse).[33]

After a brief burst of funding from the American Recovery and Reinvestment Act of 2009 (ARRA) at the beginning of the Obama administration, funding for AHRQ has been flat, increasing less than 12% between 2010 and 2021, a period during which the NIH budget increased by over 37%.[34] A new organization, the Patient-Centered Outcomes Research Institute (PCORI), which was created as part of the Affordable Care Act in 2010, now has a budget of similar magnitude. Their combined budgets amount to just over 2% of the NIH budget. Adding in all other funding of similar research by all federal agencies still amounts to less than 9% of the NIH total budget, and less than one-thousandth of what the United States spends on health care annually.[35]

Even then, much health services research is restricted by the language of the legislation that authorizes its funding. In a country that spends more of its gross domestic product on health care than any other, and has worse health outcomes, one might expect that government authorities would welcome the opportunity to learn how to contain exploding costs and invest health care dollars more wisely. Alas, even PCORI, which is funded by the federal government to understand whether the health care system is meeting the needs of the population, has not been allowed to support research that considers cost-effectiveness, which is a key analytic approach in health economics. The PCORI website specifies:

> Our founding legislation prohibits us from doing cost-effectiveness analysis. We don't consider cost effectiveness to be an outcome of importance to patients. Applications will be considered nonresponsive if the proposed research:
>
> - Conducts a formal cost-effectiveness analysis
> - Directly compares the cost of care between two or more alternative approaches to providing care
>
> Proposals that include measures of these issues may measure and report utilization of any or all health services, but they may not employ direct measurements of costs of care.[36]

After the agency was reauthorized in 2019, there was a slight modification of the language on their website. They can now consider burdens such as cost and "economic impacts" but still cannot consider cost-effectiveness or compare the costs of care of different treatments.[37]

In part, this absurd prohibition is related to the professed panic in conservative circles, and an ensuing torrent of letters from the public, that such research would result in "death panels." These imagined star chambers would judge certain treatments not to be worth the societal cost, and thence relegate robust individuals to premature demise by preventing them from getting the care that would make them better. Discourse about fixing health care is eroded by this kind of politically motivated misinformation, when the goal of cost-effectiveness research is to understand what things cost and how much benefit they produce.[38]

Apart from health services research, the broad field of behavioral and social science research gets short shrift at NIH. In a 2003 analysis, Ste-

fanek and his colleagues found that less than 10% of overall NIH research dollars went to such studies. While acknowledging that behavioral science is not absent from NIH, they raised the question, "What
would we have learned about health behavior and behavior change related to disease prevention and health maintenance if 93.8 percent
(versus 6.2 percent) of the NCI budget or 95.7 percent (versus 4.3 percent)
of NHLBI funding was dedicated to behavioral and social science research?"[39] Consistent with that hypothetical scenario, we might reasonably presume that if the NCI poured vastly more resources into
projects that test and implement strategies to curtail smoking, and NHLBI
into improving diets and physical activity, those investments might affect
health and disease rates substantially.

Moonshots

The political process of allocating funding to science inevitably is responsive to the voices that Congress hears. It is natural for people with a
particular disease (or their friends and families) to want the cure, or the
"magic bullet," especially for conditions that are troublesome, debilitating, or lethal. Many such treatments have not been effective, but the
quest goes on. Scientists feed this longing by proclaiming that a particular area of research will cure cancer, wipe out infectious diseases, prevent degenerative processes like dementia, and so on. Scientists often
pay little attention to the context of what will do the most good to help
people with cancer or some other condition.[40]

Politicians contribute to this misinformation by calling for "moonshots." Scientists have proclaimed that cancer can be beaten with genet-
ically specific treatments, by fortifying the immune system, by identifying
and treating infectious causes, and so on. While each of these might have
marginal value, none is the single approach that will solve the problem.
Yet overpromising the benefits of a particular slice of science enhances
some research budgets. Searching for solutions in the realm of genetics is
currently most popular. The advocates of this line of scientific inquiry

tried out different ways to brand it. First it was personalized medicine. Now, "precision medicine" is the preferred term. Analyze someone's genome, and you will find out what diseases they will get. Analyze the genetics of the tumor, and you will be able to treat it more effectively. Sparseness of evidence to back up such assertions is not even a relative contraindication to proclamations of the value of the work so touted. Such moonshot efforts are expanding.[41]

Flavor of the Decade

It is not surprising that scientists want more resources for what they do, regardless of whether that is society's greatest need. That point of view coincides with what enhances their programs and their careers. Driven by the appetites of the scientists, the public and politicians, the NIH has responded by prioritizing such fads, looking for the magic bullet: cancer is caused by infection, then by immunological disarray, then by genetic disturbances. All of these can contribute, but when half of cancers are attributable to smoking (discernable by looking at the rates in smokers compared to nonsmokers), should not much of our efforts be aimed at finding ways to curtail or eliminate use of tobacco?[42] Chasing scientific fads not only distorts science, but also diverts attention from the mission of improving the health of the public.

How much of a problem is it to have some of the NIH's research portfolio focused upon uncommon health problems and on seeking even better treatments for other conditions for which good ones already exist? Arguably, those are appropriate components of a scientific agenda. At worst, they may represent an inefficiency of the system, if all other needs were being attended to, but they are not. Conversely, if good and effective treatments are available but many people are not getting them, the priority should be to find ways to disseminate these approaches to those whose lives might be saved or improved by what is already known. Many people with colon cancer do not get colonoscopies or other screening procedures. Many of those with lung cancer do not get identified soon enough and often experience lethal delays before they are treated. Many people with autism who might benefit greatly from behavioral interventions do not get them.

The list is endless, but the NIH tends to prioritize other things. Putting more resources into optimizing the dissemination of effective treatments that are not these faddish "flavors" but are underutilized could same many lives. More resources should be applied to ensuring that everyone gets these treatments—if they need them—before any funds are lavished on elusive miracle cures.

For some time now, the NIH and the scientific community have been propagating, with considerable success, the notion that molecular genetics will solve many of the problems in human disease. NIH Director Francis Collins foresaw several potential benefits: explaining common diseases based on a small number of strong associations to genetic variants, using this evidence to improve detection of the diseases, basing preventive medicine on this information about risk, improving treatment decisions based on genetics, and developing new treatments (including gene therapy).[43]

The idea of precision medicine inevitably appeals to scientists who long to explain things. Why do some people get a disease but others do not? Why does a drug work for some people but not others? What causes cells to go through malignant transformation? These are all interesting questions. For example, some precision research in the area of pharmacogenomics attempts to predict response to such treatments as immunotherapy.[44] Other work has looked at predicting which people's genetic makeup indicates a higher risk for thrombophlebitis (blood clots in the veins).[45] Still other work has used neural networks to reliably read images from pathology and radiology.[46] Some have studied virtual models of disease, to test combinations of drugs in silico (in the computer), to see what is likely to work for a particular disease, and to fast-track their applications to human studies and clinical care.[47]

The promise of precision medicine is exciting to the scientist. Certainly, few would question the usefulness of identifying effective drugs more efficiently, reading images more reliably, and determining the tumor category in which a drug is most likely to be beneficial. In the case of cancer, the theory is that if you characterize the genetics of a person's tumor, you can develop an individualized treatment for it.

Even if research like that cited above does lead to personalized treatments, the evidence to date suggests that that is not going to affect the care of the vast majority of patients anytime soon.[48] There have been some noteworthy findings, such as the BRCA1 gene and HER2/neu in breast cancer as well as studies that have led to slightly more effective (but expensive) treatments for some tumors. Mostly what has been identified is lots of associations between certain genes and diseases that don't have diagnostic or therapeutic implications, at least at this point. It is inevitable that statistically significant associations will be found when one looks at thousands of possible such relationships, but many of them are chance occurrences.[49]

Nonetheless, the precision medicine industry has continued to grow and has become entrenched in academia and in the NIH. In New York City, for example, New York University has a precision immunology laboratory and the Center for Precision Health in Diverse Populations; Columbia's Institute for Genomic Medicine is part of the broader Columbia Precision Medicine Program; Weill Cornell has the Englander Institute for Precision Medicine; Mount Sinai/Icahn School of Medicine has an Institute for Personalized Medicine; and the New York Genome Center coordinates efforts across these medical schools and others in the region.

Billions of NIH dollars are being funneled into the Precision Medicine Initiative, which among other things has undertaken a 10-year, $1.5 billion "All of Us Research Project," in which they plan to recruit 1 million Americans and characterize their genomes. They then will be able to see what diseases the participants develop. There is no reason to believe that any of the participants will benefit from being study subjects. The investigators have promised to provide participants with their genetic information, but even they acknowledge that people will be unlikely to be able to use it to improve their health, given issues "such as health care delivery and variable insurance coverage." The investigators report that they are recruiting a diverse population and will consider such variables as the social determinants of health. It is far from clear that their sampling strategy and measurements will provide much useful information about such "epigenetic" factors.[50]

Critics of the initiative note that many diseases are complex, that the "effect size" of a genetic association is generally small, compared to behavioral and environmental factors. They point out that identified associations are unlikely to lead to specific therapies for most diseases (some cancers being the exception). They observe that associations of genetic data with diseases in a population are likely to be far too weak to permit prediction of disease in an individual. They also point to the abundant evidence that providing people with information that they are at risk for a disease does not often have much effect on their behavior. In the face of such considerations, some have called for applying the idea of precision to problems in public health and population health, fields that have lost funding to the "-omic" disciplines of late. Such efforts might, for example, try to discern which prevention programs work best in which populations.[51]

Are programs like the Precision Medicine Initiative the best possible investments of public monies in a society with extraordinary health expenditures and large swaths of the population having terrible health outcomes? Their outcomes are poor not because patients' genomes have not been analyzed, but because they are not getting treatments that are known to be beneficial. In reality, investigators have been studying genes and associations to disease for some time.

Where this research goes off track is in the notion that drug treatment can and should be personalized, that there should be a treatment specific to the genetic alterations in one or a small number of individuals. That may be attainable, but it ignores the population-level concern. These efforts are likely to make the bad problems in American health care even worse. Imagine developing even more drugs that cost hundreds of thousands of dollars per year or more to extend life a little for someone. The notion that we can afford medications that could take many millions of dollars to develop, and provide them to only a few people, is beyond absurd.

Medical care in the US already is insanely expensive. I can't get past the shocking fact that, with health care comprising 18% of the GDP, everyone works about seven hours a week to pay for medical care, 50% more than any other country, including all of those countries with longer life expectancy, lower infant mortality, and generally better health statistics. New medications that are not personalized sometimes cost tens of thousands of dollars per year. Personalizing medicines will only drive our medical bills even higher and create more disparities.

In America, we ration health care by denying basic services to the poorer members of society, not by limiting services for all. The Precision Medicine Initiative and programs like All of Us won't benefit all of us, not even very many of us. Instead, if precision medicine becomes a dominant approach to discovery and practice, costs will continue to mount, and effective care for many will become even more difficult to obtain. For now, precision medicine remains extremely well funded, and that does not appear likely to change. The proponents have suggested that miraculous cures will emerge from this research, and the lack of evidence of much progress has not dampened the rhetoric.[52]

A similar, entrenched subindustry in academia relates to stem cell treatments. There have been many political machinations about the ethics of such research, but the evidence of benefit is slight. I find it encouraging that the International Society for Stem Cell Research has shown some responsibility in this regard, issuing "anti-hype guidelines" and calling for more balanced discussion of the benefits (or lack thereof) of this approach.[53] Perhaps scholars in the precision medicine industry eventually will become less hyperbolic, more *precise* in their accounts about what the research has shown, and perhaps more *imprecise* and modest in their promises about where it will lead.

Patents and Royalties: The Bayh-Dole Act and Its Sequelae

A key development in the growth of science in the universities and in its prioritization of invention was the Bayh-Dole Act of 1980. This piece of legislation, proposed by a Democratic senator from Indiana (Birch Bayh) and a Republican senator from Kansas (Robert Dole), opened the floodgates to opportunities for universities and their scientists to participate in ownership of patents of products that they develop with grants from the federal government. Prior to that, the government owned the patents on products emanating from research that they funded through some (although not all) agencies and could lease out nonexclusive rights to market these products.

Some representatives from Purdue University lobbied Senator Bayh by arguing that this system was keeping products from the market: only about 5% of all government patents led to products. This claim probably overstated the problem, since many of the other 95% were military products with no meaningful public market niche (although at least some Second Amendment aficionados would contend that military-grade weaponry should be widely available). Among the 325 patents held by the Department of Health and Human Services, 23% had made it to market.[54] There also was concern that failure to patent these inventions made it more likely that they would be developed by corporations outside of the United States.

The act was approved as part of an omnibus bill in December 1980, just before Jimmy Carter left office. Congress passed it overwhelmingly, with little discussion of its implications, but academic institutions were well aware of what it meant and welcomed it. Initially, participation in patenting was limited to small businesses, but that provision was dropped a few years later. One of the reasons the senators proposed the bill was to stimulate the economy at a time of severe economic distress. There certainly was an enormous impact on patenting of such products. The number of approved patents to government grantees increased from 264 in 1979 to 3,278 in 2005.[55]

The legislation has been popular with biological and pharmacological companies, which benefited from the legislation by getting to market the fruits of science. Others have been concerned that such pass-through to corporations may not always serve the public interest. To ensure benefit for the public, the law includes a "march-in" provision, which allows the government to cancel the exclusive right to make the product if the licensee was not taking action "necessary to alleviate health or safety needs," and if the contractor refuses a request to grant a license to meet that need.[56] The NIH has not acted in any of the cases of march-in rights petitions for health care-related products, however, including two related to their high cost, one concerning the shortage of a drug, and one pertaining to cross-licensing of a product for a different application from what the original license-holder was pursuing. Thus it is not clear that the march-in provision is protecting the potential purchasers of these products in key ways.[57]

On the one hand, there is some evidence that the Bayh-Dole Act has been an engine of innovation. In that sense, it has been good for business. On the other hand, critics have voiced concern that the act has distorted the priorities of science and of universities that house the researchers, and that it is not bringing broad benefit to the population that funded the research through the government. In one analysis, Walter Valdivia found that the law, as it has been implemented over time, has failed in several measures of providing public value, including efficiency of the market (pricing), transparency, inclusion of firms prepared to produce the goods, and assurance of fair distribution of benefits.[58]

As for Bayh-Dole's impact on the priorities of science, scientists, and the institutions that hire researchers, one key issue is the overall impact on the priorities and the very nature of scholarship in the university. Researchers may be highly motivated to develop patents and augment their incomes as a result. I have known of quite a few who did that, some of whom made a great deal of money. One who did particularly well now owns the Los Angeles Times.[59] Universities are interested in sharing patent and royalty revenue. They may prioritize using discretionary resources to recruit faculty in the biological, medical, and physical sciences who offer that prospect, over those in disciplines in the humanities and the social sciences who hardly ever generate patents (or get NIH grants).

We have seen that the social sciences and humanities departments, even in leading universities in those fields, are microscopic in comparison with the burgeoning ranks of scientists and clinicians in medical schools. In these respects, the missions and priorities of the university may well have been distorted by these developments over the last four decades. At the very least, funding sources for faculty salaries that are not derived from patents or the anticipation of them, or from other corporate interests, may well need to be identified to neutralize those pernicious effects upon higher education.[60]

Conflicts of Interest between Scientists and Manufacturers

In addition to the impact of Bayh-Dole on the priorities of scientists, there is a great deal of evidence that other financial relationships between manufacturers, scientists, and academic institutions are clouding scientific objectivity and institutional priorities. Many clinical and basic scientists have economic relationships with the manufacturers of cancer drugs. Sometimes they are on "advisory" panels, sometimes they earn substantial stipends as members of speaker boards, and sometimes they own equity in the companies. For far too many of these individuals, the principal goal is pursuit of revenue, not truth, and that pursuit may well occur at the expense of truth. Some of the scientists so engaged may make millions, or even billions, of dollars if they own stock and stock options on successful products, or merely tens or hundreds of thousands if they play other roles.

Can such individuals display "disinterestedness" (be objective) about the products involved? The chief medical officer of Memorial Sloan Kettering, a preeminent cancer center in New York, was forced to resign when it became clear that he had been paid millions of dollars by product manufacturers and had failed to disclose those relationships more than 100 times in medical journals. At the same time, it became known that Sloan Kettering as an institution had made a $25 million deal with a start-up company, granting it exclusive use in its research of their invaluable archive of millions of tissue slides (from Sloan Kettering patients), with officials of Sloan Kettering and the Hospital itself having equity shares in the start-up.[61]

Many universities are attempting to limit the degree of conflicts of interest, for example, by not allowing faculty members who own substantial stock in a company to lead studies of the clinical effectiveness of the products. Medical journals have been embarrassed when it turned out that authors of review papers relating to products owned equity in those products. Many have tried to increase transparency regarding such relationships and to avoid publishing reviews by such individuals. As early as 1984, the *New England Journal of Medicine*'s editor wrote, "One does not have to assume that researchers are venal to appreciate that they may be affected (consciously or unconsciously) by economic incentives, which can influence the way they design or conduct their studies, how they interpret the results, or how and when they choose to report them."[62]

In that article, he indicated that his journal was establishing a policy whereby it *suggested* that authors routinely report their sources of funding and business relationships in articles. This suggestion did not get the job done. Ultimately, the *New England Journal of Medicine* laid down stricter rules once they understood that so many authors of their editorials and review articles continued to fail to disclose conflicts of interest. In 1996 the editors stated, "Because editorials involve interpretation and opinion, we require that authors be free of financial associations . . . with a company that stands to gain from the use of a product (or its competitor) discussed in the editorial," but a subsequent editor backed away from this improved standard in 2002 and allowed editorialists to have some financial associations with companies whose products they discuss.[63]

This issue has implications for the validity of research studies. Clinical trials published by scientists with conflicts of interest more often reported positive results when the products' manufacturers had funded the studies.[64] Academic institutions do not consistently enforce standards for their faculty that are consistent, for example, with those promulgated by the International Committee of Medical Journal Editors, including on such matters as assuring that faculty who are authors of industry-sponsored studies have access to all data from the trials.[65]

Occasionally, the payoff for scientists from their discoveries can be gloriously substantial. Research that is supported by the government fills the laboratories of medical schools. Sometimes a researcher working on one of these grants discovers something useful and then decides to leave their academic position and start a company to make money off the government-funded discovery. One such doctor who developed a cancer drug did just that and became a multibillionaire. Medical schools have been addressing this phenomenon for years by striking agreements with scientists to split the winnings, and sometimes going to court in disputes with corporations about patents and royalties.[66]

A notorious episode of the consequences of conflicts of interest occurred in the late 1990s with the drug troglitazone, developed and marketed under the name Rezulin by Parke-Davis (a subsidiary of Warner-Lambert, which later merged with pharmaceutical giant Pfizer). The drug was approved for inclusion in the Diabetes Prevention Study, a $150 million effort by the National Institute of Diabetes and Digestive and Kidney Diseases (NIDDK). The committee that approved inclusion of the drug was chaired by Jerrold Olefsky, who held patents with the manufacturer but abstained in the approval vote. Also involved was Richard Eastman, leader of NIDDK's Division of Diabetes. He received tens of thousands of dollars annually in consulting fees from the manufacturer.

When reports emerged of serious liver complications in a number of patients, British health authorities withdrew the drug from the market. In the United States, Eastman sent out a letter reassuring practitioners that it was safe to use. The US Food and Drug Administration (FDA) convened a committee to review the safety of the drug and recommended by a vote of 11 to 1 that it remain on the market, at a time when it also was withdrawn in Australia. Of note, nine of the physicians attesting to the safety of the drug at the FDA meeting were consultants for Parke-Davis. A year later, after many more deaths, the drug was finally withdrawn. The NIH director investigated the episode, and Eastman was forced out of his position.[67]

A subsequent study of advisory committee meetings of the FDA revealed that at 73% of the meetings, at least one of the committee members revealed financial conflicts of interest that were often substantial. But the individuals with these conflicts were recused from participation in the meetings in only 1% of cases.[68]

To understand the pernicious nature of commercialization, I describe two examples from the area of research in which I have worked (health services research). An academic researcher developed a measure of the behavior of persons with a chronic condition, using a standardized series of questions. The diagnostic questionnaire became popular. He patented it, and later began to insist on payment for its use. He tracked down instances where use of this set of questions was described in clinical papers and asked for substantial fees for the use of his questionnaire in their published studies, including some from researchers in poor countries where those fees were prohibitively expensive. His representative told the authors of the papers that they must pay or retract the research. Many chose the latter. Other investigators who had collected data with his measure did not even publish the results.

In another instance, I was on a committee that visited the site of an investigator who had used public funds to develop a measure of how sick patients were when in the hospital. He had published two previous versions of this measure that were open and available to all users. When version three came along, he took a different approach. Upon publication of the results, he did not include the regression coefficients that were needed to calculate this measure of physiological aberration and chronic illnesses. Those who wanted to use this measure would have to pay a large fee for it. We were perplexed and frustrated by this situation, but the investigator was unwilling to change his position. We were able to do little but suggest that future funding be contingent upon making all results and details of measurement methods freely available.

Keeping such measures private was a way to generate revenue, but it meant that others would not be able to scrutinize the method, and some would not be able to afford to use it. This was not a medical product that was to be used to treat patients, so the consequences were somewhat different, but it was relevant to health research. Any product that is not fully scrutinized may be used in situations where there are better tools, or where the one in use could be improved upon. In any event, failure to disclose methodological details has the potential to slow the advance of knowledge.[69]

Academic institutions often require lecturers to present any conflicts of interest on a slide at the beginning of a talk. Doing so does not eliminate the bias, however, and consideration of it may not come up in the talk or the discussion. In my experience, the slide with that information rarely is up on the screen long enough fully to grasp its implications for the lecture.

One scientist, who discovered a basic mechanism that may lead to useful treatments, recently gave a talk at Cornell during which he "disclosed" (as required) his conflicts of interest in his first slide. One of these conflicts was a financial relationship with a company that licensed a product derived from his research. When I asked what his view was of the outrageous pricing of newer biologics in recent years, he said that they had not yet established the right "price point." He added that he would not be involved in that decision.

Who talks about price points? Mostly, people who are trying to maximize price with respect to the likely demand for the product. There is no reprobation for such attitudes and little appetite for constraining such conflicts of interest. When I served on a committee at UCLA considering the issue, a vice chancellor, who hoped to see the university share more royalties that emanated from research, told us, "we want conflicts of interest."

The Norms, Values, and Worldview of the Biomedical Scientist

Returning to Merton's norms, discussed early in this chapter, how does the present state of biomedical science measure up? The commercialization and widespread pursuit of patents and royalties stand in stark contrast to the "communalist" ethos of scientists who only patented an invention to ensure that it was available to the public. Keeping findings secret in order to be able to profit from them is a violation of this norm. The effort to give priority to favored fads or theories of disease causation in order to increase funding for one's own area of work seems like a betrayal of the concept of "universalism."

The concept of "disinterestedness" has not disappeared. Clinical trials, for example, begin with the assumption of equipoise (treatments offered are not known to differ in effectiveness). But the problem of the difficulty of publishing negative studies, and the need to publish in prestigious journals (or else perish, academically), represents a foot on the scales, pushing scientists to spin results in more favorable ways at times, or to overstate their implications. Conflicts of interest also may lead to framing questions or measuring answers in ways favorable to sponsors, undermining the norm of "organized skepticism."

Merton's norms are an idealization of the scientific process. Some question whether they have any relationship to the work of discovery and the ways in which discovery has been applied in the real world. Nonetheless, it is sobering to consider how far modern medical science has deviated from these norms, even in comparison with several decades earlier.

Much has been written about these norms, including whether they are exclusively a domain of science, whether one needs to distinguish between the cognitive/moral/intellectual domain and the social or technical/operational domain, whether Thomas Kuhn's theory of scientific revolutions supersedes the notion of such norms, and the extent to which they would apply to both pure and applied science.[70] Nonetheless, there is wide agreement that there is an ethos ascribed to science. It is a useful framework for thinking about the role and responsibilities of medical science in contemporary society, and a testament to how far the field has strayed.

Investing to Maximize Benefit with the Tools We Already Have

Rather than allowing the NIH's large budget to continue going primarily to discovery research, we should think about whether existing treatments, if fully implemented, would solve many or most of the problems caused by a disease. If we judge that to be likely or even possible, are they reaching all of the population? If not, what can we do to change that? We may not need new pills but rather behavioral, environmental, psychological, policy, or other "treatments" that might get care to everyone.

Expanding care should be a priority if the goal of medical science is to improve the health of the population as a whole.

For example, hypertension (high blood pressure) is a common health problem. Medicines exist to control it in almost all people, but a large proportion of the population is either untreated, inadequately treated, or nonadherent with their prescribed medicines. The challenge to public health is to implement systems of care to ensure that patients are properly diagnosed and treated with sufficient medicines, as well as behavioral and policy strategies that will make it more likely that patients will take those medicines on an ongoing basis.[71]

For conditions whose existing treatments don't work well for a substantial proportion of the population, better standard treatments that are applicable to many of these people—and not just a few of them, and making sure that people take them—are likely to do more good than the quixotic search for personalized genetic approaches or magical cures with stem cells that will benefit relatively few.

Once that is accomplished, we can consider what more can be done with any remaining resources, and not just for those who can afford insanely expensive personalized medicines. Just as we do not (or should not) build roads or bridges to serve a few people when there is a need for something to serve many, health care, as a public utility, should serve the many. As it is, our expensive health care system diverts needed resources from education, infrastructure, housing, and other key needs of society. Allocating public funds to programs to develop drugs that few can afford is a misappropriation of society's resources and a distortion of both the priorities and the mission of medical science. The goal of medical science should be to preserve and improve life and health for the many, and not at the expense of other societal necessities.

Noting in 2019 that genomics have not affected any measure of public health to date, Michael Joyner and Nigel Paneth rued that pressing public health challenges such as the need to address "the toll of obesity, inactivity, and diabetes . . . the mental health problems that lead to distress and violence . . . a terrible opiate epidemic [that] ravages our country . . . We have to prepare conscientiously for the next influenza pandemic . . . Topics such as these have taken a back seat to the invest-ment of the NIH and of many research universities in a human genome-driven research agenda that has done little to solve these problems, but has offered us promises and more promises."[72]

Modern medical science cannot flourish in an austere Swiss patent of-fice, with one person thinking carefully about problems and coming up with solutions. There are staff to support, salaries to cover, facilities to build, and much more. Furthermore, scientists love the idea of discov-ery. From the perspective of the directors of successful laboratories and many other scientists, the notion that the required resources might do more good attacking problems outside of the laboratory is beside the point. They view their mission as being "To follow knowledge like a sinking star / Beyond the utmost bound of human thought."[73] That re-quires funding. To keep it flowing, scientists regularly oversell their products. The inattention to the context of the research perhaps is best represented by Tom Lehrer's lyrics: "'Once the rockets are up, who cares where they come down? / That's not my department,' says Wernher von Braun."[74]

To summarize: For reasons that have little to do with evidence of ben-efit from the investment, there has been bipartisan support for massive increases in the NIH budget for a long time. To justify ever-growing bud-gets, the scientific community has created unrealistic expectations of what their work will do for health. The NIH and the scientific organ-izations, whose members benefit from the largesse of the NIH, oversell and overpromise: cures for cancer, eradication of infectious diseases, in-creasingly effective treatments for every chronic condition. They sell their areas of research to the public and to potential funders much as any corporation might seek a market for their goods. They bear the mien of scientific respectability and credibility, but they do not present their advo-cacy in measured, scientific terms. If one-fifth of the current NIH budget were diverted each year to making sure that people get the treatments and public health interventions that we know work, that might do a lot more for health than some harebrained initiatives that keep genetics research-ers flush with cash.[75]

We have seen that medical schools, scientists, and their organizations lobby for budgets in areas that bear relatively little fruit, including genetics and personalized medicine, and that comes at the expense of working on health problems that could benefit far more people. While that goes on, only half of people with hypertension are getting their blood pressures controlled, even though standard medicines are available that could control more than 90% of hypertension cases and save many lives. Similarly, many people with diseases such as depression, HIV, many cancers, bowel diseases, and rheumatologic disorders do not get the effective standard treatments that we already have. As funders fill the coffers of scientists with resources to discover personalized treatments, care gets more expensive for everyone, and it becomes harder for many to get effective treatment for their conditions.

Are there health consequences of the NIH's blissful neglect of implementation research? Indeed, there are. Jeff Leroy and colleagues examined research grants from the NIH between 2000 and 2004 that concerned the leading causes of childhood mortality in developing countries (including diarrhea, pneumonia, malaria, HIV/AIDS, measles, birth asphyxia, sepsis, preterm birth, and tetanus), as well as a smaller portfolio of grants on the same topics from the Bill and Melinda Gates Foundation. They found that 97% of grants were directed at developing new technologies: either "predelivery research" or studies of improved diagnostic methods or of the efficacy of new treatments. They judged that these studies, if successful, had the potential to reduce child mortality by 21.5%. In contrast, only 3% of studies looked at delivery or utilization of existing technologies, even though achieving full utilization of these technologies had the potential to decrease mortality by 61.5%.[76]

A useful code of ethics for scientists was published in 1984. Among its other components, the Uppsala Code states, "The scientist has a special responsibility to assess carefully the consequences of his/her research, and to make them public . . . Scientists who form the judgment that the research which they are conducting or participating in is in conflict with this code, shall discontinue such research, and publicly state the reasons for their judgment."[77]

When advances in biomedical science tilt the health system toward treatments that are likely to benefit very few and add to the cost of the health care system, and when continued inquiry in areas likely to be of limited consequence to the health of the population diverts funding away from areas in which there is greater potential benefit, scientists are not fulfilling their ethical responsibilities. They are substituting self-interest for a commitment to the principle of disinterestedness.

Treat hypertension. Immunize against pneumonia. Help people quit smoking. Stop chasing treatments that even in the most optimistic scenarios will only benefit the well-to-do. Yet so many medical scientists who understand how great the needs are in some of these areas love the idea of precision medicine, perhaps because it's easier to get one's head around that, rather than taking on the messy task of managing disease in a population replete with social, behavioral, and psychological complexity.

Despite the crisis in disparities in health, recent declines in life expectancy, and lack of good value for extraordinary expenditures, the US deliberately avoids allowing an agency devoted to the study of outcomes of health care to accumulate information on how we could better marshal health care resources to achieve equivalent or superior results. This avoidance coincides with what many in the scientific community perceive to be their interests. Adjudicating that tension is not something that the NIH considers to be its responsibility. They see themselves as being in the business of supporting the large scientific community that has grown exponentially, as the NIH budget increased at a pace far beyond contributions to many other vital societal needs.

The responsibilities of scientists include the duty to select problems that are in society's best interest and to consider not just one's internal (self, career, institutional) needs in one's work.[78] It is fair to say that the biomedical scientific community, writ large, does not fulfill these obligations with any consistency. Increasing awareness among scientists about the need to prioritize research questions in the greater interests of society as a whole is likely to be a daunting challenge, when they are far more focused, perhaps singularly so, on obtaining funding to cover their time, their staff, and their labs.

Meaningful education for scientists and scientists-to-be in the broad ethical questions that surround the research enterprise, such as what should receive priority as an area of study (as opposed to the current treatment of ethics, which is superficial at best), might be a good place to start. That would require someone with training in these matters, and without conflicts, to lead this part of the curriculum, someone other than the research team leaders, who would be only too happy to give their imprimatur to the instruction and to the perpetuation of the status quo.[79]

Notes

1. "All Nobel Prizes in Physiology or Medicine," Nobel Prize, accessed October 10, 2021, https://www.nobelprize.org/prizes/lists/all-nobel-laureates-in-physiology-or -medicine/.

2. At times, he characterized this as the social structure of science. Robert K. Merton, "The Normative Structure of Science," in The Sociology of Science (Chicago: University of Chicago Press, 1973), 267–78, originally published as "Science and Technology in a Democratic Order," Journal of Legal and Political Sociology 1 (1942): 115–26.

3. Merton, "Normative Structure," 274; see also Walton Hamilton, Patents and Free Enterprise (Washington, DC: US Government Printing Office, 1941), 154, https://babel.hathitrust.org/cgi/pt?id=mdp.39015078692475&view=1up&seq=164. Merton used the word "communism" for this concept but did not intend it in a political sense at all. Subsequently, "communalism" has become the preferred characterization of this norm.

4. This work appeared before much of the evidence in the past 40 years that scientific misconduct, whether intentional or unintentional, is less uncommon than he thought. Wolfgang Stroebe, Tom Postmes, and Russell Spears, "Scientific Misconduct and the Myth of Self-Correction in Science," Perspectives on Psychological Science 7, no. 6 (November 2012): 670–88, https://doi.org/10.1177/1745691612460687; Douglas L. Weed, "Preventing Scientific Misconduct," American Journal of Public Health 88, no. 1 (January 1998): 125–29, https://doi.org/10.2105/ajph.88.1.125; Martin F. Shapiro and Robert P. Charrow, "Scientific Misconduct in Investigational Drug Trials," New England Journal of Medicine 312, no. 11 (March 14, 1985): 731–36, https://doi.org/10.1056/NEJM198503143121128.

5. Victoria A. Harden, "A Short History of the National Institutes of Health," accessed February 24, 2020, https://history.nih.gov/exhibits/history/index.html; "Dr. Joseph Kinyoun: The Indispensable Forgotten Man," National Institute of

Allergy and Infectious Diseases, accessed September 19, 2021, https://www.niaid.nih
.gov/about/joseph-kinyoun-indispensable-man.

6. Harden, "Short History."

7. The rates of increase were remarkable. In the decade from 1949 to 1959, the
budget increased tenfold to $291.8 million, then by another 280% by 1969 to $1.11
billion (even without the National Institute of Mental Health, which was accounted
separately from 1967 to 1992). The 1979 budget of close to $3.19 billion represented
another 187% increase in a decade. It rose by 124% to $7.14 billion by 1989, and by 91%
in the in the next 9 years to $13.7 billion in 1998. At that point, congressional appro-
priators got even more aggressive: the budget was $27.2 billion in 2003, an increase of
99% in 5 years. After that, the increases tapered off dramatically, reaching $30.3 billion
in 2015, up just 12% in 12 years. The spigot opened again after that, reaching $41.6
billion in 2020 and $42.9 billion in 2021, an increase of 42% in 6 years. Budgets in 2021
by institute in millions of dollars were as follows: NCI, 6,559; NIAID, 6,067; NHLBI,
3,665; NIA, 3,900; NIGMS, 2,992; NINDS, 2,571; NIDDK 2,282; NIMH, 2,106; NICHD,
1,858; NIDA, 1,480; NIEHS, 897; NCATS, 855; NEI, 836; NIAMS, 634; NHGRI, 616;
NIAAA, 555; NIDCD, 498; NIDCR, 485; NLM, 462; NIBIB, 411; NIMHD, 392; NINR,
175; NCCAH, 151; 2,284 was allocated to the Office of the Director and an innovations
account. "National Institutes of Health (NIH) Funding: FY1996-FY2022, Updated
June 29, 2021," Congressional Research Service, accessed September 12, 2021,
https://sgp.fas.org/crs/misc/R43341.pdf. See also "Appropriations (Section 1),"
National Institutes of Health, NIH Almanac, accessed May 3, 2021, https://www.nih
.gov/about-nih/what-we-do/nih-almanac/appropriations-section-1; "Actual Total
Obligations by Institute and Center FY 2001–FY 2019," National Institutes of Health,
accessed May 30, 2020, https://officeofbudget.od.nih.gov/pdfs/FY21/spending-hist
/Actual%20Obligations%20By%20IC%20FY%202000%20-%20FY%202019%20(V).pdf.

8. Harden, "Short History."

9. "Mission and Goals," National Institutes of Health, accessed April 12, 2020,
https://www.nih.gov/about-nih/what-we-do/mission-goals.

10. "Mission and Goals."

11. "List of NIH Institutes, Centers, and Offices," National Institutes of Health,
accessed April 12, 2020, https://www.nih.gov/institutes-nih/list-nih-institutes
-centers-offices.

12. "Survey of Earned Doctorates: Doctorate Recipients by Major Field of Study:
Selected Years, 1988–2018," National Science Foundation, accessed February 24,
2020, https://ncses.nsf.gov/pubs/nsf20301/data-tables.

13. The overall increase across all disciplines was 65% (33,497 to 55,195). In
biological/biomedical disciplines, the increase was 114% (4,111 to 8,801), in other
health sciences 187% (from 882 to 2534), and in bioengineering/biomedical engineering 895% (from 114 to 1,134). In all other fields, numbers increased 50% (28,490 to
42,726). "Survey of Earned Doctorates."

14. In addition to the funding that went to the respective medical schools, other
components received substantial NIH funding, including $245 million to Johns
Hopkins ($152 million for the School of Public Health) and $66 million to the

University of California, San Francisco ($29 million for their School of Nursing) in 2019, some of which also was for infrastructure/indirect costs. Robert Roskoki Jr. and Tristam G. Parslow, "Ranking Tables of NIH Funding to U.S. Medical Schools in 2020, Table 2 (Schools of Medicine) and Tables for Schools of Public Health and Schools of Nursing," Blue Ridge Institute for Medical Research, accessed September 11, 2021, http://www.brimr.org/NIH_Awards/2020/default.htm; idem, "Ranking Tables of NIH Funding to U.S. Medical Schools in 2019, Table 2 (Schools of Medicine) and Tables for Schools of Public Health and Schools of Nursing," Blue Ridge Institute for Medical Research, accessed September 11, 2021, http://www.brimr.org/NIH _Awards/2019/NIH_Awards_2019.htm.

15. See, e.g., "IU School of Medicine Continues Record-Setting Research Trend; Up 5 Spots in National Institutes of Health Rankings," Indiana University School of Medicine Newsroom, accessed September 20, 2020, https://medicine.iu.edu/news /2020/01/iu-school-of-medicine-continues-record-setting-research-trend-up-5-spots -in-national-institutes-of-health-rankings; "Emory School of Medicine Receives Record NIH Funding in 2019," Emory News Center, accessed September 20, 2020, http://news.emory.edu/stories/2020/02/emory_som_record_nih_funding/.

16. This is set to match the salary of a deputy secretary of a cabinet department (ES Level II), which in 2021 was $199,300.

17. Paul Cleary, personal communication, around 1997.

18. Mark J. Lerchenmueller, Olav Sorenson, and Anupam B. Jena, "Gender Differences in How Scientists Present the Importance of Their Research: Observational Study," BMJ 367 (December 16, 2019): l6573, https://doi.org/10.1136/bmj.l6573; Reshma Jagsi and Julie K. Silver, "Gender Differences in Research Reporting," BMJ 367 (December 16, 2019): l6692, https://doi.org/10.1136/bmj.l6692.

19. Neil Greenspan, "Too Much Optimism at NIH: Opinion," The Scientist, July 22, 2009, https://www.the-scientist.com/daily-news/too-much-optimism-at -nih-opinion-44007; Gardiner Harris, "Pick to Lead Health Agency Draws Praise and Some Concern," New York Times, July 9, 2009, https://www.nytimes.com/2009/07 /09/health/policy/09nih.html?searchResultPosition=1.

20. Michael Weinstein, "Stop AIDS Vaccine Research," Los Angeles Times, April 4, 2008, https://www.latimes.com/opinion/la-oew-weinstein4apr04-story.html; Donald G. McNeil Jr., "Another H.I.V. Vaccine Fails a Trial, Disappointing Researchers," New York Times, February 4, 2020, https://www.nytimes.com/2020/02/04 /health/hiv-vaccine.html.

21. Daniel S. Greenberg, Science, Money, and Politics: Political Triumph and Ethical Erosion (Chicago: University of Chicago Press, 2001), 197–201.

22. Stephanie J. Bird, "Socially Responsible Science Is More Than 'Good Science,'" Journal of Microbiology and Biology Education 15, no. 2 (December 15, 2014): 169–72, https://doi.org/10.1128/jmbe.v15i2.870.

23. Gregory A. Petsko, "Goodbye, Columbus," Genome Biology 13, no. 5 (May 19, 2012): 155, https://doi.org/10.1186/gb-2012-13-5-155; Alexander A. Berezin, "The Perils of Centralized Research Funding Systems," Knowledge, Technology and Policy 11 (1998): 5–26, https://doi.org/10.1007/s12130-998-1001-1.

24. "2019 NIH Director's Awards for High-Risk, High-Reward Research Program Announced," news release, National Institutes of Health, October 1, 2019, https://www.nih.gov/news-events/news-releases/2019-nih-directors-awards-high-risk-high-reward-research-program-announced.

25. Mikko Packalen and Jay Bhattacharya, "NIH Funding and the Pursuit of Edge Science," *Proceedings of the National Academy of Sciences of the United States of America* 171, no. 22 (June 2, 2020): 12,011–16, https://doi.org/10.1073/pnas.1910160117.

26. Greenberg, *Science, Money, and Politics*, 439.

27. Rachel Kahn Best, "Disease Politics and Medical Research Funding: Three Ways Advocacy Shapes Policy," *American Sociological Review* 77 (September 30, 2012): 780–803, https://doi.org/10.1177/0003122412458509; Deepak Hegde and Bhaven Sampat, "Can Private Money Buy Public Science? Disease Group Lobbying and Federal Funding for Biomedical Research," *Management Science* 61, no. 10 (October 2015): 2281–98, https://doi.org/10.1287/mnsc.2014.2107.

28. Sara Reardon, "U.S. Mental-Health Agency's Push for Basic Research Has Slashed Support for Clinical Trials," *Nature* 546, no. 7658 (June 13, 2017): 339, https://www.nature.com/news/us-mental-health-agency-s-push-for-basic-research-has-slashed-support-for-clinical-trials-1.22145; Steven Breckler, "The Strategic Plan of NIMH," American Psychological Association Psychological Science Agenda, January 2008, https://www.apa.org/science/about/psa/2008/01/ed-column.

29. The study found that at NIMH, the number fell from 192 projects in 2005 to 66 in 2016. At the NCI, the number dropped from 91 to 49. At NIDA, it fell from 58 to 41. Other institutes increased funding during that time (NIA from 38 to 66 projects, NIDDK from 22 to 30, and NLM from 4 to 15). Others varied widely: NHLBI rose from 32 to 70 projects, then fell to 24, then finished at 51; NINDS rose from 5 to 23 projects, then fell to 3. Other institutes had little or no interest (NIAID funded 1 to 7 projects per year). Overall, the 21 institutes and centers funded 630 projects in 2005 and 586 in 2016. Most received $500,000 in direct costs or less per year. Janet Weiner, "NIH Funding of Health Services Research," Leonard Davis Institute of Health Economics, June 8, 2017, https://ldi.upenn.edu/healthpolicysense/nih-funding-health-services-research; Lisa A. Simpson et al., "Show Me the Money! Trends in Funding for Health Services Research," *Health Services Research* 53, suppl. 2 (October 2018): 3967–75, https://doi.org/10.1111/1475-6773.13040.

30. Simpson, "Show Me the Money!"

31. See, e.g., Robert M. Kaplan, *More Than Medicine: The Broken Promise of American Health* (Cambridge, MA: Harvard University Press, 2019).

32. Bradford H. Gray, Michael K. Gusmano, and Sara R. Collins, "AHCPR and the Changing Politics of Health Services Research," *Health Affairs* (Millwood) 22, suppl. 1 (June 2003): W3-283-307, https://doi.org/10.1377/hlthaff.w3.283; Richard A. Deyo et al., "The Messenger under Attack—Intimidation of Researchers by Special-Interest Groups," *New England Journal of Medicine* 336, no. 16 (April 17, 1997): 1177–80, https://doi.org/10.1056/NEJM199704173361611.

33. The clearinghouse is no longer available on AHRQ's website and is not being updated anymore, but its contents can be obtained from the Alliance for the Implemen-

tation of Clinical Practice Guidelines. "About NGC and NQMC," Agency for Healthcare Research and Quality, accessed October 24, 2021, https://www.ahrq.gov/gam/about/index.html; "NGC Summaries Archive," Alliance for the Implementation of Clinical Practice Guidelines, accessed March 2, 2020, https://aicpg.org/ngc-summaries/.

34. "National Institutes of Health (NIH) Funding."

35. AHRQ received $397 million in 2010, $416.6 million in 2017, and $436.5 million in 2021. They also receive some transfers from the PCORI budget. PCORI received $466.1 million in 2017 and projected $420 million of support in 2020. Combined support for these agencies, about $857 million in 2020, was approximately 2.1% of the NIH's budget of $41.6 billion in 2020. By one estimate, about $1.77 billion (5.6% of the NIH's budget in 2017) went to similar research. Accounting for such funding in all federal agencies, including Veterans Affairs and the CDC, total expenditures in 2017 were $2.973 billion, still less than the individual budgets of several of the institutes. Simpson, "Show Me the Money!"; "Operating Plan for Fiscal Year 2021," Agency for Healthcare Research and Quality, accessed May 3, 2021, https://www.ahrq.gov/cpi/about/mission/operating-plan/index.html; "PCORI 2019 Annual Report," Patient-Centered Outcomes Research Institute, accessed May 3, 2021, https://www.pcori.org/sites/default/files/PCORI-Annual-Report-2019.pdf.

36. "What Is PCORI's Official Policy on Cost and Cost-Effectiveness Analysis?," PCORI Help Center, accessed July 12, 2020, https://help.pcori.org/hc/en-us/articles/213716587-What-is-PCORI-s-official-policy-on-cost-and-cost-effectiveness-analysis-.

37. "What Is PCORI's Official Policy." While some cost-effectiveness analyses are conducted by private insurers and by the government's Center for Medicare and Medicaid Services, it is a loss not to support such studies by experts who do not have potential or actual conflicts of interests in their outcome.

38. David M. Frankford, "The Remarkable Staying Power of 'Death Panels,'" Journal of Health Politics, Policy, and Law 40, no. 5 (October 2015): 1087–101, https://doi.org/10.1215/03616878-3161212.

39. Michael Stefanek, Stephanie Hess, and Wendy Nelson, "Behavioral and Social Science Research at the National Institutes of Health," Association for Psychological Science Observer, January 19, 2005, https://www.psychologicalscience.org/observer/behavioral-and-social-science-research-at-the-national-institutes-of-health.

40. Geoffrey Kabat, "A 'Cancer Moonshot' Is the Wrong Analogy," Forbes, February 10, 2016, https://www.forbes.com/sites/geoffreykabat/2016/02/10/a-cancer-moonshot-is-the-wrong-analogy/#7b0156f3d68f.

41. In 2021, the Biden administration proposed creation of a new agency, ARPA-H (for Advanced Research Projects Agency for Health), within NIH to manage, initially, moonshot efforts directed at cancer, diabetes, and Alzheimer disease with an initial budget of $6.5 billion. It is to be funded through a contract mechanism based on deliverables, rather than on grants. Jocelyn Kaiser, "Biden Wants $6.5 Billion for New Agency to Speed Treatments," Science, April 9, 2021, https://www.science.org/news/2021/04/biden-wants-65-billion-new-health-agency-speed-treatments.

42. Health services researchers similarly advocate for more funding for their field as well, but rarely with much effect; they have no magic bullets to proffer, just earnest efforts to make some progress against important public health problems.

43. Francis S. Collins, "Shattuck Lecture—Medical and Societal Consequences of the Human Genome Project," *New England Journal of Medicine* 341, no. 1 (July 1, 1999): 28–37, https://doi.org/10.1056/NEJM199907013410106.

44. Bhavneet Bhinder and Olivier Elemento, "Towards a Better Cancer Precision Medicine: Systems Biology Meets Immunotherapy," *Current Opinion in Systems Biology* 2 (April 2017): 67–73, https://doi.org/10.1016/j.coisb.2017.01.006.

45. Marta Crous-Bou, Laura B. Harrington, and Christopher Kabrhel, "Environmental and Genetic Risk Factors Associated with Venous Thromboembolism," *Seminars in Thrombosis and Hemostasis* 42, no. 8 (November 2016): 808–20. https://doi.org/10.1055/s-0036-1592333.

46. Pierre Courtoi et al., "Deep Learning-Based Classification of Mesothelioma Improves Prediction of Patient Outcome," *Nature Medicine* 25, no. 10 (October 2019): 1519–25, https://doi.org/10.1038/s41591-019-0583-3.

47. Wei Du et. al., "Effective Combination Therapies for B-Cell Lymphoma Predicted by a Virtual Disease Model," *Cancer Research* 77, no. 8 (April 15, 2017): 1818–30, https://doi.org/10.1158/0008-5472.CAN-16-0476. There are several other examples. Studies of whole-genome sequencing of individuals with cancer (as well as sequencing of the tumors) have found unusual mutations, for example, in bladder and uterine tumors, that are more common in breast tumors. This has led to use in those other tumors of a treatment that is effective in breast cancers with the same mutation. Britt K. Erickson et al., "Targeting Human Epidermal Growth Factor Receptor 2 (HER2) in Gynecologic Malignancies," *Current Opinion in Obstetrics and Gynecology* 32, no. 1 (February 2020): 57–64, https://doi.org/10.1097/GCO.0000000000000599. Others have identified some mutations in blood cells that occur years before people with those mutations develop acute myelogenous leukemia. Pinkal Desai et al., "Somatic Mutations Precede Acute Myeloid Leukemia Years before Diagnosis," *Nature Medicine* 24, no. 7 (July 2018): 1015–23, https://doi.org/10.1038/s41591-018-0081-z. Still other studies have found high rates of alteration in DNA repair in some cancers (including almost a quarter of breast cancers) that are prognostically relevant because they are associated with more aggressive tumors. Laura Keren Urbina-Jara et al., "Landscape of Germline Mutations in DNA Repair Genes for Breast Cancer in Latin America: Opportunities for PARP-Like Inhibitors and Immunotherapy," *Genes (Basel)* 10, no. 10 (October 2019): 786, https://doi.org/10.3390/genes10100786.

48. Jennifer Couzin-Frankel, "Genetics: The Promise of a Cure: 20 Years and Counting," *Science* 324, no. 5934 (June 19, 2009): 1504–7, https://doi.org/10.1126/science.324_1504.

49. Statistical significance most often is defined as an association that would occur by chance no more than 1 time in 20.

50. The All of Us Research Program Investigators, "The 'All of Us' Research Program," *New England Journal of Medicine* 381, no. 7 (August 2019): 668–76, https://doi.org/10.1056/NEJMsr1809937.

51. Muin J. Khoury and Sandro Galea, "Will Precision Medicine Improve Population Health?," JAMA 316, no. 13 (October 2016): 1357–58, https://doi.org/10.1001/jama.2016.12260; The "-omic" disciplines include genomics, epigenomics, transcriptomics, proteomics, metabolomics, and microbiomics. Yehudit Hasin, Marcus Seldin, and Aldons Lusis, "Multi-omics approaches to disease," Genome Biology 18, no. 1 (May 2017): 83, https://doi.org/10.1186/s13059-017-1215-1.

52. Nathaniel Comfort and Aeon, "The Overhyping of Precision Medicine," The Atlantic, December 12, 2016, https://www.theatlantic.com/health/archive/2016/12/the-peril-of-overhyping-precision-medicine/510326/; Meg Barbor, "Precision Medicine: Hope or Hype?" ASCO Post, February 10, 2018, https://www.ascopost.com/issues/february-10-2018/precision-medicine-hope-or-hype/; "Does the Hype Exceed Reality for Precision Medicine?," Knowledge@Wharton, accessed May 30, 2020, https://knowledge.wharton.upenn.edu/article/does-the-hype-exceed-reality-for-precision-medicine/.

53. Michael J. Joiner, Nigel Paneth, and John P. A. Ioannidis, "What Happens When Underperforming Big Ideas in Research Become Entrenched?," JAMA 316, no. 13 (October 4, 2016): 1355–56, https://doi.org/10.1001/jama.2016.11076. The FDA has sued and shut down physicians doing autologous stem cell transplants for unproven indications under a provision of the Public Health Service Act that allows the government to prevent interstate transmission of disease. "Statement from FDA Commissioner Scott Gottlieb, M.D. on the FDA's New Policy Steps and Enforcement Efforts to Ensure Proper Oversight of Stem Cell Therapies and Regenerative Medicine," US Food and Drug Administration, August 28, 2017, https://www.fda.gov/news-events/press-announcements/statement-fda-commissioner-scott-gottlieb-md-fdas-new-policy-steps-and-enforcement-efforts-ensure.

54. Howard Markel, "Patents, Profits, and the American People—The Bayh-Dole Act of 1980," New England Journal of Medicine 369, no. 9 (August 29, 2013): 794–96, https://doi.org/10.1056/NEJMp1306553.

55. Aaron S. Kesselheim and Rahul Rajkumar, "Who Owns Federally Funded Research? The Supreme Court and the Bayh–Dole Act," New England Journal of Medicine 365, no. 13 (September 29, 2011): 1167–69, https://doi.org/10.1056/NEJMp1109168.

56. "35 U.S. Code 203—March-In Rights," Legal Information Institute, accessed September 11, 2021, https://www.law.cornell.edu/uscode/text/35/203.

57. Carolyn L. Treasure, Jerry Avorn, and Aaron S. Kesselheim, "Do March-In Rights Ensure Access to Medical Products Arising from Federally Funded Research? A Qualitative Study," Milbank Quarterly 93, no. 4 (December 2015): 761–87, https://doi.org/10.1111/1468-0009.12164; Arthur M. Feldman, "The Bayh-Dole Act: A Lion without Claws," Clinical and Translational Science 8, no. 1 (February 2015): 3–4, https://doi.org/10.1111/cts.12262. The government has failed to pursue other legal pathways for ensuring fair pricing of drugs developed with federal grants. Alfred B. Engelberg, Jerry Avorn, and Aaron S. Kesselheim, "A New Way to Contain Unaffordable Medication Costs—Exercising the Government's Existing Rights," New England Journal of Medicine 386, no. 12 (March 24, 2022): 1104–6, https://10.1056/NEJMp2117102.

58. Walter D. Valdivia, "The Stakes in Bayh-Dole: Public Values beyond the Pace of Innovation," *Minerva* 49, no. 1 (March 2011): 25–46, https://doi.org/10.1007/s11024-011-9162-6.

59. "A New List of America's Richest: #89 Patrick Soon-Shiong," *Forbes*, accessed October 24, 2021, https://www.forbes.com/profile/patrick-soon-shiong/?sh=2fea78bf1fee.

60. Nicola Mazzarotto, "Competition and Market Incentives in Higher Education," Social Science Research Network, December 12, 2007, http://dx.doi.org/10.2139/ssrn.1059881.

61. Katie Thomas and Charles Ornstein, "Memorial Sloan Kettering's Season of Turmoil," *New York Times*, December 31, 2018, https://www.nytimes.com/2018/12/31/health/memorial-sloan-kettering-conflicts.html?action=click&module=Top%20Stories&pgtype=Homepage; Charles Ornstein and Katie Thomas, "Sloan Kettering's Cozy Deal with Start-Up Ignites a New Uproar," *New York Times*, September 20, 2018, https://www.nytimes.com/2018/09/20/health/memorial-sloan-kettering-cancer-paige-ai.html; Charles Ornstein and Katie Thomas, "Memorial Sloan Kettering Leaders Violated Conflict-of-Interest Rules," *New York Times*, April 4, 2019, https://www.nytimes.com/2019/04/04/health/memorial-sloan-kettering-conflicts-.html.

62. Arnold S. Relman, "Dealing with Conflicts of Interest," *New England Journal of Medicine* 310, no. 12 (September 19, 1984): 1182–83, https://doi.org/10.1056/nejm198405033101809.

63. Arnold S. Relman, "New 'Information for Authors'—and Readers," *New England Journal of Medicine* 323, no.1 (July 5, 1990): 56, https://www.doi.org/10.1056/NEJM199007053230111; Marcia Angell and Jerome P. Kassirer, "Editorials and Conflicts of Interest," *New England Journal of Medicine* 335, no. 14 (October 3, 1996): 1055–56, https://doi.org/10.1056/NEJM199610033351410; Sarah Ramsay, "NEJM Conflict-of-Interest Policy under Scrutiny," *Lancet* 354, no. 9189 (October 30, 1999): 1536, https://doi.org/10.1016/S0140-6736(05)76577-6; Marcia Angell, "Is Academic Medicine for Sale?," *New England Journal of Medicine* 342, no. 20 (May 18, 2000): 1516–18, https://doi.org/10.1056/NEJM200005183422009; Jeffry M. Drazen and Gregory D. Curfman, "Financial Associations of Authors," *New England Journal of Medicine* 346, no. 24 (June 13, 2002): 1901–2, https://doi.org/10.1056/NEJMe020074.

64. Roy H. Perlis et al., "Industry Sponsorship and Financial Conflict of Interest in the Reporting of Clinical Trials in Psychiatry," *American Journal of Psychiatry* 162, no. 10 (October 2005): 1957–60, https://doi.org/10.1176/appi.ajp.162.10.1957; Thomas Bodenheimer, "Uneasy Alliance—Clinical Investigators and the Pharmaceutical Industry," *New England Journal of Medicine* 342, no. 15 (May 18, 2000): 1539–44, https://doi.org/10.1056/NEJM200005183422024. Conflicts of interest are widespread, and universities and their medical schools are often complicit. Justin E. Bekelman, Yan Li, and Cary P. Gross, "Scope and Impact of Financial Conflicts of Interest in Biomedical Research," *JAMA* 289, no. 4 (January 22–29, 2003): 454–65, https://doi.org/10.1001/jama.289.4.454.

65. Kevin A. Schulman et al., "A National Survey of Provisions in Clinical-Trial Agreements between Medical Schools and Industry Sponsors," *New England Journal*

of Medicine 347, no. 17 (October 24, 2002): 1335–41, https://doi.org/10.1056/NEJMsa020349.

66. See, e.g., "Board of Trustees of the Leland Stanford Junior Univ. v. Roche Molecular Systems, Inc. 563 U.S. 776 (2011)," Justia US Supreme Court, accessed October 24, 2011, https://supreme.justia.com/cases/federal/us/563/776/.

67. David Willman, "Drug Maker Hired NIH Researcher," *Los Angeles Times*, December 7, 1998, https://www.latimes.com/archives/la-xpm-1998-dec-07-mn-51498-story.html; David Willman, "NIH Director Calls for Review of Scientist's Ties to Firm," *Los Angeles Times*, December 16, 1998, https://www.latimes.com/archives/la-xpm-1998-dec-16-mn-54649-story.html; see also Jerome P. Kassirer, *On the Take: How Medicine's Complicity with Big Business Can Endanger Your Health* (New York: Oxford University Press, 2005); Jerry Avorn, *Powerful Medicines: The Benefits, Risks, and Costs of Prescription Drugs* (New York: Knopf, 2004).

68. Peter Lurie et al., "Financial Conflicts of Interest Disclosure and Voting Patterns at Food and Drug Administration Drug Advisory Committee Meetings," *JAMA* 295, no. 16 (April 26, 2006): 1921–28, https://doi.org/10.1001/jama.295.16.1921. Advisory committees are not required by law and are supposed to be balanced, but including individuals with financial conflicts of interests make it less likely that the advice given will be only the disinterested judgment of experts.

69. Martin F. Shapiro, "Is the Spirit of Capitalism Undermining the Ethics of Health Services Research?," *Health Services Research* 28, no. 6 (February 1994): 661–72, PMID 8113051.

70. Ragnvald Kalleberg, "A Reconstruction of the Ethos of Science," *Journal of Classical Sociology* 7, no. 2 (July 2007): 137–60, https://doi.org/10.1177/1468795X07078033; Nico Stehr, "The Ethos of Science Revisited: Social and Cognitive Norms," *Sociological Inquiry* 48, no. 3–4 (1978): 172–96, https://doi.org/10.1007/978-3-319-76995-0_10.

71. Paul K. Whelton, "The Elusiveness of Population-Wide High Blood Pressure Control," *Annual Review of Public Health* 36 (March 2015): 109–30, https://doi.org/10.1146/annurev-publhealth-031914-122949; Pragna Patel et al., "Improved Blood Pressure Control to Reduce Cardiovascular Disease Morbidity and Mortality: The Standardized Hypertension Treatment and Prevention Project," *Journal of Clinical Hypertension (Greenwich)* 18, no. 12 (December 2016): 1284–94, https://doi.org/10.1111/jch.12861.

72. Michael J. Joyner and Nigel Paneth, "Promises, Promises, and Precision Medicine," *Journal of Clinical Investigation* 129, no. 3 (March 1, 2019): 946–48, https://doi.org/10.1172/JCI126119.

73. Alfred, Lord Tennyson, "Ulysses," available at the Poetry Foundation website, accessed May 5, 2022, https://www.poetryfoundation.org/poems/45392/ulysses.

74. Tom Lehrer, "Wernher von Braun," track 13 on *That Was the Year That Was*, Reprise / Warner Bros., 1965.

75. Kaplan, *More Than Medicine.*

76. Jeff L. Leroy et al., "Current Priorities in Health Research Funding and Lack of Impact on the Number of Child Deaths per Year," *American Journal of Public Health* 97, no. 2 (February 2007): 219–23, https://doi.org/10.2105/AJPH.2005.083287.

77. Bengt Gustafsson et al., "Focus On: The Uppsala Code of Ethics of Scientists," *Journal of Peace Research* 21, no. 4 (1984): 311–16, https://doi.org/10.1177/002234338402100401.

78. David B. Resnik and Kevin C. Elliott, "The Ethical Challenges of Socially Responsible Science," *Accountability in Research* 23, no. 1 (2016): 31–46, https://doi.org/10.1080/08989621.2014.1002608.

79. Catherine C. Elgin, "Science, Ethics, and Education," *Theory and Research in Education* 9, no. 3 (November 14, 2011): 251–63, https://doi.org/10.1177/1477878511419559.

Dialogue #7

Student: Medical science sure has become closely entwined with the business of medical practice and the interests of the pharmaceutical companies, but we need to be careful about what we say, especially with some politicians and members of the public prepared to reject science altogether for ideological reasons.

Professor (reading): We do lay out some serious concerns about the way biomedical science operates and sets priorities without rejecting its potential value. Is that sufficient?

Student: Well, I do worry about it. But I also agree that this stuff is important, and not just the topics they study. Conflicts of interest, overselling their findings, and the priorities of the universities are big deals. We can't ignore them.

Professor: I totally agree. We've learned a lot. And we can see some linkages to issues affecting doctors, medical educators, and hospitals and health systems. But there are some more elements of health care that we need to think through.

Student: Right. After analyzing hospital corporations and the business of science, I am sure you'll agree that this is the right time to look at pharmaceutical corporations. I think they're among the worst actors on the health care scene.

Professor: Don't go after them like a hungry predator. These are great industries. We need to acknowledge all that they contribute.

Student: Professor, we can't give them a free ride!

Professor: I am confident that you won't let that happen. And let's be sure to poke around and see what other kinds of corporations are getting involved in health care and how they're behaving.

Student: I'll leave no corporate cornerstone unturned.

9

"Doing Everything for Money"

The Producers of Health Care Products

Don't think money does everything or you are going to end up doing everything
for money.
—Voltaire

Early on the morning of June 1, 1992, my colleague Michael Wilkes telephoned me.

"Our paper on drug advertising just came out," he said. "It is causing
a firestorm. It is on the front pages of the *New York Times* and the *Washington Post*."

Michael, who did some broadcast journalism in addition to his clinical
and research work, was clearly pleased by this development. But how could
any scientific paper about a topic as innocuous as drug ads be so controversial? Read on. First, a bit of context; then, I'll share the rest of the story.

The producers of health care goods include manufacturers of pharmaceutical and biological products; fabricators of implantable medical devices such as stents, joints, and pacemakers; suppliers of disposable
health care products; and the manufacturers of medical machines large
(magnetic resonance scanners) and small (microscopes, monitors). Their
products are essential components of care, but their primary mission as
corporations is to produce profits for their shareholders. Increased sales
and newer, more expensive devices may sometimes enhance health, but
that is a secondary concern. Corporations are in the business of inducing
and satisfying demand.[1]

Manufacturing health care products hasn't always been big business, but it has grown enormously over the past century or two. Through much of human history, physicians and other healers had little to offer that improved health outcomes, and the technologies employed were not complex. There was a demand for bandages, plasters for broken bones, and the like. Apothecaries or chemists provided compounds intended to treat patients' ailments, but many were ineffective, and most others had limited usefulness.

Since the nineteenth century, knowledge about diseases and how to diagnose and treat them has exploded. Advances have included simple preventive measures, such as removing the pump handle from a contaminated well and having doctors wash their hands before delivering a baby. Others have involved new equipment, supplies, and substances for diagnosing and treating diseases. These developments have transformed public health and medical care, although the benefits have been applied unevenly across and within societies. Consider the realm of diagnostic technology. René Laënnec, a French physician who carved his own flutes, invented the first stethoscope in 1816, in part to preserve the modesty of women when physicians were listening to the heart and lungs.[2] And physicians have analyzed urine for thousands of years to draw inferences about health and disease. Until relatively recently, the principal analytic techniques were observation and tasting the urine. Now, much can be learned from sophisticated microscopic, chemical, and microbiological analyses.[3]

Scientific advances led to revolutions in diagnosis and treatment. As physiologists, biochemists, immunologists, and bacteriologists began to understand the mechanisms of diseases, new diagnostic tests and treatments soon followed. French scientist Louis Pasteur's germ theory of disease, along with the work of German researchers Ferdinand Cohn and Robert Koch on such infectious diseases as anthrax, tuberculosis, and typhus, provided practical value to the use of the microscope and led to the introduction of laboratories to analyze and culture specimens to diagnose bacterial illnesses.

Advances in Therapeutics

Therapies, too, improved dramatically. Increasingly effective treatments for specific diseases began to appear in the second half of the eighteenth century, such as lime juice for scurvy and digitalis for heart failure. The first quarter of the nineteenth century saw the isolation of morphine to treat pain, colchicine for gout, and quinine for malaria, as well as the introduction of blood transfusion. The synthesis of chloroform in 1831 made possible its use 15 years later as a general anesthetic.[4] While there were some companies selling chemicals to treat medical conditions that mostly had emerged from apothecary shops in the Middle Ages, business was limited. Even late in the nineteenth century, the general consensus was that relatively few such treatments were essential to the practice of medicine.

Around the time of the US Civil War, new products became available, and some entrepreneurs saw new opportunities. Pfizer, which began as a chemical company, grew during the Civil War in response to demand for pain killers and antiseptics. A Union soldier, Eli Lilly was a chemist who started a pharmaceutical company a decade after the war, using advanced manufacturing methods and introducing a component of research and development. Edward Squibb, who had served in the Mexican American War in the late 1840s, recognized the poor quality of medicines provided to the military and set up a business in 1858 to produce better products.

In the next 50 years, chloral hydrate and barbiturates became available to induce sleep; salicylic acid, phenacetin, and acetanilide were developed to manage pain and fever; and antitoxins were introduced to treat diphtheria and tetanus. The first Nobel Prize in Medicine or Physiology was awarded in 1901 to Emil von Behring for his 1880 discovery that made possible passive immunization against diphtheria. In the first 25 years of the twentieth century, new treatments appeared for syphilis, epilepsy, malaria, and edema.

The most stunning breakthrough was the isolation in Toronto of insulin from a cow's pancreas, a discovery that led to effective treatment for diabetes in 1921, for which Frederick Banting and J. J. R. Macleod received a Nobel Prize two years later. Type I diabetes previously had been untreatable, and the cure was perceived as miraculous. In order to meet the broad demand, Banting and his colleagues partnered with Connaught Laboratories in Canada and Eli Lilly Company in the United States to mass-produce the medicine.[5]

After that came enormous numbers of breakthroughs in medications, including such hormonal treatments as parathyroid extract (1924), estrogen and adrenal extract (1929), oxytocin to induce labor (1930), testosterone (1935) adrenocorticotrophic hormone, or ACTH (1948), vitamins (vitamin D in 1927, riboflavin in 1933, thiamin in 1934, niacin in 1937, folic acid in 1943, and B_{12} in 1948), anti-infectious agents (plasmoquin for malaria in 1921, sulfonamides for pneumonia and other infections in 1934, penicillin for gram positive infections in 1941, streptomycin for tuberculosis in 1944, and chloramphenicol for typhoid and gram negative infections in 1947), and treatments for psychosis (chlorpromazine in 1951).[6]

Scottish bacteriologist Alexander Fleming's discovery of penicillin, and elucidation of its value in infections in research at Oxford University by Australian-born Howard Florey and German-born Ernst Chain, was at least as important as insulin in catapulting the industry forward. The need for penicillin was enormous for treatment of wounded soldiers during World War II and provided a boost to the burgeoning pharmaceutical industry when the government collaborated with Merck (the American firm that emerged from a German company at the time of World War I), Pfizer, and Squibb to mass-produce the drug for the military. The three scientists were awarded a Nobel Prize in 1945 for this work.[7]

All of these advances led to new expenditures for medical care. By 1980, annual costs for medicines in most Western, industrialized countries was about $50 per person. Costs have risen steadily since, but at far different rates in different countries. American expenditures were in line with those in other developed countries until the late 1990s but began to rise more rapidly then, about the time that direct-to-consumer advertising became much more common.[8]

By 2015, average retail spending on pharmaceuticals (excluding spending on medications dispensed directly by physicians and hospitals) averaged about $400 per person in Austria, Netherlands, Norway, and Sweden; between $500 and $600 in the United Kingdom and France; a little less than $700 in Canada and Germany; and nearly $800 Switzerland. In the United States, the per person cost was $1,011 in 2015 and has continued to rise since then. The disparities are even greater for some of the newer, popular medications.[9] In the first six months of 2019, 3,400 drug prices were raised an average of 10.5% in the US, or five times that year's inflation rate.[10]

As of 2021, the US government had not allowed Medicare to negotiate drug prices with the manufacturers, and prices for almost all medications continued to be higher in the US than elsewhere. There are frequent reports of Americans going to Canada to fill prescriptions for medications like insulin, for which US prices have skyrocketed. One analysis found that for new drugs, the US price was about 80% higher than the average price in other countries for the 28% of medicines that are dispensed directly by physicians and hospitals.[11]

A government analysis of the prices of all dispensed medications found increases of as much as 12% in some years, significantly higher than the increase in overall costs of care, with the proportion of personal health expenses going to medications reaching 16.7% in 2015, amounting to $457 billion. When researchers broke down the increases in costs, they found that 30% was a result of more prescriptions per person, 30% from increasing prices, 10% attributable to population growth, and 30% from overall inflation.[12]

Pharmaceutical advertising and price gouging were critical drivers of the increased costs, abetted by heavily lobbied members of the executive and legislative branches of government. Worldwide revenue from pharmaceutical products increased from $390 billion to $1.42 trillion (nearly half of the expenditure being in North America) between 2001 and 2021.[13]

Advertising

The pharmaceutical industry advertises to providers and patients.[14] The industry contends that its products extend life and improve quality of life and convenience. It shows little regard for real benefits to health or costs, whether economically or in terms of adverse effects. Advertising aimed at medical practitioners often inflates the benefits and minimizes the adverse effects of treatments and misrepresents the populations for whom such treatments are appropriate.[15] Our UCLA study of drug advertising, referenced at the beginning of this chapter, made it clear that criticism of the marketing approaches of the pharmaceutical industry is not welcome.

My colleagues and I were troubled by slickness and misrepresentation in drug ads in medical journals. We conducted a study in which we randomly selected such ads from medical journals in several specialties and then asked researchers who reviewed for those journals to review the ads. We asked them to comment on any features of the ad that might lead to misinterpretation of who benefits from taking the drug, what the side effects are, any contraindications to taking it, how well the drug worked, images in the ad, and so on. We also asked them to make summary judgments about the ad as they would for a scientific article: accept as is, request minor revisions, request major revisions, or reject. The reviewers recommended rejection or major revision for 57% of the ads. The paper was published in a leading journal with accompanying and supportive editorials by the commissioner of the US Food and Drug Administration (FDA) and by the journal's editors. At the same time, the inspector general of the Department of Health and Human Services published a parallel analysis of our data.[16] The two reports received considerable media attention. Several weeks later, 13 US senators signed a letter to the FDA, "urging that the FDA act quickly and decisively to ensure that prescription drug advertisements in medical and pharmaceutical journals meet regulatory standards for quality and integrity as established by the agency."

The pharmaceutical industry was furious. It obtained our data and had them reanalyzed by outside researchers. The researchers whom they hired found no meaningful errors that compromised the findings, but they took issue with minor methodological points, such as whether reviewers should have rated on a five-point or four-point scale. It soon became clear, however, that the industry chose to punish the journal, substantially reducing advertising in it.[17]

Alongside about $20 billion per year now being spent on advertising to physicians and health plans, the industry spends substantially on direct-to-consumer advertising. This spending exploded once the FDA removed certain restrictions in the late 1990s. From 1997 to 2016, manufacturer spending more than quadrupled from $2.1 billion to $9.6 billion per year on advertisements aimed at consumers, promoting drugs for depression, testosterone replacement, hair loss, erectile dysfunction, cancer, inflammatory bowel disease, psoriasis, schizophrenia, and many other conditions.[18] As part of this effort, corporations have enlisted celebrity spokespeople from the worlds of politics, entertainment, and sports to promote their products to the public.[19]

The manufacturers insist that they only are trying to promote conversations between patients and their doctors. But such conversations often lead to prescription of a specific drug when there is a less expensive alternative available or when no medication is indicated. For example, patients requesting a drug for depression were significantly more likely to get one, even when they had adjustment disorders that do not respond to antidepressants.[20] Such advertising has also led to increased prescribing of androgen replacement therapy, notwithstanding concerns that it is overused.[21]

In cancer treatment, companies advertise heavily for new products that are expensive, generally giving short shrift to adverse effects and even to amount of long-term benefit, while failing to acknowledge the availability of less expensive alternatives. These advertisements can raise unrealistic expectations in patients desperate for a cure.[22] These kinds of considerations have led to many voices, including those of such organizations as the American College of Physicians, suggesting that direct-to-consumer advertising can leave patients confused and misinformed and do more harm than good.[23]

Exorbitant Pricing and Its Apologists

The industry pursues extremely inflated pricing of new (and even old) products,[24] raising prices or extending patents with minor modifications and squashing competition. For some new medications for rare conditions, prices as high as $2 million have been established.[25] As the industry has raised these prices aggressively in recent years, they have recruited respected academicians, mostly economists, to help them make the argument for high prices and lack of regulation of these prices.

One successful business in this regard is Precision Health Economics (PHE), which conducts analyses of the benefits of the new drugs. Most of its funding comes from pharmaceutical companies. One of the company's founders has testified against regulation, saying, "We have to ensure access to future innovation, and that's going to require some recognition that if someone develops an innovative drug, they're going to charge a lot for it."[26] Papers published in scholarly journals by academicians affiliated with PHE on work conducted under PHE's aegis (and almost always funded by pharmaceutical or biologics companies) do not consistently acknowledge ties to the consulting firm, and not all journals require such disclosure. In the view of some critics, the assumptions in their economic models tend to bias findings in ways favorable to the manufacturers and their pricing strategies. The company's researchers advocate for pricing a drug based on its value to society. The late economist Uwe Reinhardt of Princeton criticized this model, arguing, "If you did value pricing and say it's OK for the drug companies to charge up to what the patient values his or her life to be, you are basically saying that the pharmaceutical companies can take your savings. American society will not stand for that."[27]

Such pricing of drugs for cancer, psoriasis, and other conditions often leads to list prices of tens or hundreds of thousands of dollars for a course of treatment. For example, adalimumab (marketed as Humira), which is used to treat chronic conditions such as rheumatoid arthritis, had a retail price in 2021 of $77,000 for a year of treatment, which is 470% more than it cost when it was introduced in 2003, yielding revenue of $16 billion in the United States for AbbVie. Some insurers are able to negotiate discounts on these prices.[28] Clinicians who prescribe cancer drugs dispense them at a price that is a set percentage above the list price, giving them an incentive to prescribe more expensive medications. Manufacturers recognized this as an opportunity, and "launch prices" for cancer drugs increased by about 10% per year between 1995 and 2013.[29]

Even more worrisome, although insurance covers some of these costs for many patients, these relentlessly rising prices can lead to denial of coverage, particularly in state-run Medicaid programs that are strapped for funds. Critics of the pharmaceutical industry have even questioned the role of the industry in innovation, as many of these new drugs were developed with federal grants but then licensed to pharmaceutical companies whose contributions were largely limited to obtaining FDA approval (and sometimes to funding the phase 3 clinical trials, which can cost tens of millions of dollars), then packaging and marketing the products.[30]

A recent study found that of 210 "new molecular entities" approved by the FDA between 2010 and 2016, all 210 had received National Institutes of Health (NIH) grants for their basic and/or applied research, which produced over 600,000 research publications related to these drugs, amounting to 29% of all publications relating to them. The grants for the products that were the first ones in their classes of drugs had received NIH funding amounting to more than $64 billion. None of the proceeds from sales of these products were repaid to the NIH or to the federal government in recognition of their role.[31] Presumably, an argument for an unregulated market is undermined when much of the innovation has been paid for by someone other than the company establishing the price and collecting the revenue.

The corporate pharmacy benefit managers negotiate private sector prices but receive commissions proportional to price, thereby lacking an incentive to maximally lower prices.[32] Of 36 commonly prescribed drugs available since 2012 in one large insurance database, 44% more than doubled in price, and 78% increased by 50% or more by 2017.[33]

Lobbying

The pharmaceutical industry spends far more on lobbying than any other industry, a total of $4.45 billion from January 1998 to March 2020.[34] As a result, they successfully prevented the government from negotiating prices in the Medicare Part D program, thereby ensuring higher prices in the US than elsewhere, even for medications produced in the United States.[35] They have also worked vigorously to prevent government intervention to bring down the prices of common, essential medications such as insulin.

The pharmaceutical industry claims that it needs the revenue from its price structure to be able to invest in research and development. But it is far from clear that that is the case. Profits in the pharmaceutical sector are higher than in most other manufacturing sectors. Pharmaceutical and biologic manufacturers enjoy large profit margins.[36] At least one private equity firm has been buying royalties on future sales of popular drugs. With prices of approved drugs surging, the firm has amassed about $15 billion in this way.[37]

Regulatory Failure

The Food and Drug Administration is responsible for regulating entry of new pharmaceutical products into the US market. After an episode in which more than 100 people died as a consequence of taking the anti-infectious agent sulfanilamide contaminated with diethylene glycol (which is used for antifreeze), Congress passed a law in 1938 that required corporations to submit formal applications to the FDA for approval of new drugs demonstrating their safety.[38] In 1960, an application for approval of thalidomide as a sleeping aid and treatment of morning sickness in pregnant women came across the desk of FDA's Dr. Frances Kelsey. The drug had been developed in Germany and was in widespread use in several other countries.

The manufacturer lobbied heavily for US approval, but Kelsey was concerned that the application contained no hard data on the drug's safety and included an implausible claim that there was no lethal dose. Kelsey came across a letter in the *British Medical Journal* about cases of peripheral neuritis (nerve damage) in some patients who had taken it, and she questioned why the company had failed to report that. She also asked about safety to the fetus. The unhappy manufacturer went to her supervisor, who backed Kelsey. Kelsey rejected the application four times in a year and a half. When reports emerged in other countries linking the drug to missing or malformed limbs, ultimately identified in some 8,000 newborns, the application was withdrawn. In this famous case, US regulation had been effective.[39]

It may have been a proud accomplishment of the FDA, but the regulatory process has not always been nearly so successful. In ensuring the safety of medical products, the FDA has often been far too deferential to industry. In 1971, for example, there were reports of 150 cases of septicemia and 9 deaths in patients receiving intravenous fluids produced by Abbott Laboratories. But a collaborative response to these reports from the FDA, Abbott, and the Centers for Disease Control stated that "these solutions are essential for patient care and cannot be withdrawn before a replacement is in hand." They recommended continued use but stopping treatment if patients developed signs of septicemia.

Dr. Sidney Wolfe, who worked at NIH, heard about this situation and wrote a letter with Ralph Nader to the FDA commissioner demanding immediate removal of the product from the market, stating that the "FDA is in possession of clear, unequivocal evidence and is not using its powers to get a documented serious hazard off the market." The FDA finally acted the next day, but by the time all cases of septicemia, including fatalities, were accounted for, there had been an estimated 2,000 to 8,000 instances of blood infections with the rare organism *Enterobacter cloacae*, with about 10% of recipients dying.

Wolfe left the NIH to create a Health Research Group in affiliation with Nader's Public Citizen organization. They have challenged the undue deference to industry by the regulators at the FDA. Relying on research, petitions to regulators, litigation, and public advocacy and education, they have had a role in getting banned or limiting the use—sometimes after many years of effort—of 34 unsafe prescription drugs, including those that had been used for pain relief, diabetes, depression, dementia, diet, and sedation.

The pharmaceutical industry and advocacy groups for some diseases (sometimes funded by the pharma companies) have loudly complained about the pace of the approval process in the United States and pressed for streamlining the regulatory process. In response, Congress passed the 1992 Prescription Drug User Fee Act (PDUFA), which further complicated the relationship between the FDA and industry in a number of ways.

For starters, it mandated that the FDA collect fees from producers of drugs and biologics to support its review process. In the beginning, this was a relatively small fraction of the FDA budget devoted to regulatory review. In President Biden's budget for 2021, these "user fees" constituted two-thirds of the $2.022 billion allocation for the Division of Drugs.[40] These funds enable the FDA to hire more staff and upgrade its data systems. But FDA is now financially dependent upon the industry it regulates, a clear conflict of interest.

The industry expects prompt service. FDA scientists feel that they're under pressure to speed up the review process at the cost of weakening standards.[41] PDUFA creates hard deadlines for approval once a New Drug Application is judged to be complete (10 months for many drugs, 6 months for those selected for priority review). This has cut the average approval time in half, from about 13 months to 6.5. As a result, far more drugs are being approved earlier in the US than in other countries with advanced economies. Advocacy groups and the pharmaceutical industry approve of this change. But critics are concerned that by accelerating the review process, the FDA is now more of a partner of the industry than an organization that regulates it and withholds approval when there is uncertainty about safety and effectiveness, as Frances Kelsey once did.[42]

More worrisome, it also has led to an increase in the proportion of drugs later withdrawn because of dangerous adverse effects or for which "black box warnings" to consumers about potentially dangerous complications must appear on packaging.[43] The hard "PDUFA dates" (deadlines for approval) contribute to this situation: drugs approved in the weeks just prior to their PDUFA dates were more likely to be withdrawn or issued black box warnings.[44]

Finally, far more products are being approved, many without evidence that they represent any improvement over existing treatments. The International Society of Drug Bulletins has issued a declaration clarifying that not all new products represent advances that benefit health. They describe three types of "innovation": commercial innovation (a me-too product, or new indications or formulations for an old one); technological innovation (a new delivery system such as a spray or patch, or a new isomer or metabolite carrying the active ingredient); and, most importantly, a therapeutic advance, in which the product actually benefits patients and is superior to other available options. Many new products are designed to extend patents or capture market share from existing successful drugs, rather than to help patients.[45]

The Departments of Health and Human Services and Justice do issue fines to pharmaceutical companies for unlawful promotion, overcharging government programs, monopoly practices, kickbacks, and other offenses, amounting to $3 to $4 billion per year recently. But this is rounding error for industry, and like the user fees, it is a small price to pay for questionable but lucrative business practices.[46] The industry also lines the pockets of thousands of physicians and the institutions in which they work with funding for consultations, participation on advisory boards, speaker bureaus, and the like. As with the PDUFA fees and the fines that they pay, these payments (that are in a searchable database back to January 2014) are all in a day's work.[47]

Marketing of Advances in Medical Technology

Breakthroughs in medical technology have also had important impact on the practice of medicine. Wilhelm Röntgen submitted a paper in 1895 that described a technique for obtaining images of the inside of the human body by sending electrical current through a cathode tube that was partly evacuated to produce a kind of radiation that he called "x-rays." The finding amazed scientists, clinicians, and the general public. Within the year, major institutions like New York Hospital had purchased one of the machines.[48] Willem Einthoven, who introduced the term "electrocardiogram" in 1893, developed a practical device in 1901 and worked out the physiology of what it was measuring. This device, too, rapidly became popular.[49] Both of these inventors received Nobel recognition: Röntgen receiving the first physics prize in 1901, and Einthoven receiving the physiology or medicine prize in 1924.

Since then, there has been enormous expansion in the role of technology in medicine, including diagnostic technologies such as computed tomography (CT), magnetic resonance imaging (MRI), and positron emission tomography (PET), myriad diagnostic laboratory tests, the introduction of robotic surgery, cardiac pacemakers, all of the machines associated with intensive care units, dialysis devices, heart-lung machines for cardiac surgery, and so on.

By some accounts, the introduction of such technologies has contributed the most to increasing the cost of care.[50] No one is suggesting that it all be thrown away. Some of it has saved lives. At the same time, not all increase in life expectancy is attributable to such advances: much more is related to better nutrition, clean water, vaccines, and sanitation.

What is needed is careful assessment of the extent to which such technologies enhance health, and of ways to ensure that they are allocated primarily in situations where they are likely to advance health, rather than being used profligately in other clinical circumstances in which they have little or no value. Indeed, many of these technologies are used much more in the United States (and often cost much more per use). That has not led to better health outcomes in the US than elsewhere. Clinicians, health systems, and manufacturers all benefit financially from greater use of these technologies, however.

Equipment manufacturers induce demand in part by counting on pressure from competing providers in their communities who tout acquisition of their latest toy.[51] There is evidence that acquisition of such technologies may increase the share of a clinical market for a hospital or medical provider group,[52] although some argue that this reflects competition to provide better quality of care.[53]

Some advertising is directed to consumers, highlighting the dazzling technology available at the nearby hospital or clinic. This, too, induces demand among patient populations for procedures using these machines.[54] Abetted by effective marketing, such technology use often spreads rapidly, even in the absence of convincing evidence of its long-term benefit.[55]

Once such a device is acquired, the new owners are motivated to pay it off by maximizing use, thereby generating additional costs. Both the increase in the supply of such technologies and direct-to-consumer advertising of the new equipment are associated with increase in use. The advertising does not consistently provide information on costs versus benefits and risks. Such is the case of imaging studies such as MRIs and CT scans.[56] Accordingly, advertising is effective in inducing demand for particular procedures or devices.[57] The many concerns about the effects of direct-to-consumer advertising of both medications and medical devices and technologies has led the American Medical Association to call for a ban on such advertising.[58]

In addition to other forms of promotion, the medical device companies are fully engaged, along with the pharmaceutical industry (to which they often are linked), in making payments to physicians and hospitals. Between 2013 and 2016, the declared payments by all such corporations totaled more than $9 billion. Genentech was the leader, with payments of $1.088 billion (the great majority for license fees and royalties), but payments by many others exceeded $100 million.[59] Some of the recipients are individual physicians, but many of them are leading academic medical centers.

As discussed previously, beyond the actual cost of machines and devices, health care systems generate other charges every time they are used: a procedure fee; a fee for the doctor who reads the result; fees for performing biopsies, processing pathology specimens, and reading biopsy slides (as in the case of colonoscopies and upper endoscopies); a fee for an anesthesiologist to administer treatments (for procedures in which sedation or anesthesia is used); a fee for the facility where the procedure is done; and charges for medications given to sedate or anesthetize the patient or treat other symptoms. If the procedure produces a result that leads to the need for another test, the cycle is repeated. Multiply this by usage over the entire population, and the expenses can be substantial. As Illinois Senator Everett Dirksen famously said in another context, "A billion here, a billion there, and pretty soon you're talking about real money."

Electronic Health Records

When supervising a hospital ward, I would often spend an hour or more over the course of the day looking for the charts. Medical records were compiled on paper until the 1960s. Sharing of information was labor-intensive and inconsistent. Even within one health system it was often challenging. That began to change in the 1960s, when Lockheed developed a clinical information system that was maintained electronically. In the 1970s, the US government followed suit, introducing an electronic medical record into Veterans Affairs. Other initiatives followed, and in 1991, the Institute of Medicine (now the National Academy of Medicine) recommended that an electronic medical record should be adopted widely. The government established the Office of the National Coordinator (of health information technology) in 2004.

In February 2009, the Health Information Technology for Economic and Clinical Health Act was signed into law as part of the economic stimulus package that the Obama administration introduced to confront the recession. As part of this act, providers would receive higher payments from the government if they met "meaningful use criteria" (using the electronic medical record and meeting some other technical parameters).[60]

The incentives to convert to electronic health records (EHRs) were substantial, and the industry producing them grew explosively. In 2004, about 21% office-based physicians used any kind of electronic record system. That proportion reached 42% in 2008 and 86% in 2017, with 80% meeting the federal standard for such systems.[61] Adoption of such systems by nonfederal acute care hospitals increased from 9% with basic EHR systems in 2008 to 96% with certified systems in 2017.[62]

A few manufacturers of systems for electronic medical records control the majority of the market: in 2021, three companies (EPIC, Cerner, and Meditech) had 72% of the market of more than 5,400 acute care hospitals, representing 84% of all hospital beds. Their market share has been increasing, in part because of consolidation of hospital systems in recent years.[63] These companies acquire smaller vendors, reducing competition. Government policy has pushed almost 90% of practices to acquire these systems, and prices are prohibitive, presenting enormous financial challenges for small groups or individual practices.

The cost to health systems for these products is extraordinary. For example, Mass General Brigham in Boston and the Mayo Clinic in Minnesota each spent more than $1 billion on EPIC systems in the past few years. The New York Health and Hospitals system spent close to $800 million. The US Veterans Affairs health system spent about $10 billion for Cerner's electronic health record rollout in their system.[64]

The electronic record systems used in the private sector prioritize efficient billing over enhancing the quality and efficiency of care. Their lack of user-friendliness erodes clinician face time and eye contact with patients,[65] and aggravates the multifactorial problems of professional dissatisfaction and burnout for benefits in quality of care that are yet to be definitively forthcoming.[66] The electronic records also allow cutting and pasting of prior notes by clinicians in lieu of eliciting careful histories from patients.

Instead, they are designed primarily to improve the efficiency of billing at the highest possible rates, and there is no doubt that they have been successful in this regard. And the electronic health record industry continues to grow rapidly. The global EHR market was valued at about $23.6 billion in 2016 and at $30.6 billion in 2020. It is projected to reach $63.8 billion by 2030.[67]

The producers of medicines, devices, and electronic record systems are not diabolical entities. Certainly, there is much good that emanates from what they produce. But they are not fundamentally in the business of doing good. They are enterprises that seek to maximize their market shares and to extract all that they can from the market, through inducing demand, maximizing revenue, and minimizing any form of regulation that would affect their ability to generate revenue, although not necessarily that which would act as a barrier to smaller companies entering the market. Sometimes, as in the overselling of opioids,[68] they do things that are unmistakably horrible, in ways obvious to everyone. On other occasions, as when the manufacturer worked the regulatory system to gain approval of aducanumab for Alzheimer disease in the absence of clinical trials demonstrating that it delays progression of the disease, then set the price at over $50,000 per year, the harmful consequences of their business practices may be less obvious but are no less serious.[69]

Modern medicines and medical machines can do a great deal of good. Maximizing their benefit to society as a whole is far from the central concern of the corporations that produce these products.

Notes

1. Roberta Labelle, Greg Stoddart, and Thomas Rice, "A Re-examination of the Meaning and Importance of Supplier-Induced Demand," *Journal of Health Economics* 13, no. 3 (October 1994): 347–68, https://doi.org/10.1016/0167-6296(94)90036-1.

2. Ariel Roguin, "Rene Theophile Hyacinthe Laënnec (1781–1826): The Man behind the Stethoscope," *Clinical Medicine and Research* 4, no. 3 (September 2006): 230–35, https://doi.org/10.3121/cmr.4.3.230.

3. J. A. Armstrong, "Urinalysis in Western Culture: A Brief History," *Kidney International* 71, no. 5 (March 1, 2007): 384–87, https://doi.org/10.1038/sj.ki.5002057; Joel D. Howell, *Technology in the Hospital: Transforming Patient Care in the Early Twentieth Century* (Baltimore: Johns Hopkins University Press, 1995), 69–71.

4. Edmund D. Pellegrino, "The Sociocultural Impact of Twentieth Century Therapeutics," in *The Therapeutic Revolution: Essays in the Social History of American Medicine*, ed. Morris J. Vogel and Charles E. Rosenberg (Philadelphia: University of Pennsylvania Press, 1979), 245–66.

5. "Emergence of Pharmaceutical Science and Industry: 1870-–930," *Chemical and Engineering News*, June 20, 2005, https://cen.acs.org/articles/83/i25/EMERGENCE -PHARMACEUTICAL-SCIENCE-INDUSTRY-1870.html; Robin Walsh, "A History of the Pharmaceutical Industry," Pharmaphorum, October 1, 2010, https:// pharmaphorum.com/articles/a_history_of_the_pharmaceutical_industry/; "1920s & 1930s: Salving with Science," in "The Pharmaceutical Century: Ten Decades of Drug Discovery," American Chemical Society, accessed September 10, 2019, http://www3 .uah.es/farmamol/The%20Pharmaceutical%20Century/Ch2.html.

6. Pellegrino, "Sociocultural Impact."

7. Walsh, "History of the Pharmaceutical Industry"; "The Nobel Prize in Physiology or Medicine 1945," Nobel Prize, accessed September 19, 2021, https://www.nobelprize .org/prizes/medicine/1945/summary/.

8. Dana O. Sarnak et al., "Paying for Prescription Drugs around the World: Why Is the U.S. an Outlier?," Issue Brief (Commonwealth Fund) (October 2017): 1–14, https://www.commonwealthfund.org/sites/default/files/documents/___media_files _publications_issue_brief_2017_oct_sarnak_paying_for_rx_ib_v2.pdf.

9. Sarnak et al., "Paying for Prescription Drugs"; Austin Frakt, "Something Happened to U.S. Drug Costs in the 1990s," *New York Times*, November 12, 2018, https://www.nytimes.com/2018/11/12/upshot/why-prescription-drug-spending -higher-in-the-us.html.

10. Aimee Picchi, "Drug Prices in 2019 Are Surging, with Hikes at 5 Times Inflation," CBS News Moneywatch, July 1, 2019, https://www.cbsnews.com/news /drug-prices-in-2019-are-surging-with-hikes-at-5-times-inflation/.

11. "Comparison of U.S. and International Prices for Top Medicare Part B Drugs by Total Expenditures," US Department of Health and Human Services, Office of the Assistant Secretary for Planning and Evaluation, October 24, 2018, https://aspe.hhs .gov/reports/comparison-us-international-prices-top-medicare-part-b-drugs-total -expenditures. One contributing factor is that providers are permitted to charge Medicare 106% of the listed retail price of the drug for medications they dispense directly, while the listed retail price often is substantially greater than what an insurer or government would negotiate or what a hospital and its clinicians would pay. Such discounts are reported to substantially increase profits for hospitals from the cancer drugs they administer. Jeff Lagasse, "Report Claims 340B Hospitals Are Leveraging Discounts to Increase Profits from Cancer Drugs," Healthcare Finance, September 16, 2021, https://www.health carefinancenews.com/news/report-claims -340b-hospitals-are-leveraging-discounts-increase-profits-cancer-drugs.

12. "Observations on Trends in Prescription Drug Spending," ASPE Issue Brief, US Department of Health and Human Services, Office of the Assistant Secretary for Planning and Evaluation (ASPE), March 8, 2016, https://aspe.hhs.gov/system/files /pdf/187586/Drugspending.pdf.

13. Matej Mikulic, "Revenue of Worldwide Pharmaceutical Market from 2001 to 2021 (in Billion U.S. Dollars)," Statista, July 27, 2022, https://www.statista.com /statistics/263102/pharmaceutical-market-worldwide-revenue-since-2001/.

14. Bo Wang and Aaron S. Kesselheim, "The Role of Direct-to-Consumer Advertising in Patient Consumerism," *Virtual Mentor* 15, no. 11 (November 1, 2013): 960–65, https://doi.org/10.1001/virtualmentor.2013.15.11.pfor1-1311.

15. Michael S. Wilkes, Bruce H. Doblin, and Martin F. Shapiro, "Pharmaceutical Advertisements in Leading Medical Journals: Experts' Assessments," *Annals of Internal Medicine* 116, no. 11 (June 1, 1992): 912–19, https://doi.org/10.7326/0003-4819 -116-11-912; David A. Kessler, "Addressing the Problem of Misleading Advertising," *Annals of Internal Medicine* 116, no. 11 (June 1, 1992): 950–51, https://doi.org/10.7326 /0003-4819-116-11-950.

16. Richard P. Kusserow, *Prescription Drug Advertisements in Medical Journals*, OEI-01-90-00482 (Washington, DC: Department of Health and Human Services, Office of Inspector General, June 1992), https://oig.hhs.gov/oei/reports/oei-01-90 -00482.pdf.

17. Wilkes et al., "Pharmaceutical Advertisements"; Kessler, "Addressing the Problem"; Robert H. Fletcher and Suzanne W. Fletcher, "Pharmaceutical Advertisements in Medical Journals," Annals of Internal Medicine 116, no. 11 (June 1, 1992): 951–52, https://doi.org/10.7326/0003-4819-116-11-951; Edward J. Huth and Kathleen Case, "Annals of Internal Medicine at Age 75: Reflections on the Last 25 Years," Annals of Internal Medicine 137, no. 1 (July 2, 2002): 34–45, https://doi.org/10.7326/0003-4819-137-1-200207020-00010; Spencer Rich, "Medical Journal Ads Called Misleading," Washington Post, June 1, 1992, https://www.washingtonpost.com/archive/politics/1992/06/01/medical-journal-ads-called-misleading/1b584e0c-19cc-4ae7-8bd2-c62b636f3e0b/; Lawrence K. Altman, "Study Says Drug Ads in Medical Journals Frequently Mislead," New York Times, June 1, 1992, https://www.nytimes.com/1992/06/01/us/study-says-drug-ads-in-medical-journals-frequently-mislead.html; Alexander C. Tsai, "Conflicts between Commercial and Scientific Interests in Pharmaceutical Advertising for Medical Journals," International Journal of Health Services 34, no. 4 (October 1, 2003): 751–68, https://doi.org/10.2190/K0JG-EXG1-FB12-0ANF.

18. Lisa M. Schwartz and Steven Woloshin, "Medical Marketing in the United States, 1997–2016," JAMA 321, no. 1 (January 1, 2019): 80–96, https://doi.org/10.1001/jama.2018.19320; see also Robert P. Charrow, "Advertising Prescription Drugs," Science 220, no. 4602 (June 10, 1983): 1106, https://doi.org/10.1126/science.6857235.

19. Chris Elkins, "Celebrities Team with Big Pharma to Promote Drugs, Disease Awareness," Drugwatch, November 9, 2015, https://www.drugwatch.com/news/2015/11/09/celebrity-and-big-pharma-drug-promotion/.

20. Richard L. Kravitz et al., "Influence of Patients' Requests for Direct-to-Consumer Advertised Antidepressants: A Randomized Controlled Trial," JAMA 293, no. 16 (April 27, 2005): 1995–2002, https://doi.org/10.1001/jama.293.16.1995; Sara J. Becker and Miriam M. Midoun, "Effects of Direct-to-Consumer Advertising on Patient Requests and Physician Prescribing: A Systematic Review of Psychiatry-Relevant Studies," Journal of Clinical Psychiatry 77, no. 10 (October 2016): e1293–e1300, https://doi.org/10.4088/JCP.15r10325.

21. J. Bradley Layton et al., "Association between Direct-to-Consumer Advertising and Testosterone Testing and Initiation in the United States, 2009–2013," JAMA 317, no. 11 (March 21, 2017): 1159–66, https://doi.org/10.1001/jama.2016.21041; Richard L. Kravitz, "Direct-to-Consumer Advertising of Androgen Replacement Therapy," JAMA 317, no. 11 (March 21, 2017): 1124–25, https://doi.org/10.1001/jama.2017.1364.

22. Lowell E. Schnipper and Gregory A. Abel, "Direct-to-Consumer Advertising in Oncology Is Not Beneficial to Patients or Public Health," JAMA Oncology 2, no. 11 (November 1, 2016): 1397–98, https://doi.org/10.1001/jamaoncol.2016.2463.

23. Arthur G. Lipman, "Direct to Consumer Prescription Drug Advertising: More Harm Than Good," Journal of Pain and Palliative Care Pharmacotherapy 30, no. 3 (September 2016): 176–77, https://doi.org/10.1080/15360288.2016.1210714.

24. Robert Pearl, "The Immorality of Prescription Drug Pricing in America," Forbes, September 24, 2018, https://www.forbes.com/sites/robertpearl/2018/09/24/nostrum/#3f2f1ee64fb1.

25. Katie Thomas, "This New Treatment Could Save the Lives of Babies. But It Costs $2.1 Million," *New York Times*, May 24, 2019, https://www.nytimes.com/2019/05/24/health/zolgensma-gene-therapy-drug.html.

26. Annie Waldman, "Big Pharma Quietly Enlists Leading Professors to Justify $1000-per-Day Drugs," ProPublica, February 23, 2017, https://www.propublica.org/article/big-pharma-quietly-enlists-leading-professors-to-justify-1000-per-day-drugs.

27. Waldman, "Big Pharma."

28. Committee on Oversight and Reform, US House of Representatives, *Drug Price Investigation: AbbVie—Humira and Imbruvica*, staff report (Washington, DC: Committee on Oversight and Reform, May 2021), https://oversight.house.gov/sites/democrats.oversight.house.gov/files/Committee%20on%20Oversight%20and%20Reform%20-%20AbbVie%20Staff%20Report.pdf.

29. David H. Howard et al., "Pricing in the Market for Anticancer Drugs," *Journal of Economic Perspectives* 29, no. 1 (2015): 139–62, https://doi.org/10.1257/jep.29.1.139.

30. Marcia Angell, *The Truth about the Drug Companies: How They Deceive Us and What to Do about It* (New York: Random House, 2004), 52–73.

31. Ekaterina Galinka Cleary et al., "Contribution of NIH Funding to New Drug Approvals 2010–2016," *Proceedings of the National Academy of Sciences of the United States of America* 115, no. 10 (March 6, 2018): 2329–34, https://doi.org/10.1073/pnas.1715368115.

32. John Arnold, "Are Pharmacy Benefit Managers the Good Guys or the Bad Guys of Drug Pricing?," Statnews, accessed June 30, 2019, https://www.statnews.com/2018/08/27/pharmacy-benefit-managers-good-or-bad/.

33. Nathan E. Wineinger, Yunyue Zhang, and Eric J. Topol, "Trends in Prices of Popular Brand-Name Drugs in the United States," *JAMA Network Open* 2, no. 5 (May 3, 2019): e194791, https://doi.org/10.1001/jamanetworkopen.2019.4791.

34. Jake Frankenfield, "Which Industry Spends the Most on Lobbying?," *Investopedia*, May 7, 2020, https://www.investopedia.com/investing/which-industry-spends-most-lobbying-antm-so/. Pfizer, Amgen, and Eli Lilly led the way among 12 companies spending more than $100 million each. These companies also made millions of dollars each in contributions to political campaigns. Olivier J. Wouters, "Lobbying Expenditures and Campaign Contributions by the Pharmaceutical and Health Product Industry in the United States, 1999–2018," *JAMA Internal Medicine* 180, no. 5 (May 1, 2020): 688–97, https://doi.org/10.1001/jamainternmed.2020.0146.

35. So-Yeon Kang et al., "Using External Reference Pricing in Medicare Part D to Reduce Drug Price Differences with Other Countries," *Health Affairs* (Millwood) 38, no. 5 (May 2019): 804–11, https://doi.org/10.1377/hlthaff.2018.05207.

36. Matej Mikulic, "2021 Ranking of the Global Top 10 Biotech and Pharmaceutical Companies Based on Net Income (in Billion U.S. Dollars)," Statista, October 25, 2021, https://www.statista.com/statistics/272720/top-global-biotech-and-pharmaceutical-companies-based-on-net-income/.

37. Randall Smith, "The Private Equity Firm That Quietly Profits on Top-Selling Drugs," *New York Times*, July 8, 2017, https://www.nytimes.com/2017/07/08/business/dealbook/drug-prices-private-equity.html.

38. If the FDA did not disapprove or put a hold on the application within a short interval, the product could be marketed.

39. Stephen Phillips, "How a Courageous Physician-Scientist Saved the U.S. from a Birth-Defects Catastrophe," UChicago Medicine, March 9, 2020, https://www .uchicagomedicine.org/forefront/biological-sciences-articles/courageous-physician -scientist-saved-the-us-from-a-birth-defects-catastrophe.

40. "Human Drugs," in *Justification of Estimates for Appropriations Committees, Fiscal Year 2021* (Washington, DC: Department of Health and Human Services Food and Drug Administration, 2020), 73, https://www.fda.gov/media/135078/download.

41. Sidney M. Wolfe, "Does $760M a Year of Industry Funding Affect the FDA's Drug Approval Process?," BMJ 349 (August 5, 2014): g5012, https://doi.org/10.1136 /bmj.g5012.

42. Michael Gabay, "The Prescription Drug User Fee Act: Cause for Concern?," *Hospital Pharmacy* 53, no. 2 (April 2018): 88–89, https://doi.org/10.1177 /0018578718757519; Jimmy J. Zhuang, "A Legal Challenge of the Prescription Drug User Fee Act," *Journal of Law and Health* 29, no. 1 (October 2016): 85–94, PMID 30866592. By some accounts, employees who approve drugs fare better in the FDA culture than those who reject them, and many move on to industry when they leave the FDA. Farhad Manjoo, "America Desperately Needs a Much Better FDA," *New York Times*, September 2, 2021, https://www.nytimes.com/2021/09/02/opinion/fda-drug -approval-trust.html?searchResultPosition=1).

43. Cassie Frank et al., "Era of Faster FDA Drug Approval Has Also Seen In- creased Black-Box Warnings and Market Withdrawals," *Health Affairs* (Millwood) 33, no. 8 (August 2014): 1453–59, https://doi.org/10.1377/hlthaff.2014.0122.

44. Daniel Carpenter, Evan James Zucker, and Jerry Avorn, "Drug-Review Deadlines and Safety Problems," *New England Journal of Medicine* 358, no. 13 (March 27, 2008): 1354–61, https://doi.org/10.1056/NEJMsa0706341.

45. Gaurav Dwivedi, Sharanabasava Hallihosur, and Latha Rangan, "Evergreen- ing: A Deceptive Device in Patent Rights," *Technology in Society* 32, no. 4 (Novem- ber 2010): 324–30, https://doi.org/10.1016/j.techsoc.2010.10.009; Randall S. Stafford, Todd H. Wagner, and Philip W. Lavori, "New, but Not Improved? Incorporating Comparative-Effectiveness Information into FDA Labeling," *New England Journal of Medicine* 361, no. 13 (September 24, 2009): 1230–33, https://doi.org/10.1056 /NEJMp0906490.

46. "Twenty-Five Years of Pharmaceutical Industry Criminal and Civil Penalties: 1991–2015," Public Citizen, March 31, 2016, www.citizen.org/hrg2311; see also "Fraud Statistics—Overview: October 1, 1986–September 30, 2018," Civil Division, US Department of Justice, accessed March 14, 2022, https://www.justice.gov/civil/page /file/1080696/download; "2020 Year-End False Claims Act Update," Gibson Dunn, January 27, 2021, https://www.gibsondunn.com/2020-year-end-false-claims-act -update/.

47. The database of payments to doctors and hospitals is accessible at the Open Payments website, last updated June 2022, https://openpaymentsdata.cms.gov /search.

48. Howell, *Technology in the Hospital*, 103.

49. Howell, *Technology in the Hospital*, 132.

50. Corinna Sorenson, Michael Drummond, and Beena Bhuiyan Khan, "Medical Technology as a Key Driver of Rising Health Expenditure: Disentangling the Relationship," *ClinicoEconomics and Outcomes Research* 5 (May 30, 2013): 223–24, https://doi.org/10.2147/CEOR.S39634.

51. Dominique Thomas et al., "Direct-to-Consumer Advertising for Robotic Surgery," *Journal of Robotic Surgery* 14 (2020): 17–20, https://doi.org/10.1007/s11701-019-00989-0.

52. Ajay Aggarwal et al., "Effect of Patient Choice and Hospital Competition on Service Configuration and Technology Adoption within Cancer Surgery: A National, Population-Based Study," *Lancet Oncology* 18, no. 11 (November 2017): 1445–53, https://doi.org/10.1016/S1470-2045(17)30572-7.

53. Sean A. Fletcher et al., "Adoption of Robotic Surgery: Driven by Market Competition or Desire to Improve Patient Care?," *Lancet Oncology* 19, no. 2 (February 2018): e66, https://doi.org/10.1016/S1470-2045(18)30021-4.

54. Judy Illes et al., "Advertising, Patient Decision Making, and Self-Referral for Computed Tomographic and Magnetic Resonance Imaging," *Archives of Internal Medicine* 164, no. 22 (December 13–27, 2004): 2415–19, https://doi.org/10.1001/archinte.164.22.2415.

55. Dragan Ilic et al., "Laparoscopic and Robotic-Assisted versus Open Radical Prostatectomy for the Treatment of Localized Prostate Cancer," *Cochrane Database of Systemic Reviews* 9, no. 9 (September 12, 2017): CD009625, https://doi.org/10.1002/14651858.CD009625.pub2.

56. Edson de Oliveira Andrade, Elizabeth Nogueira de Andrade, and José Hiran Gallo, "Case Study of Supply Induced Demand: The Case of Provision of Imaging Scans (Computed Tomography and Magnetic Resonance) at Unimed-Manaus," *Revista da Associacão Médica Brasiliera* 57, no. 2 (March–April 2011): 138–43, https://doi.org/10.1590/s0104-42302011000200009; Illes, "Advertising."

57. Mohamad J. Halawi and Wael K. Barsoum, "Direct-to-Consumer Marketing: Implications for Patient Care and Orthopedic Education," *American Journal of Orthopedics* 45, no. 6 (September/October 2016): E335–36, https://cdn.mdedge.com/files/s3fs-public/ajo04509335e.PDF.

58. "AMA Calls for Ban on DTC Ads of Prescription Drugs and Medical Devices," AMA Press Center, November 17, 2015, https://www.ama-assn.org/press-center/press-releases/ama-calls-ban-dtc-ads-prescription-drugs-and-medical-devices; Michael McCarthy, "US Physician Group Calls for Ban on Direct to Consumer Drug Advertising," *BMJ* 351 (November 18, 2015): h6230, https://doi.org/10.1136/bmj.h6230.

59. Medtronic, a device manufacturer, spent $431 million through three companies (Medtronic USA, Medtronic Vascular, and Medtronic Sofamor Danek USA). DePuy Synthes, a purveyor of orthopedic and neurosurgical devices and a subsidiary of Johnson and Johnson, dispensed $309 million. Stryker Corporation, whose devices include implantable joints, surgical and endoscopic equipment, and communication systems, handed out $217 million. Zimmer Biomet, which was spun

off from Bristol Myers Squibb and makes orthopedic devices, sent along $309 million during that time. Mike Tigas, Ryann Grochowski Jones, and Charles Ornstein, "Dollars for Docs," ProPublica, accessed September 23, 2019, https://projects .propublica.org/docdollars/. Data for 2018 show that many of these companies have further increased these outlays. In that year, for example, Genentech spent $478 million, Zimmer Biomet $109 million, and Stryker $91.9 million. Mike Tigas et al., "Dollars for Docs: How Industry Dollars Reach Your Doctors," ProPublica, October 17, 2019, https://projects.propublica.org/docdollars/.

60. Gabby Marquez, "The History of Electronic Health Records (EHRs)," *Elation Health*, August 4, 2017, https://www.elationhealth.com/clinical-ehr-blog/history -ehrs/.

61. "Office-Based Physician Electronic Record Adoption," Office of the National Coordinator for Health Information Technology, January 2019, https://dashboard .healthit.gov/quickstats/pages/physician-ehr-adoption-trends.php.

62. "Non-Federal Acute Care Hospital Electronic Health Record Adoption," Office of the National Coordinator for Health Information Technology, September 2017, https://dashboard.healthit.gov/quickstats/pages/FIG-Hospital-EHR -Adoption.php.

63. The respective shares were: EPIC with 31% of hospitals and 42% of hospital beds, Cerner with 25% of hospitals and 27% of hospital beds, and Meditech with 16% of hospitals and 15% of hospital beds. Rajiv Leventhal, "The Top EHR Vendors by Hospital Market Share," KLAS Healthcare Innovation, June 9, 2021, https://www .hcinnovationgroup.com/finance-revenue-cycle/health-it-market/news/21226099 /the-top-ehr-vendors-by-hospital-market-share-klas; Mandy Roth, "In EMR Market Share Wars, Epic and Cerner Triumph Yet Again," HealthLeaders Media, April 30, 2019, https://www.healthleadersmedia.com/innovation/emr-market-share-wars- epic-and-cerner-triumph-yet-again; Heather Landl, "Epic, Cerner Growing EHR Market Share with Increased Hospital Consolidation: KLAS," Fierce Healthcare, April 30, 2019, https://www.fiercehealthcare.com/tech/epic-cerner-growing-ehr -market-share-increased-hospital-consolidation-klas.

64. "8 Epic EHR Implementations with the Biggest Price Tags in 2015," Becker's Health IT & CIO Report, July 1, 2015, https://www.beckershospitalreview.com /healthcare-information-technology/8-epic-ehr-implementations-with-the-biggest -price-tags-in-2015.html; Kate Monica, "Top 5 Most Expensive EHR Implementa- tions of 2017," EHR Intelligence, November, 29, 2017, https://ehrintelligence.com /news/top-5-most-expensive-ehr-implementations-of-2017; Bill Siwicki, "NYC Health + Hospitals Adds $289 Million Revenue Cycle System to Epic EHR," Health- care Finance, May 5, 2017, https://www.healthcarefinancenews.com/news/nyc -health-hospitals-adds-289-million-revenue-cycle-system-epic-ehr.

65. Danielle Ofri, "Empathy in the Age of the Electronic Medical Record," *Lancet* 394, no. 10201 (September 7, 2019): 822–23, https://doi.org/10.1016/S0140 -6736(19)32036-7.

66. Atul Gawande, "Why Doctors Hate Their Computers," *New Yorker*, November 12, 2018, https://www.newyorker.com/magazine/2018/11/12/why-doctors-hate

-their-computers; Philip J. Kroth et al., "Association of Electronic Health Record Design and Use Factors with Clinician Stress and Burnout," *JAMA Network Open* 2, no. 8 (August 2, 2019): e199609, https://doi.org/10.1001/jamanetworkopen.2019.9609; Mary K. Pratt, "EHR Market Consolidation and the Impact on Physicians," *Medical Economics*, January 2, 2019, www.medicaleconomics.com/business/ehr-market-consolidation-and-impact-physicians; Erica Fry and Fred Schulte, "Death by a Thousand Clicks: Where Electronic Health Records Went Wrong," *Fortune*, March 18, 2019, https://fortune.com/longform/medical-records/.

67. "Electronic Health Records Market Overview," Allied Market Research, February 2022, https://www.alliedmarketresearch.com/electronic-health-records-EHR-market; "Global Electronic Health Records Market Share and Trends Expected to Reach USD 40 Billion by 2026: Facts and Figures," Global Newswire, June 1, 2021, https://www.globenewswire.com/en/news-release/2021/06/01/2239627/0/en/Global-Electronic-Health-Records-Market-Share-Trends-Expected-to-Reach-USD-40-Billion-by-2026-Facts-Factors.html.

68. Melissa Healy, "Who's to Blame for the Nation's Opioid Crisis? Massive Trial May Answer That Question," *Los Angeles Times*, September 18, 2019, https://www.latimes.com/science/story/2019-09-17/opioid-lawsuit-who-is-to-blame; Washington Post Staff, "The Opioid Files: Follow the *Post*'s Investigation of the Epidemic," *Washington Post*, January 24, 2020, https://www.washingtonpost.com/national/2019/07/20/opioid-files/?arc404=true.

69. Elisabeth Rosenthal, "Why We May Never Know Whether the $56,000 Alzheimer's Drug Actually Works," *Washington Post*, July 7, 2021, https://www.washingtonpost.com/opinions/2021/07/07/why-we-may-never-know-whether-56000-alzheimers-drug-actually-works/.

Dialogue #8

Student: These corporations are shameless. The business model is to gain control of the market, induce demand, name your price point, then complain that any government constraint will stifle innovation.

Professor: With profit margins that are among the highest in any industry, they are many orders of constraint away from ceasing to want to develop new products. And raising prices on older products is hardly the kind of innovation that society needs.

Student: Professor, speaking of corporate misbehavior, we should look at the insurance industry.

Professor: Absolutely, and while we do that, we also should explore the many ways in which the structure and financing of the system and even the behavior of governments cause American health care to fall far short of what the population needs.

Student: Ah, yes. But why group government with the insurance industry. Government isn't part of the problem. Government is the solution.

Professor: I know you believe that. But think for a moment of government not as an immutable abstract idea, but rather as a diverse set of actors implementing policies, or failing to do so, over time.

Student: I can see that governments may not always do the right thing.

Professor: Keep in mind that we are interested in why the United States is where it is, in terms of the relative roles of governments and the private sector, in providing insurance or covering the costs of care. We need to examine past failed efforts to address these challenges. How do you think that we should approach this topic?

Student: Maybe we should describe some of the problems with the ways in which Americans finance health care, then assemble information on how other countries got to a different system. That may help us understand why the United States didn't go down the same road.

Professor: That's an excellent idea. We shouldn't idealize those efforts abroad. Indeed, we might learn something from how they have addressed problems that they have encountered. Just as there are positive and negative actions by all the other players we've been considering, I suspect we'll find that's the case for governments as well.

Student: Problems in the US with health care financing, issues with governments and insurers, and reforms efforts abroad and in the US. We may need two chapters to cover all that.

10

Human Rights and Wrong Turns

Some Problems with Health Care Financing, American Style

Justice will not be served until those who are unaffected are as outraged as those who are.
—Benjamin Franklin

I will not reproduce here the considerable documentation of how scandalously bad American health care is. It costs far more per capita than care in any other country. It fails to cover the entire population. Health outcomes (including life expectancy) are poor compared to many countries at similar levels of affluence. At the same time, particular features of this intractable system are especially problematic and deserve mention.

Copayments
Penalty

I had a chronic skin problem called atopic dermatitis, or eczema, for which I had been treated since early childhood. It was well controlled with steroid cream, so I only went to a dermatologist about once a year. As I was getting ready to head off to university late one summer, I scheduled my dermatology appointment. When I went to the office for my appointment, the receptionist told me that I owed $4.

"For what?" I asked.

"It is a penalty for missing your last appointment a year ago."

"OK. I will send the payment in."

"The doctor will not see you unless you make this payment now."

"I don't have any money with me," I told her. (This was 1970, and I did not have a credit card.)

"Well, then, you will have to come back when you have the payment."

"But I am leaving tomorrow for Montreal. Medical school is starting in a few days," I said. "I really need to see him."

The receptionist went into the back room, returning a few minutes later. "He will see you."

I was greatly relieved and proceeded to the doctor's examining room. He was looking at a chart as I entered and did not look up. "I understand that you are in medical school," he said.

I was fumbling with the zipper on my pants. It was stuck. I knew that he booked four patients every 15 minutes, so I was concerned that I might not get my pants down to reveal the rash on my leg in my aliquot of 3 minutes and 45 seconds. "Yes, I am."

"Well, that is the only reason that I will see you today," he said.

That experience has stayed me all these years. I would have survived without the dermatology appointment, but I realized that even what may seem like a minor financial barrier can stand in the way of medical care.

Skin in the Game

In many countries, health care is considered a basic right. While there are certain gaps in some programs (prescription medicines in Canada, for example), basic services tend to be covered, often with no associated charges. When I came to the United States to study health care delivery, I heard the word "copayment" for the first time. Although I had spent time in my training studying health care delivery and access (and even had worked on a government policy document in Manitoba), I had never come across that word until I attended a seminar at UCLA, given by an economist from the RAND Corporation. As I then learned, the US system is built on the assumption that having "skin in the game" (and not only on visits to a dermatologist), by paying part of the cost out-of-pocket, will deter people from using medical care when they don't really need it, while not causing harmful effects.

Granted, there was debate about whether copayments were harmful to patients. Having come from Canada, which had just completed adoption a few years earlier of a universal health insurance program, in which there were no deductibles or copayments (except for medications), I was surprised to learn that serious consideration was being given in the US to making people continue to pay part of the cost. At the time, there was an expectation that the United States was moving toward adopting universal coverage. The question was, What would that coverage look like? Would it mean free care, as in Canada or the United Kingdom? There was at least some evidence emerging that even small payments could be harmful, by impeding access for some to needed care.

Copayments obviously can matter a lot to people who have little or no money. A study in Utah found that $2 copayments for Medicaid patients led to reduction in doctor visits and that $3 copayments reduced use of doctor visits even more. The study also found that $2 copayments for medicines reduced use of prescription drugs.[1] Another study in Quebec, Canada, found that when the government introduced copayments for medications among welfare recipients (capped at $200 per year), there was a reduction in use of nonessential medications and a reduction in the use of medicines that are essential to either treat or prevent disease. Associated with this change, there was an 88% increase in visits to emergency rooms and a 78% increase in hospitalizations.[2]

A study of TennCare (Tennessee Medicaid) found that when copayments were imposed in the program, 20% could not make the copayments for doctor visits, 22% were unable to do so for medications, and that two-thirds of those unable to afford the medication copayments went without those medications.[3] These findings were not at all surprising. An earlier study of a $1 copayment in New Hampshire Medicaid, instituted in 1982, found that the $1 fee reduced the number of prescriptions filled by 30%. The decrease was largest for medications judged to be ineffective (58%), but there was also a significant drop for medicines essential to health, including a 28% drop for insulin.[4] It is hard to imagine that people who were taking insulin did not really need it.

The most influential study of the impact of copayments on costs and outcomes of health care was conducted in the late 1970s by researchers at the RAND Corporation. This was a randomized trial of different kinds of insurance coverage for health care: free versus various levels of copayments or deductibles, at six US locations.[5] The RAND study reported that free care cost a lot more because people used more care. In their initial reports, they also found only modest evidence of an effect on health. There are numerous reasons to question the generalizability of their findings.

First, they did not study the effect of free care throughout a community, which would have been too expensive to study and unwieldy to undertake as an experiment (which requires comparing two randomly assigned treatments in a population at the same time). In most of the study sites, a small proportion of the population participated. In a real-world setting, if everyone had free care, use might have increased somewhat, but it would have run into the problem of the supply of providers. In the absence of unused capacity, or of doctors and nurses working longer hours, there might well have been little increase in use and somewhat longer waiting times for appointments.

Second, other economists observed that when people in this study were randomized to free care or copayment, more of the copayment patients dropped out when they learned that they did not get free care; the ones who stayed in that group may have been less motivated to use a lot of care. The copayment group also may have been less likely to report their expenditures for the care they used if they had not yet covered the deductible (costs that the patient pays before insurance kicks in).[6] Third, countries with systems in which people can get care without making copayments have done a better job of controlling costs than the United States, notably by limiting the rates of procedures of little or no value and by limiting what the service providers get paid.[7]

Fourth, they carefully evaluated health outcomes, but the study excluded people who were completely disabled or older than 62 because those people would qualify for Medicare coverage during the study. Thus those participating were a relatively healthy population. Participants were only studied for three to five years, probably not long enough to see harmful effects, such as development of chronic diseases, in a relatively young and healthy population. For acute problems like strokes, heart attacks, and severe bleeding, people might well seek emergency care regardless of insurance coverage.

Even so, the study did report some differences. Those with copayments had worse vision, worse blood pressure control, and a worse calculated risk of dying among those that began the study in the lowest 20% of both health status and income.[8] For families making copayments, children had more anemia and dental problems, and decreased use of outpatient care, for both prevention and acute illness episodes.[9] Copayments decreased adult outpatient visits, but at comparable rates for serious symptoms (like chest pain and passing out) and minor ones, and were associated with an increase by the end of the study in the rate of serious symptoms among those who began the intervention with low income and poor health.[10]

Notwithstanding such concerns, the RAND study has been cited as evidence in support of copayments much larger than any that the RAND investigators ever envisioned, and that now can amount to thousands of dollars with some kinds of insurance. Many patients who declare bankruptcy report that health care expenses and lost income due to illness were the main cause. Their numbers appear to be increasing: from 46.2% in a five-state 2001 study to 62.1% in a 2007 national survey in which 29% cited medical bills as a reason for bankruptcy and 40% mentioned income loss due to illness (some specified both). In a similar survey in 2013–16, 66.5% cited a medical cause as contributing to their bankruptcy, among whom 58.5% mentioned medical expenses and 44.3% lost income due to illness).[11] Another study estimated that in early 2020, $140 billion in medical debt was in the hands of collection agencies in the US and that 17.8% of individuals had medical debt, with the rate being highest in the southern states, in states that did not expand Medicaid, and in zip codes with the lowest incomes.[12]

Choosing between Health Care and Other Basic Necessities

The comedian Jack Benny, whose stage persona was parsimonious in the extreme, had a famous routine in which a gun-wielding robber accosts him on the street, demanding "your money or your life." Benny responds with silence. His assailant, increasingly impatient, repeats his demand. "I'm thinking," Benny replies at last. In modern medical care, commodified to the gills, everyone is asked to make the same choice. Ironically, patients tend not to know how much their care is going to cost because pricing is not transparent. Few would buy an automobile without knowing the cost and what others are charging for it. Yet many medical acts, particularly those involving hospitalization, are far more expensive than cars, and the patients have no idea what they will have to pay.[13]

In American health care, people are being asked all the time to choose between their health care and other basic needs. In a study of persons with HIV disease in the United States, fully 11.5% of those in care for HIV reported that they had gone without health care to address other necessities such as food, clothing, or housing, and 7.6% had gone without those necessities in order to pay for health care.[14] Nor are such findings limited to those with HIV. In poor populations, such as those attending free clinics, an even higher proportion confront a trade-off analogous to that faced by Jack Benny.[15]

Private Insurance and Its Sequelae
Cost of Insurance

Most Americans who have health insurance coverage get it from private insurance policies, whether through their employer or private purchase. There are a number of problems with these policies. One is that they cost a lot and don't provide particularly good value. Insurers do offer some products that are less expensive, but many of those have high deductibles and copayments, as well as limitations to coverage. The Affordable Care Act (ACA) addressed insurance cost for a proportion of the population. The expense of policies that are not subsidized by employers or ACA programs is an important contributor to the high rate at which Americans continue to be uninsured. Are these prices inevitable? The forces driving up utilization in American health care also drive up the cost of health insurance, but other factors also contribute to this situation. Insurance corporations extract large profits from their businesses and have substantial administrative costs that contribute to putting health insurance out of reach for many.

Administrative Costs and Their Consequences

The health insurance industry has blossomed into a big business in the United States. In 2020, 1,096 such corporations were on file with the National Association of Insurance Commissioners, up from 864 in 2009, with net revenue of $31.4 billion, representing 3.8% of premiums of $824 billion. They reported that administrative costs plus surplus revenue was 17.2% of the health insurance premiums, as written in 2020 (compared to 14.2% in 2009).[16]

Health services researchers David Himmelstein and Steffie Woolhandler of City University of New York and Harvard and Terry Campbell of the University of Ottawa compared administrative costs in US and Canadian health care in 2017. They noted that industry overhead expenses are only part of the administrative costs of dealing with health insurance in the United States. Other components include the expenses of hospitals, nursing homes, hospices, doctors' offices, and home care organizations in billing for services. They estimate that these costs amount to $812 billion in the US, or $2,457 per capita, compared to $551 per capita in Canada. Their estimates (based on national data from both countries) include insurer overhead ($844 per capita in the US, $146 in Canada); hospital administration ($933 in the US, $196 in Canada); nursing home, home care, and hospice administration ($255 in the US, $123 in Canada); and physician insurance-related costs ($465 in the US, $87 in Canada).

Overall, these administrative costs amounted to about 34% of health care expenditures in the US and 17% in Canada in 2017. The researchers reported that administrative costs in the US had grown as a percentage of health care costs by 3.2 percentage points since 1999, of which three-quarters was attributable to increased overhead in the private insurance sector.

Much of the difference in the administrative costs of hospitals and doctors' offices involves the challenge of interacting with insurers and collecting payments from patients. To assess doctors' costs, they used estimates from another study that the average doctor's staff spends about 80 hours per week interacting with payers (insurers and patients) in the US, compared to about 21 hours per week in Canada.[17]

What is gained by all of this? Insurance companies protest that they provide many jobs. They do, as did the railroads when they employed workers to shovel coal to power their engines. Having the insurance sector derive profit from what they do makes health care more expensive. Being inefficient makes care more expensive. At one time, there were major not-for-profit insurers, but they have since become for-profit companies. Insurance is a commodity to sell, as is health care.

Complexity of Policies

One frustrating feature of health insurance in the United States is its complexity. There are copayments (what you pay when you go for care to a doctor's office, or to purchase a prescription), deductibles (what you must spend before insurance kicks in), coinsurance (the percentage of the cost of care that you pay personally once you have met your deductible, which may be different, e.g., between primary care settings and the emergency department), out-of-pocket limits (the most you have to pay in a year for care), annual or lifetime limits for certain services, charges for out-of-network care, pharmaceutical benefits, hospital care charges, and so on. The purchaser of insurance also needs to figure out which providers are in or out of their network. This requires a set of skills that are not needed in other countries to nearly the same extent, if at all: so-called health insurance literacy.[18]

Insurers do provide enrollees with statements about all of these details, but they are impenetrable even to sophisticated readers. When a person participates in a research study, they receive an informed consent form to read and sign. The form is typically aimed at the level of a person with a ninth-grade education. Health insurance policies are a long way from passing muster in this regard.

In- and Out-of-Network

Even when you figure out which primary care doctors or specialists are in your network, there is no guarantee that you will be able to go to that doctor for an extended period. Doctors contract with insurers, often as part of a medical group. If that group does not negotiate a renewal of the contract with an insurer, you can't keep going to that doctor at the much lower cost for in-network providers. Defenders of the current system in the United States often say that the US preserves "freedom of choice" for patients to go to their preferred doctor. The reality is that a country like Canada has much more freedom of choice. As long as you can get an appointment there, you can go to virtually any doctor. In the US, this is not the case.[19]

US insurance clinical networks are associated with even more problems when people are hospitalized. Even if you see a surgeon in-network, the anesthesiologist may be out-of-network. If you go to a hospital that is in-network, they may have doctors working in the emergency room who are not part of the network. One study of privately insured patients who were admitted to an in-hospital network found that 11.8% of the anesthesiology charges, 12.3% of pathologist charges, 5.6% of radiology care, and 11.3% of times in which an assistant surgeon was involved were billed as out-of-network. These are situations in which the patient has no control over who participates in their care, yet the out-of-pocket consequences can be substantial.[20] Efforts to rein in these "surprise bills" have not yet been successful.[21]

Denial of Coverage

When my wife was pregnant, she had an amniocentesis, an entirely appropriate and covered procedure, but coverage was denied at the time the amniocentesis was performed. It took many hours of calls, arguments, and pursuit of additional documentation to get it covered. We absolutely questioned whether it was worth that effort, frustration, and lost opportunities to spend the time doing other things (work, visiting with friends, playing with children, etc.) to deal with the hassle.

Denial of insurance payment is an enormous problem in American medicine. Sometimes, patients learn about it after the fact, when the fine print in their policy does not identify their treatment as a "covered service." On other occasions, the service is coverable, but not, in the judgment of the person processing the claim, for the patient's particular problem or level of disease severity. Still other times, the insurer may refuse to pay for a particular act even if it meets every conceivable requirement for coverage. The insurers create bureaucratic barriers to rectifying errors that lead to the refusal to reimburse the patient. My wife and I both have had medical educations and knew that her amniocentesis qualified for coverage. We also had enough flexibility in our work circumstances to take the time to address this issue.

While some people overcome these nefarious obstacles, many do not because they don't have the time, the assertiveness, or the sophistication to challenge denials of coverage, or even the understanding that they can contest them. Insurers vary in their frequencies of claims denials, but for some it may be as much as 40% of the time. If even a portion of these ultimately are not paid, they represent a financial gain for the insurance company.[22]

Separate and Unequal
Good Insurance, Bad Insurance, or No Insurance

Most would agree that the persistent large number of people lacking insurance in the United States is a bad thing. But insurance in itself is no guarantee of decent medical care in this country. The benefits associated with such care are severely stratified. In particular, the 74 million people covered by Medicaid have inferior access to the care available to most others with health insurance. Many doctors will not see someone covered by Medicaid because reimbursement is much lower. In one recent analysis, only 67.3% of primary care physicians in the United States were accepting new Medicaid patients, even after the Affordable Care Act legislation increased the fees for primary care for a short period.

The low participation levels may have been related to the fact that the increase in the fees for primary care of Medicaid patients was temporary. In 2015, the year after the fee increase went away, participation fell to 63.7%. By comparison, primary care doctors were accepting Medicare and privately insured patients at substantially higher rates (82.4% and 84.5%, respectively, in 2015).[23] Even in the states with relatively generous Medicaid reimbursement, it is still second-class insurance, and there is no guarantee that a doctor will accept your Medicaid coverage for payment.

When politicians talk about the US having the greatest health care in the world, they can't seriously contend that that is true for everyone. When we examined who received lifesaving treatment for HIV disease in the United States shortly after highly acting antiretroviral therapy became available, we found that it tracked strongly with type of insurance: those with private insurance fared the best, and Medicare beneficiaries did next best. Those with Medicaid coverage lagged far behind and tracked more closely with those who lacked any insurance than with those covered by private insurance or Medicare.[24]

In another particularly poignant situation, the difference between good and bad insurance can mean the difference between life and death: liver, heart, and lung transplantation. Once someone is on a transplant list, they are eligible for a replacement organ, although retired baseball superstars, computer billionaires, and gangsters from abroad have been guilty of cutting in line.[25] The biggest challenge is getting on that list. Often, people are denied because they are judged to lack the social support to adhere appropriately to treatment. Those of lower socioeconomic status and people with Medicaid insurance are more likely to have that judgment rendered against them and to have their prospects for staying alive extinguished.

For example, patients with liver cancer who had Medicaid insurance were much less likely to get a liver transplant, surgical resection of the tumor, or intraarterial ablation than were those with private insurance.[26] African Americans also were less likely to be listed or to receive liver transplants when they had liver failure.[27] Among patients with heart failure that is so severe that they need a left ventricular assist device to stay alive, Medicaid patients were more than 50% more likely than those with private insurance to die while waiting for a heart transplant.[28]

Someone Else's Problem

While hospitals in many states are obliged to provide some care to anyone who enters through the emergency room, many of them meet the bare requirements of that obligation, but do no more, when it comes to patients covered by Medicaid (and, of course, those who do not have insurance). Anti-dumping laws in many states do not allow them to throw patients out onto the street. But ongoing follow-up care (which has been shown to decrease serious complications and readmissions) is something else.[29]

Sometimes, these hospitals will provide one follow-up visit to such patients, but sometimes not even that, however unstable their condition. As for ongoing care, the attitude is YOYO (you're on your own): Many patients are expected to go to a public clinic or a free clinic, where continuity often is challenging because clinics depend upon on the contributed labor of volunteer clinicians. Access to needed specialty care in such situations is highly problematic.[30]

The variable generosity of reimbursement by insurance type allows providers and health systems to make socially regressive and unethical decisions at some remove from the consequences of their actions. For doctors who do not accept insurance, hospitals that do not contract with Medicaid, and health care systems that do not provide specialty care in selected clinical areas to the Medicaid beneficiary or to the uninsured individual, each such policy involves a decision to make more money by avoiding patients for whom they are paid less. The ethics are problematic but are never challenged because the health care executive and even the clinical service chief may never be face-to-face with the patient or even with others who deal with the patient.

The structure of the system invites unethical or immoral acts. It makes the providers less honorable people. Even though they may feel that the decision is out of their control, the act of choosing to work in such settings reflects their ethical choices and, in the end, their character. As for teaching hospitals, where students and postgraduate trainees learn about the norms of acceptable professional behavior, we have already seen that the institutions that do take on patients with less desirable insurance generally relegate their ongoing care to the residents and fellows.

The Uninsured, the Underinsured, and Where the Poor Must Go

How consequential is it that many people lack health insurance and have to seek overcrowded public facilities or free clinics for their medical care? When Mitt Romney was running for president, he said that the poor could go to emergency rooms when they were sick.[31] Care for chronic diseases requires something more than that. To what extent is acute disease care equitable (as implied by Romney), given the potential for admission to the hospital? First, not all acute illnesses need to be treated in a hospital. Second, preventative treatment, such as early diagnosis of infections, can avert worse complications. Third, part of acute care is what happens after the admission to the hospital. Poor people are more likely to die of strokes after they have been hospitalized because they get less of the supportive care that can be lifesaving.[32]

Specifying that people can go to the emergency department when they are acutely ill does not begin to address the problem. Poor people die at younger ages from the consequences of chronic diseases. Rules that guarantee emergency department and hospital access in acute illness are no more than a smokescreen for a system that tolerates the death of the "undeserving" poor.

As for the public hospitals and clinics, *care that is separate is not equal*, and it will never be even close to comparable. As discussed previously, public hospitals are intended for the poor. Other people end up there almost only in emergency situations. The creature comforts are fewer. The sophisticated equipment is less available. The staffing is not as good. These hospitals do take care of patients with Medicaid, along with the uninsured. Once people reach the age at which they qualify for Medicare, the vast majority go elsewhere. The same is true of those who eventually obtain private insurance (generally through a job).

When living in Los Angeles, I hosted a visiting journalist from Toronto who was doing a series of newspaper articles on the American health care system. When we talked about the tiers in the system, she wanted to see what that looked like. I took her to two emergency rooms, one at Los Angeles County / University of Southern California Hospital, which is the largest of three general hospitals run by the County of Los Angeles. It takes care of a poor population, many of whom lack any health insurance or are covered by Medicaid. The other, UCLA Hospital (now bearing the name of Ronald Reagan), is publicly owned (by the University of California) and caters largely to people with private insurance and Medicare who live nearby.

On the day we visited UCLA, a man came in with an injury to his orbit (the bones around the eye). He had been hit in the face by a ball when playing handball. When we went to LA County Hospital, we saw a man come in with virtually the same injury: trauma and bleeding around the orbit. This man was in handcuffs, however, and was accompanied by the police.

Even though emergency departments (EDs) are supposed to be available to all who come, public hospital EDs care almost exclusively for the disadvantaged, while voluntary hospital EDs in the better neighborhoods generally attract a different clientele. The care of disadvantaged populations is inevitably more complex. Even when the presenting problems are the same, social context and its consequences are often different.

The Disparities Keep Growing

In the United States, there is rationing of the supply and the quality of care for those who do not have "good" insurance coverage. Each community and state have responsibility for their uninsured populations, which while diminished by the Affordable Care Act, persist in large numbers. Most have public hospitals that are intended to care for them. But these facilities do not have nearly the resources of many private sector hospitals, and this has predictable implications for the quality of care that they can provide. The latter often have donor bases and high operating margins that put them in a position to acquire high-quality facilities and equipment. During the COVID-19 pandemic, the differences across hospitals in the US in their ability to respond to the surge in sick patients was apparent.[33]

Different Boats

Because Americans obtain coverage for health care services from a variety of public and private sources, the decisions made by all levels of government affect them differentially.

The Relentless Rise in Public Program Costs

Understandably, governments at all levels in the United States are anxious to limit expenditures. From the time that Medicare and Medicaid were implemented, costs have increased enormously. When Medicaid was introduced in the US in 1966, the budget the first year was less than $0.9 billion. In 2018, it cost $629.3 billion. Given that Lyndon Johnson agreed to it as a last-minute add-on to the Medicare bill as an attempt to do something for the poor, he could hardly have imagined how much the program would grow.[34]

Medicare in the United States costs about as much as Medicaid, reaching $776 billion in 2020. Whereas 75% of Medicare expenditures in

1970 were covered by payroll taxes and premiums and 25% had to be covered by general government revenues, by 2020, general revenues were needed to cover 47% of the costs because of a decline in the proportion that payroll taxes were available to cover. Part of the explanation for this situation is that the Medicare payroll tax is a flat tax of 2.9% on income, of which the employer and employee each pay half. On income above $200,000, individuals pay an additional 0.9%. Were it treated as a progressive income tax, more revenue could be generated without penalizing the lowest-income earners.[35]

The rising cost of health care has been a major burden in the United States. For all programs that federal, state, and local governments run, they need at least a plan of how they intend to generate revenue to cover their costs over time. Governments averse to revenue generation (taxes) are not inclined to fund the programs at a high level. They look for ways to limit spending. Some of the mechanisms for achieving that goal, such as copayments that deter use of services by those who need them, limiting coverage, and limiting eligibility, can be harmful, as we have seen. Other strategies, such as methods to increase efficiency (by eliminating services that are of low value, incentivizing patients and providers to use less care, or cutting payments to providers), also have the potential to affect populations differentially.

All of these potential policy levers can have some effect on costs, but they also have the potential to harm some patients, depending on how they are implemented. In the United States, there is justifiable concern that these kinds of interventions could increase racial, ethnic, and socioeconomic disparities in care, and they have faced vigorous opposition from groups concerned about this possibility.[36] In the end, the governments muddle through, in accordance with their political priorities and general philosophies and the extent of the pushback from interested groups of patients, providers, insurers, and producers. What is almost always the case is that the allocation decisions are only infrequently based primarily on what will optimize health.

Who Cares about Health Care for the Poor?
Variation in State Programs

In the face of the enormous increase in the cost of public programs, political attitudes in the states affect what the state governments are willing to fund. This is notably different from the situation in Canada, where government resources differ by province but there is a recognized obligation to take care of the entire population, all of whom are covered by provincial insurance programs with the same basic characteristics.

Medicaid is a nationwide, state-run program that receives substantial funding from the US government. Many of the states seriously underfund their Medicaid programs by limiting eligibility for enrollment to the poorest, by paying much less for the services (which leads many doctors not to participate), and by limiting generosity of benefits (kinds of medications, kinds of procedures allowed, etc.). The parsimonious politicians responsible for these relative deprivations do not seem to suffer electorally, since the poor have relatively few champions in the state assemblies and almost no lobbyists to make their case.

With the implementation of the Affordable Care Act, all states had an opportunity to expand the income eligibility threshold for Medicaid from 100% to 138% of the Federal Poverty Level (FPL), with the federal government paying 100% of the cost of the expansion initially, then 90% after that. As of October 2021, 12 states still have not agreed to the expansion. Three other states—Missouri, Nebraska, and Oklahoma—had only implemented expansion in 2020 and 2021 after their hands were forced by ballot initiatives approving the expansion. Of the 12 non-expansion states, only one—Wisconsin—was covering families up to the prior allowable threshold of 100% of the FPL. The other 11 continue to be far more restrictive, with eligibility thresholds as low 18% of FPL in Alabama, 16% in Texas, 30% in Florida, and 33% in Georgia.[37]

Beyond that, some of the states that limit eligibility also pay a much smaller share of their Medicaid costs. In the original Medicaid program, the federal government paid up to half the cost but often pays more than that. By 2015, only 14 states were paying 50%, and 10 were paying 33% or less of their costs related to the original (pre-expansion) Medicaid program.[38]

The states also vary dramatically in their spending for the people who are enrolled. Thus, in 2014, spending per enrollee nationwide averaged $5,736. In Alabama, however, spending was two-thirds of that number ($3,837), while in 15 jurisdictions it was over $7,000.[39]

Some states have sought to trim Medicaid costs by introducing a requirement that some "able-bodied" enrollees document that they have applied for work. Many beneficiaries have been unable to provide documentation, which can be challenging. The courts have blocked some of those requirements at least temporarily.[40] Thus, while some states make a good-faith effort to provide a semblance of decent (albeit second-class) care in their Medicaid programs, others brazenly throw a few crumbs to the poor at best. The undeserving poor.

Regional Variations in Needs and in the Ability to Address Them

A potential problem in implementing programs in a federal system also follows from the fact that responsibility for them resides at the community or state level. Some communities, states, or provinces have the resources to build more facilities, to pay providers better, to handle more persons who lack coverage, and to fund programs focused on problems that are particularly bothersome in their jurisdictions (such as homelessness, strokes, etc.). Other jurisdictions lack the resources to do so. When occurrence of a problem and the resources to address it are not distributed homogeneously, at least some resources must be provided from another source, as occurs after hurricanes and other disasters.

In the United States, where commitment to equity in health care varies from sporadic to nonexistent, many states are unable to meet such needs, and no one else is available to address them. Alabama, the Carolinas, Georgia, and Tennessee all lack state health budgets even as generous as those in some other regions but face enormous challenges in the burden of chronic diseases, with rates of stroke more than 50% higher than those in the northeastern states. Other states like Arkansas, Kentucky, and

Mississippi have much higher rates of obesity and fewer resources to address its consequences.[41]

In the case of COVID-19, states varied substantially in the burden of cases at different times. This affected both the ability to provide care and availability of financial resources to address the need for a range of services. The states in the Northeast bore the brunt of the early phase of the pandemic, initially lacking the health care facilities needed fully to address the crisis while experiencing substantial shortfalls in tax revenue. Initially, the federal government was reluctant to distribute the needed resources. As the disease spread, additional states faced the problem of resource shortfalls in intensive care beds and equipment, as well as in funds to address the consequences of the economic collapse. By the summer of 2021, the differential rates of vaccine uptake led to explosion of cases in such states as Alabama and Idaho, which even then were unprepared for the fiscal and health care crunch. Throughout the US, states laid off workers and froze or cut other programs as they dealt with decreasing revenues and increasing costs related to COVID-19.[42] The lack of a comprehensive national program to pay for health care and other services for patients and to fund the full costs accruing to hospitals and other components of health systems makes it difficult to ensure equitable implementation of efforts to address differential impact of a serious health threat.

Political Constraints on Care and Research

Other issues regarding services reflect values of the politicians. For example, federal Medicaid funds in the United States are not allowed by law to cover the cost of an abortion. Among the states, 16 cover the cost of abortion with other state funds, and 34 do not.[43] The funding decisions regarding technologies have direct implications for clinical decision-making. In a jurisdiction with few magnetic resonance imaging (MRI) scanners, the medical community needs to adapt their indications for the procedure in relation to the availability of the technology. When the government is involved, it can do a great deal of mischief. Circumcision (which can protect against HIV disease) is covered by many Medicaid programs, but not those in 16 states. One study found that the overall rate of circumcision among Medicaid patients is substantially lower in the states where Medicaid does not cover the procedure.[44]

In seeming contradiction to the propensity of public officials to refuse to fund their public health care delivery systems at a level that would optimize health, meet the needs of patients, and save some money, the federal government has been unable to do much to mobilize scholars and analysts to identify approaches to reducing the financial burden of care that can be undertaken safely. As noted in chapter 8, Congress threatened to shut down the Agency for Healthcare Research and Quality after it promulgated a guideline that would discourage certain back surgeries in situations where they provide no benefit[45] and has passed laws prohibiting research on the cost-effectiveness of care.[46] At the same time, leading politicians advocate and approve substantial new funding for dramatic initiatives to cure cancer, Alzheimer's disease, and the like,[47] while failing to provide adequate funding for basic programs to provide health care to the population with those and other conditions.

The Limited Reach and Unintended Effects of Employment-Based Insurance

Much of the health insurance system in the United States is tied to employment. Many see this as a strength of the system, but even though more than 50% of Americans have obtained their health insurance from their employment in recent years, these policies are far from a panacea, even for those who have such coverage.

Many workers don't get health insurance through their jobs. In spite of implementation of the Affordable Care Act, which provided a modest boost, the proportion of the nonelderly population with employer-based coverage fell from 67% in 1998 to 58% in 2018. Such coverage varied remarkably by income. While 85% of workers earning more than 400% of the FPL had such coverage, that was the case for only 24% of full-time workers with incomes below the FPL and 48% of those earning 100% to 250% of the FPL. While 68% of workers now are offered health insurance by their employers, many lower-income workers do not opt to enroll, presumably because of the affordability of the plans.[48]

A second problem is so-called job lock: When your health insurance is tied to your employment, that benefit weighs heavily on decisions about where to work, whether to look for a new job, and whether to leave a job that is not ideal. This is particularly an issue for older workers and for those who have had serious illnesses, but other workers may be concerned about retaining health benefits, especially as they consider retirement. In one survey, conducted on behalf of America's Health Insurance Plans (AHIP, a lobbying group for the insurance industry), 46% of workers who had health insurance through their employer said that health benefits were an important factor in the decision to take their current job, and 56% said that it affected their decisions to stay at that employer.[49]

An economic analysis estimated that health insurance benefits reduced job turnover by one-quarter, from 16% to 12%.[50] In another study, among persons who depended on their employers for health insurance, chronic illness reduced job mobility by 40%, compared to those who did not rely on their employers for coverage.[51]

Retirement health benefits (that may include secondary insurance even after Medicare kicks in) also are affected by job lock. I worked for many years at the University of California, which provides good health insurance for employees and retirees, but they can only keep that insurance after departing from the university if they "retire" (start drawing their pension) within a short interval after they separate (leave their job). No one can retire before age 50 or 55 even if they leave, and pension benefits are reduced substantially if they retire before age 60.

Thus anyone moving to another job before age 50 will lose the opportunity to receive that health insurance benefit, as will anyone in their fifties who defers retirement to age 60 in order to maximize their pension benefit. Someone who is over 60 and retires can take another job with health benefits, then return to the University of California retirement program for health insurance coverage as soon as they leave that new job.[52]

A third problem with employer-sponsored insurance is that it is not taxed. As such, it represents a greater tax saving for high-income earners than for low-income earners, in comparison to receiving the employer payments in cash and paying premiums out-of-pocket. For example, someone with an income high enough to pay 40% in taxes would save $6,000 in taxes on a benefit of $15,000, compared with receiving the $15,000 in compensation. In contrast, a lower-wage person who earned enough, even with the additional compensation, to pay 10% in taxes would receive a benefit of only $1,500 in tax savings.

A fourth problem is the impact of loss of employment on health insurance coverage. This was strikingly evident during the COVID-19 pandemic, when tens of millions of Americans lost their jobs. While there is a provision called COBRA (for Consolidated Omnibus Reconciliation Act) that allows an individual to extend health benefits after leaving a job, by paying out-of-pocket for some time, that benefit is expensive and often not affordable to people who have lost their jobs. According to a 2009 study, the insurance premium for a COBRA plan would absorb 84% of the average unemployment insurance benefit.[53]

During the COVID-19 pandemic, the federal government announced that all people who had been laid off or otherwise lacked insurance could receive coverage for the costs of testing and treatment for COVID-19 if they were infected. But going for care in order to ascertain a diagnosis was not necessarily going to be covered if the individual was found to have a different problem. Thus, unlike other countries where insurance is not dependent upon employment, Americans who lost their jobs also lost access to health care as the pandemic raged. One study estimated that up to 27 million workers and family members were affected, although many would qualify for Medicaid or subsidized policies through the Affordable Care Act programs.[54] Estimates vary considerably as to the overall effect on insurance coverage. Many of those who lost coverage became uninsured, but there were also more than 4.3 million new Medicaid enrollees during that period, presumably among those who lost job-related coverage.[55]

A fifth issue with employment-based insurance is that some employers seek to impose their personal values on the contents of the health plans. For example, some do not wish to cover abortion or birth control-related services. This issue has been litigated through the courts,[56] and the US Supreme Court in July 2020 affirmed the right to deny such coverage on religious or moral grounds.[57]

Finally, at the margin, it is cheaper for the employer to offer a stingier plan. A plan that includes higher deductibles and copays is likely to cost the employer less. The Affordable Care Act puts limits on stinginess, but it does not eliminate parsimony. When there are cost implications for the employee for more generous plans, employers will often seek to offer options for stingier plans at low premiums.

Their lower-paid workers will likely default to those lower-cost plans, if they can afford to enroll at all, rather than opting for more generous ones with higher premiums that such workers are unlikely to be able to afford. When not everyone is in the same plan, disparities in accessibility of care are inevitable. If such care is effective, it will differentially affect the health of the lower-income workers.[58]

Living in fear of financial ruin from complications of health problems is not only an unnecessary burden. It is also a propellant toward thinking of one's health care as a commodity from which you should extract as much as you can. Stanford economist Victor Fuchs has said that "to make U.S. health care more equitable and less costly, begin by replacing employment-based insurance."[59]

Is There a Path to a Solution?

America's system, with an array of private insurance plans, a pretty good Medicare program for the elderly with some gaps, inferior coverage for many others with Medicaid, and lots more left uninsured, is chock full of problems. Do other countries do any better? If so, how did they arrive at such programs, what problems have they encountered, and why has the United States failed to move in that direction? We will consider these questions in chapter 11.

Notes

1. Leighton Ku, Elaine Deschamps, and Judi Hilman, "The Effects of Copayments on the Use of Medical Services and Prescription Drugs in Utah's Medicaid Program," Center on Budget and Policy Priorities, November 2, 2004, https://www.cbpp.org /research/the-effects-of-copayments-on-the-use-of-medical-services-and-prescription -drugs-in-utahs#_ftn3.

2. Robyn Tamblyn et al., "Adverse Events Associated with Prescription Drug Cost-Sharing among Poor and Elderly Persons," JAMA 285, no. 4 (January 24/31, 2001): 421–29, https://doi.org/10.1001/jama.285.4.421; Leighton Ku, "Charging the Poor More for Health Care: Cost-Sharing in Medicaid," Center on Budget and Policy Priorities, May 7, 2003, https://www.cbpp.org/archiveSite/5-7-03health.pdf.

3. Celia O. Larson et al., TennCare and Enrollee Cost-Sharing: A Survey of Previously Uninsured and Uninsurable Enrollees in Davidson County (Nashville, TN: Metropolitan Health Department of Nashville and Davidson County, 1996).

4. Stephen B. Soumerai et al., "Payment Restrictions for Prescription Drugs under Medicaid: Effects on Therapy, Costs, and Equity," New England Journal of Medicine 317, no. 9 (August 27, 1987): 550–56, https://doi.org/10.1056 /NEJM198708273170906.

5. They included 7,706 individuals in 2,756 families in Seattle, Washington; Dayton, Ohio; Charleston, South Carolina, and two other communities. In Seattle, there also was an option of a health maintenance organization (HMO). Joseph P. Newhouse et al., "Some Interim Results from a Controlled Trial of Cost Sharing in Health Insurance," New England Journal of Medicine 305, no. 25 (December 17, 1981): 1501–7, https://doi.org/10.1056/nejm198112173052504.

6. The authors of this analysis concluded that there is "price elasticity" (people use more when it costs less), as the study had reported, but there is considerable uncertainty about the magnitude of this effect. Aviva Aron-Dine, Liran Einav, and Amy Finkelstein, "The RAND Health Insurance Experiment, Three Decades Later," Journal of Economic Perspectives 27, no. 1 (Winter 2013): 197–222, https://doi.org/10 .1257/jep.27.1.197.

7. Victor R. Fuchs, "How to Make US Health Care More Equitable and Less Costly," JAMA 320, no. 20 (November 27, 2018): 2071–72, https://doi.org/10.1001/jama.2018.16475.

8. Robert H. Brook et al., "Does Free Care Improve Adults' Health? Results from a Randomized Controlled Trial," New England Journal of Medicine 309, no. 23 (December 8, 1983): 1426–34, https://doi.org/10.1056/NEJM198312083092305.

9. Arleen Leibowitz et al., "Effect of Cost-Sharing on the Use of Medical Services by Children: Interim Results from a Randomized Controlled Trial," Pediatrics 75, no. 5 (May 1985): 942–51, PMID 3991283; Robert B. Valdez et al., "Consequences of Cost-Sharing for Children's Health," Pediatrics 75, no. 5 (May 1985): 952–61, PMID 3991284; Howard L. Bailit et al., "Dental Insurance and the Oral Health of Preschool Children," Journal of the American Dental Association 113, no. 5 (November 1986): 773–76, https://doi.org/10.14219/jada.archive.1986.0272.

10. Martin F. Shapiro, John E. Ware Jr., and Cathy Donald Sherbourne, "Effects of Cost Sharing on Seeking Care for Serious and Minor Symptoms: Results of a

Randomized Controlled Trial," *Annals of Internal Medicine* 104, no. 2 (February 1986): 246–51, https://doi.org/10.7326/0003-4819-104-2-246.

11. David U. Himmelstein et al., "Medical Bankruptcy: Still Common Despite the Affordable Care Act," *American Journal of Public Health* 109, no. 3 (March 2019): 431–33, https://doi.org/10.2105/ajph.2018.304901; David U. Himmelstein et al., "Medical Bankruptcy in the United States, 2007: Results of a National Study," *American Journal of Medicine* 122, no. 8 (August 1, 2009): 741–46, https://doi.org/10.1016/j.amjmed.2009.04.012.

12. Raymond Kluender et al., "Medical Debt in the US, 2009–2020," *JAMA* 326, no. 3 (July 20, 2021): 250–56, https://doi.org/10.1001/jama.2021.8694.

13. In January 2021, the US government issued a rule requiring hospitals "to provide clear, accessible pricing information online about the items and services they provide" including "a display of shoppable services in a consumer-friendly format." "Hospital Price Transparency," Center for Medicare and Medicaid Services, January 1, 2021, https://www.cms.gov/hospital-price-transparency. At least in the early months of the program, however, only a small proportion of hospitals were complying with it. Suhas Gondi et al., "Early Hospital Compliance with Federal Requirements for Price Transparency," *JAMA Internal Medicine* 181, no. 10 (October 1, 2021): 1396–97, https://doi.org/10.1001/jamainternmed.2021.2531.

14. William E. Cunningham et al., "The Impact of Competing Subsistence Needs and Barriers on Access to Medical Care for Persons with Human Immunodeficiency Virus Receiving Care in the United States," *Medical Care* 37, no. 12 (December 1999): 1270–81, https://doi.org/10.1097/00005650-199912000-00010.

15. Martin F. Shapiro et al., "Impact of a Patient-Centered Behavioral Economics Intervention on Hypertension Control in a Highly Disadvantaged Population: A Randomized Trial," *Journal of General Internal Medicine* 35, no. 1 (January 2020): 70–78, https://doi.org/10.1007/s11606-019-05269-z.

16. National Association of Insurance Commissioners, *U.S. Health Insurance Industry: 2020 Annual Results* (Washington, DC: National Association of Insurance Commissioners, 2021), https://content.naic.org/sites/default/files/inline-files/2020-Annual-Health-Insurance-Industry-Analysis-Report.pdf.

17. David U. Himmelstein, Terry Campbell, and Steffie Woolhandler, "Health Administration Costs in the United States and Canada, 2017," *Annals of Internal Medicine* 172, no. 2 (January 21, 2020): 134–42, https://doi.org/10.7326/M19-2818; Dante Morra et al., "US Physician Practices versus Canadians: Spending Nearly Four Times as Much Money Interacting with Payers," *Health Affairs* (Millwood) 30, no. 8 (August 2011): 1443–50, https://doi.org/10.1377/hlthaff.2010.0893.

18. "Health Insurance Complexity Leads to Consumer Wasteful Spending," University of Connecticut Health Disparities Institute Policy Brief, February 6, 2019, https://health.uconn.edu/health-disparities/wp-content/uploads/sites/260/2019/02/HDI_HIL-Brief-2-6-19-FINAL.v3.pdf; George Loewenstein et al., "Consumers' Misunderstanding of Health Insurance," *Journal of Health Economics* 32, no. 5 (September 2013): 850–62, https://doi.org/10.1016/j.jhealeco.2013.04.004; Saurabh Bhargava and George Loewenstein, "Choosing a Health Insurance Plan: Complexity

and Consequences," JAMA 314, no. 23 (December 15, 2015): 2505–6, https://doi.org/10.1001/jama.2015.15176; Victor G. Villagra et al., "Health Insurance Literacy: Disparities by Race, Ethnicity and Language Preference," *American Journal of Managed Care* 25, no. 3 (March 2019): e71–e75, PMID 30875174.

19. Joseph S. Ross and Allan Detsky, "Health Care Choices and Decisions in the United States and Canada," JAMA 302, no. 16 (October 28, 2009): 1803–4, https://doi.org/10.1001/jama.2009.1566.

20. Zack Cooper et al., "Out-of-Network Billing and Negotiated Payments for Hospital-Based Physicians," *Health Affairs* (Millwood) 39, no. 1 (January 2020): 24–32, https://doi.org/10.1377/hlthaff.2019.00507.

21. Mark A. Hall et al., "Reducing Unfair Out-of-Network Billing—Integrated Approaches to Protecting Patients," *New England Journal of Medicine* 380, no. 7 (February 14, 2019): 610–12, https://doi.org/10.1056/NEJMp1815031.

22. Douglas Schoen, "Too Many Americans with Insurance Are Being Denied Coverage," The Hill, August 15, 2017, https://thehill.com/blogs/pundits-blog/healthcare/346652-too-many-americans-with-insurance-are-being-denied-coverage.

23. Sandra L. Decker, "No Association Found between the Medicaid Primary Care Fee Bump and Physician-Reported Participation in Medicaid," *Health Affairs* (Millwood) 37, no. 7 (July 2018): 1092–98, https://doi.org/10.1377/hlthaff.2018.0078.

24. Martin F. Shapiro et al., "Variations in the Care of HIV-Infected Adults in the United States: Results from the HIV Cost and Services Utilization Study," JAMA 281, no. 24 (June 23–30, 1999): 2305–15, https://doi.org/10.1001/jama.281.24.2305.

25. Judith Randal, "Mantle's Transplant Raises Delicate Issues about Organ Allocation," *Journal of the National Cancer Institute* 88, no. 8 (April 17, 1996): 484–85, https://doi.org/10.1093/jnci/88.8.484; Tara Parker-Pope, "How Did Steve Jobs Get a Liver Transplant?," *New York Times*, June 23, 2009, https://well.blogs.nytimes.com/2009/06/23/how-did-steve-jobs-get-a-liver-transplant/; John M. Glionna and Charles Ornstein, "Japanese Gang Figures Got New Livers at UCLA," *Los Angeles Times*, May 30, 2008, https://www.latimes.com/archives/la-xpm-2008-may-30-me-ucla30-story.html.

26. Lindsay A. Sobotka, Alice Hinton, and Lanla F. Conteh, "Insurance Status Impacts Treatment for Hepatocellular Carcinoma," *Annals of Hepatology* 18, no. 3 (May–June 2019): 461–65, https://doi.org/10.1016/j.aohep.2018.10.001.

27. Russell Rosenblatt et al., "Black Patients Have Unequal Access to Listing for Liver Transplantation in the United States," *Hepatology* 74, no. 3 (September 2021): 1523–32, https://doi.org/10.1002/hep.31837.

28. Sitaramesh Emani et al., "Impact of Insurance Status on Heart Transplant Wait-List Mortality for Patients with Left Ventricular Assist Devices," *Clinical Transplantation* 31, no. 2 (February 2017): e12875, https://doi.org/10.1111/ctr.12875.

29. Emily J. Cherlin et al., "Features of High Quality Discharge Planning for Patients following Acute Myocardial Infarction," *Journal of General Internal Medicine* 28, no. 3 (March 2013): 436–43, https://doi.org/10.1007/s11606-012-2234-y.

30. Stephen L. Isaacs and Paul Jellinek, "Is There a (Volunteer) Doctor in the House? Free Clinics and Volunteer Physician Referral Networks in the United States,"

Health Affairs (Millwood) 26, no. 3 (May–June 2007): 871–72, https://doi.org/10.1377/hlthaff.26.3.871.

31. Rachel Weiner, "Romney: Uninsured Have Emergency Rooms," *Washington Post*, September 24, 2012, https://www.washingtonpost.com/news/post-politics/wp/2012/09/24/romney-calls-emergency-room-a-health-care-option-for-uninsured/.

32. Martin F. Shapiro et al., "Mortality Differences between New York City Municipal and Voluntary Hospitals, for Selected Conditions," *American Journal of Public Health* 83, no. 7 (July 1983): 1024–26, https://doi.org/10.2105/ajph.83.7.1024.

33. Michael Schwirtz, "One Rich N.Y. Hospital Got Warren Buffett's Help. This One Got Duct Tape," *New York Times*, April 26, 2020, https://www.nytimes.com/2020/04/26/nyregion/coronavirus-new-york-university-hospital.html?action=click&module=Spotlight&pgtype=Homepage.

34. It rose to $13.1 billion in 1975, $41.3 billion in 1985, $159.5 billion in 1995, $315.9 billion in 2005, $549.1 billion in 2015, and $639.4 billion in 2019. Jenny Yang, "Total Medicaid Expenditure from 1966 to 2019 (in Billion U.S. Dollars)," Statista, September 8, 2021, https://www.statista.com/statistics/245348/total-medicaid-expenditure-since-1966/.

35. "Budget Basics: Medicare," Peter G. Peterson Foundation, September 2, 2021, https://www.pgpf.org/budget-basics/medicare; "Question and Answers for the Additional Medicare Tax," Internal Revenue Service, accessed June 19, 2020, https://www.irs.gov/businesses/small-businesses-self-employed/questions-and-answers-for-the-additional-medicare-tax.

36. Thomas Rice, "The Impact of Cost Containment Efforts on Racial and Ethnic Disparities in Care: A Conceptualization," in *Unequal Treatment: Confronting Racial and Ethnic Disparities in Health Care*, ed. Brian D. Smedley, Adrienne Y. Stith, and Alan R. Nelsons (Washington DC: National Academies Press 2006), 699–721.

37. For the other states not participating in the Medicaid expansion by October 2021, eligibility levels were 38% of the FPL in Kansas, 25% in Mississippi, 39% in North Carolina, 67% in South Carolina, 46% in South Dakota, 88% in Tennessee, and 50% in Wyoming. In the states that expanded eligibility in 2020 and 2021, eligibility levels prior to that had been 21% of the FPL in Missouri, 63% in Nebraska, and 67% in Oklahoma. "Medicaid Income Eligibility Limits for Adults as a Percent of the Federal Poverty Level as of January 1, 2022," Kaiser Family Foundation State Health Facts, accessed April 16, 2022, https://www.kff.org/health-reform/state-indicator/medicaid-income-eligibility-limits-for-adults-as-a-percent-of-the-federal-poverty-level/?currentTimeframe=0&selectedDistributions=parents-in-a-family-of-three--other-adults-for-an-individual&sortModel=%7B%22coIId%22:%22Location%22,%22sort%22:%22asc%22%7D.

38. Thirteen states were paying 33.1% to 40%; the other 13 states were paying more than 40% but less than 50%. Of the 15 states not accepting the Medicaid expansion prior to 2020, 8 (Alabama, Georgia, Mississippi, Missouri, North Carolina, Oklahoma, South Carolina, and Tennessee) were paying 40% or less of their unexpanded Medicaid costs. Laura Snyder and Robin Rudowitz, "Medicaid Financing: How Does It Work and What Are the Implications?," Kaiser Family Foundation Medicaid, May 20, 2015, https://www.kff.org/medicaid/issue-brief/medicaid-financing-how-does-it-work-and-what-are-the-implications; "Status of

State Medicaid Expansion Decisions: Interactive Map," Kaiser Family Foundation Medicaid, April 19, 2022, https://www.kff.org/medicaid/issue-brief/status-of-state -medicaid-expansion-decisions-interactive-map/.

39. "Medicaid Spending per Enrollee (Full or Partial Benefit) FY2014," Kaiser Family Foundation State Health Facts, accessed April 24, 2020, https://www.kff.org /medicaid/state-indicator/medicaid-spending-per-enrollee/?currentTimeframe =0&sortModel=%7B%22colId%22:%22Location%22,%22sort%22:%22asc%22%7D.

40. "Status of Medicaid Expansion and Work Requirement Waivers," Common-wealth Fund, September 2, 2021, https://www.commonwealthfund.org/publications /maps-and-interactives/2020/apr/status-medicaid-expansion-and-work-requirement -waivers.

41. Centers for Disease Control and Prevention, "State-Specific Mortality from Stroke and Distribution of Place of Death—United States, 1999," MMWR Morbidity and Mortality Weekly Report 51, no. 20 (May 24, 2002): 429–33, https://www.cdc.gov /mmwr/preview/mmwrhtml/mm5120a1.htm; Christina Bethell et al., "National, State, And Local Disparities in Childhood Obesity," Health Affairs (Millwood) 29, no. 3 (March–April 2010): 347–56, https://doi.org/10.1377/hlthaff.2009.0762.

42. Sarah M. Bartsch et al., "The Potential Health Care Costs and Resource Use Associated with COVID-19 in the United States," Health Affairs (Millwood) 39, no. 6 (April 23, 2020): 927–35, https://doi.org/10.1377/hlthaff.2020.00426; David Frum, "Why Mitch McConnell Wants States to Go Bankrupt," The Atlantic, April 25, 2020, https://www.theatlantic.com/ideas/archive/2020/04/why-mitch-mcconnell-wants -states-go-bankrupt/610714/; Louise Sheiner and Sophia Campbell, "How Much Is COVID-19 Hurting State and Local Revenues?," Brookings: The Hutchins Center Explains, September 24, 2020, https://www.brookings.edu/blog/up-front/2020/09 /24/how-much-is-covid-19-hurting-state-and-local-revenues/; Anshu Siripurapu and Jonathan Masters, "How COVID-19 Is Harming State and City Budgets," Council on Foreign Relations, March 19, 2021, https://www.cfr.org/backgrounder/how-covid -19-harming-state-and-city-budgets; Joshua Cohen, "In Idaho and Other States, the Delta COVID-19 Surge Is Forcing Hospitals to Ration ICU Beds," Forbes, September 7, 2021, https://www.forbes.com/sites/joshuacohen/2021/09/07/delta-surge-of-covid -19-is-forcing-hospitals-to-ration-icu-beds-in-parts-of-the-us/?sh=415632725841.

43. Alina Salganicoff et al., "Coverage for Abortion Services in Medicaid Marketplace Plans and Private Plans," Kaiser Family Foundation Women's Health Policy, June 24, 2019, https://www.kff.org/womens-health-policy/issue-brief /coverage-for-abortion-services-in-medicaid-marketplace-plans-and-private-plans/.

44. Arleen A. Leibowitz, Katherine Desmond, and Thomas Belin, "Determinants and Policy Implications of Male Circumcision in the United States," American Journal of Public Health 99, no. 1 (January 2009): 138–45, https://doi.org/10.2105/AJPH.2008.134403.

45. Casey Ross, "This Federal Agency That Aims to Make Health Care More Effective Is on the Chopping Block, Again," Statnews, March 30, 2017, https://www .statnews.com/2017/03/30/ahrq-budget-trump-nih/.

46. "What Is PCORI's Official Policy on Cost and Cost-Effectiveness Analysis?," Patient-Centered Outcomes Research Institute, accessed April 26, 2020, https://help

.pcori.org/hc/en-us/articles/213716587-What-is-PCORI-s-official-policy-on-cost-and
-cost-effectiveness-analysis-.

47. "Cancer Moonshot," National Cancer Institute, accessed April 26, 2020,
https://www.cancer.gov/research/key-initiatives/moonshot-cancer-initiative;
Thomas Sullivan, "Senate Aging Committee Takes on Alzheimer's," Policy and
Medicine, July 4, 2018, https://www.policymed.com/2018/07/senate-aging
-committee-takes-on-alzheimers.html.

48. Matthew Rae et al., "Long-Term Trends in Employer-Based Coverage,"
Peterson-KFF Health System Tracker, April 3, 2020, https://www
.healthsystemtracker.org/brief/long-term-trends-in-employer-based-coverage/.

49. Stephen Miller, "Employees Are More Likely to Stay If They Like Their Health
Plan," Society for Human Resources Management, February 14, 2018, https://www.shrm
.org/resourcesandtools/hr-topics/benefits/pages/health-benefits-foster-retention.aspx.

50. Bridgette C. Madrian, "Employment-Based Health Insurance and Job
Mobility: Is There Evidence of Job-Lock?," Quarterly Journal of Economics 109, no. 1
(February 1994): 27–54, https://doi.org/10.2307/2118427.

51. Kevin T. Stroupe, Eleanor D. Kinney, and Thomas J. J. Knieser, "Chronic
Illness and Health Insurance-Related Job Lock," Journal of Policy Analysis and
Management 20, no. 3 (June 2001): 525–44, https://doi.org/10.1002/pam.1006.

52. "Eligibility to Continue Health and Welfare Benefits," in Retirement Handbook
for UCRP Members (Berkeley: University of California, 2020), 15–16, ucnet.universityof
california.edu/forms/pdf/retirement-handbook.pdf.

53. Leah Nylen, "Study: COBRA Insurance Too Expensive for Unemployed,"
Commonwealth Fund, January 9, 2009, https://www.commonwealthfund.org
/publications/newsletter-article/study-cobra-insurance-too-expensive-unemployed.

54. Rebecca Pifer, "27M Americans May Have Lost Job-Based Health Insurance Due
to COVID-19 Downturn," Healthcaredive, May 13, 2020, https://www.healthcaredive
.com/news/27m-americans-may-have-lost-job-based-health-insurance-due-to-covid
-19-down/577852/.

55. Daniel McDermott et al., "How Has the Pandemic Affected Health Coverage in
the U.S.?," Kaiser Family Foundation Policy Watch, December 9, 2020, https://www
.kff.org/policy-watch/how-has-the-pandemic-affected-health-coverage-in-the-u-s/.

56. Adam Liptak, "Supreme Court to Consider Limits of Contraception Coverage," New York Times, January 17, 2020, https://www.nytimes.com/2020/01/17/us
/supreme-court-contraception-coverage.html.

57. Little Sisters of the Poor Saints Peter and Paul Home v. Pennsylvania et al.,
available at the US Supreme Court website, accessed May 5, 2022, https://www
.supremecourt.gov/opinions/19pdf/19-431_5i36.pdf.

58. Linda J. Blumberg, Employer-Sponsored Health Insurance and the Low-Income
Worker: Limitations of the System and Strategies for Increasing Coverage (Washington,
DC: Urban Institute, 2007), 4, https://www.urban.org/sites/default/files/publication
/46676/411536-Employer-Sponsored-Health-Insurance-and-the-Low-Income
-Workforce.PDF.

59. Fuchs, "How to Make."

11

Protagonists, Pitfalls, and Lessons from Abroad

The Tortuous Path to Health Care for All

Writing laws is easy, but governing is difficult.
—Leo Tolstoy, *War and Peace*

The best laid schemes o' Mice an' Men / Gang aft agley.
—Robert Burns, "To a Mouse"

When I was a medical student, I had the opportunity to work with the deputy minister of health in the province of Manitoba on a policy paper about the future of health policy in the province.[1] It was a wonderful experience; Manitoba recently had elected a government led by the New Democratic Party, who were social democrats. The government was intent on making a difference in health care. My boss, Deputy Health Minister Ted Tulchinsky, was idealistic and progressive.

On one occasion, I attended a major meeting that involved three cabinet ministers in discussions of issues that had arisen in the draft report. One was the challenge of creating an integrated health system that included all major hospitals. The board of directors of the Catholic hospital in Winnipeg (Manitoba's capital) was not cooperating.

As the group pondered what to do, I offered, "why not just dissolve the board of that hospital?" Saul Miller, the government minister who was chairing the meeting and was a longtime socialist, turned to me and said, "Son, the board of that hospital will be around long after you are dead."

That was a shock to my young, idealistic self, but it was also a valuable learning experience. It proved to be useful preparation for grappling with how hard it has been to ensure that everyone in the United States has access to health care as well as a way to pay for it. Even when you have a clear vision of what needs to happen to make the world a better place, lots of things can get in the way.

Making change in health care systems never is easy. As we have seen, many groups of participants in the world of health care—clinicians, patients, educators, health systems, and other corporate providers, manufacturers, insurers, unions, employers, and scientists—contribute to the problems that manifest in health care and often resist efforts to address them. Who can intercede and tackle these issues effectively on behalf of society as a whole? Is government a potential solution? Some would hold, as did Ronald Reagan in his inaugural address, "government is not the solution to our problem; government is the problem." Notwithstanding such ideological abhorrence of government's role in health care, there is considerable agreement that certain aspects of promoting the well-being of the population are the proper province of the government.

Yet efforts to develop a government role in health and health care have encountered formidable obstacles, in both the health sector and the world of politics, particularly, although not exclusively, in the United States. A major challenge has been insuring the population to cover the costs while providing access to and high quality of care. There is broad consensus in advanced, industrialized countries that the government has key roles in prevention of disease, sanitation, promotion of physical and mental well-being in the population as a whole, and managing the spread of infectious diseases in the population. The issue of insurance coverage and who should provide it often has been more divisive.

It is illuminating to consider these issues in the broader context of the ways in which other societies have worked out issues pertaining to both public health services (such as water, sewage, and epidemic control) and individual health care services. In this chapter, I draw on some insights from Western Europe and Canada to frame the consideration of health insurance and the role of government in the United States.

Government Involvement in Public Health
Public Health in Europe

It long has been recognized (even as far back as ancient Greece) that some aspects of well-being of any population require interventions at the level of the community. The French Revolution augured in an era in which health was considered, at least to some degree, to be a right of the citizen. It took a while for various countries to operationalize that right in terms of policies.[2] Even prior to that revolution, some countries developed models through which "medical police" sought to improve well-being through improved environment (typically sanitation), quarantines, and regulation of both drugs and the practice of medicine.[3]

France

After the French Revolution determined health to be a right of citizenship (although not listing it explicitly as such in the 1789 Declaration of the Rights of Man and Citizen, or in the subsequent constitutions), there was at least an intellectual commitment to the problem of the health of the public. Accordingly, France was at the forefront of giving academic respectability to public health after 1815, but the country did not do much to change the central government's approach, which was based on surveillance. A journal of public hygiene and legal medicine was established in 1829. Even so, this evidence that the French were conscious of the importance of public health did not lead to policies to address it for some time. It was left to each community to develop programs that accorded with the national ideal.

Each town had responsibility for public hygiene, but there was no national legislation to back it up. In the Department of the Seine (which included Paris and environs), there was an active health council from 1802. This council investigated such problems as sewage, industries that emitted sickening pollutants, and epidemics. Their role was only advisory, and they had no enforcement authority. The Paris Health Council produced reports with health statistics, which became a model for such councils elsewhere. The issues of public health emerged in the failed 1848 revolution and again in 1870. After that, the Third Republic made an explicit commitment to public health, reinforced by Louis Pasteur's sensational bacteriology discoveries. In the 1890s, the government resuscitated the principles of the 1789 revolution and began to act more programmatically. Health care for the poor ceased to be a relief program and became a system of national insurance. An 1893 law required the departments and towns to provide medical care to the poor. Another law came into effect in 1904, requiring all communities to meet national standards for sanitation, vaccination, and notification.[4]

Sweden

The medical police in Sweden, introduced in the eighteenth century, had an impact on mortality and enabled growth of the population. Early on, much of this work was done by volunteer physicians. In 1813, a National Board of Health gave the Swedish medical profession some public authority. In 1867, the Swedish parliament created the first professorship of public health. Bacteriology (following Louis Pasteur's discoveries) gave public hygiene a higher profile. In 1874, a Public Health Act established boards for public health throughout the country, with responsibility for the water supply and sewage disposal.[5]

Germany

In Germany, the Prussian state established the role of the district doctor in 1817. They instituted a program of "state medicine," which comprised some public health measures as well as forensics, but there was little authority associated with it. Local health committees were often dominated by civil servants with no relevant expertise. Radical doctors such as Rudolf Virchow contended that poverty was contributing to ill health and advocated radical change. He argued that medicine (by which he meant both clinical practice and public health) had to become political and affect policy. Although the revolutions of 1848 failed, the point of view espoused by Virchow and some others eventually affected government. After German unification in 1871, an Imperial Health Office was established in 1873, along with a national Society of Public Health. The bacteriologist Robert Koch codirected the Imperial Health Office for several years. In 1899, Prussia implemented a system of full-time officers of health, and the political class gave much more attention to what they characterized as "social hygiene."[6]

United Kingdom

The United Kingdom established a health ministry in 1848 with the passage of a Public Health Act, which put in place a Central Health Board for England and Wales to address matters relating to sewage, water supply, and living standards. This act was stimulated by Edwin Chadwick's self-published 1842 report, *The Sanitary Condition of the Labouring Population of Great Britain*, but was finally precipitated by an 1848 cholera outbreak. A second act in 1875 gave the local health authorities much more power, including over creation and repair of sewers, control of water supplies, regulation of lodging houses, and establishment of standards for streets.[7]

Public Health in the United States

Unlike the French Revolution, the ideology of the American Revolution did not encompass a right to health (rather to life, liberty, and pursuit of happiness). Health boards were formed early on in response to epidemic diseases but tended not to be functional at other times. The New York City Board of Health had a budget of only $500 in 1819. It had responsibility to organize annual street cleanings. Boston's board was more active. Created in 1798, it had representatives from all city wards and authority to remove nuisances (things that represented threats to the health or safety of the population). In New Orleans, a health board was activated for a yellow fever epidemic one year and a flood more than a decade later. In each case, the business community had it dismissed after the emergency had ended. Similar patterns were seen in other cities. There was a need for clean water, and supplies were piped in, but the role of public health authorities was limited. During the Civil War, many of the soldiers died from dysentery due to unsanitary conditions in the camps.

A movement for sanitary reform in the military ultimately succeeded, and the sanitary programs affected civilian populations as well. John Henry Griscom in New York and Lemuel Shattuck in Boston had been advocating for more systematic health efforts, and these began to take hold. Griscom published a report on the health of the laboring classes of New York in 1845, modeled after Chadwick's report on public health in Britain from a few years earlier.[8]

Shattuck, the founder of the American Statistical Association who also revolutionized procedures for the US Census, led a commission that published the Report of a General Plan for the Promotion of Public and Personal Health for Massachusetts in 1850.[9] The book included 50 recommendations for the organization of health agencies, locally and statewide, as well as for the collecting of data related to public health that remain standard public health procedures today.[10]

The industrial revolution and advances in bacteriology heightened the awareness of ongoing problems and of things that could be done about them, as in Europe. Both the federal government and the local authorities played increasingly larger roles in public health as the nineteenth century drew to a close.

The Growth of Government Involvement in Clinical Services in Europe

Establishing a role for the government in the financing, delivery, and organization of personal health services followed a more perilous route.

The medical profession was fiercely independent and protective of its professional prerogatives in all countries. Payments (except in the case of the indigent) were made directly by patients to providers. Health insurance did not emerge as a recognized need in Europe until late in the nineteenth century. In reality, development of sewers and a clean water supply, as well as the management of epidemics with quarantine along with vaccination, were the most useful tools available to augment health, apart from the treatment of injuries. It was not until the diagnostic and therapeutic revolutions—including anesthesia and antiseptic surgery, and the associated explosion of knowledge about the pathogenesis diseases and of treatments for them—that it mattered a great deal to be able to get to a doctor. Different countries approached this challenge in rather different ways.

Germany: From Sickness Funds to Universal Coverage in 124 Years

The modern idea of health insurance emerged in what became Germany. There had been a tradition of mutual-aid societies in Germany that began with guilds in the Middle Ages. Starting with miners in Prussia in 1849, there was movement toward mandatory health insurance coverage for workers. The most dramatic development occurred in 1883, when Chancellor Otto von Bismarck introduced and implemented a Health Insurance Law. This law mandated health insurance coverage for all industrial workers throughout Germany who earned less than a specified income level. The program was intended to stabilize income and keep workers healthy and productive. The program also had a political intent: curbing enthusiasm for the leftist Social Democratic Party.

This legislation instituted a program of social insurance, which included "sickness funds" (organized at the community, corporate, or occupational level) as well as funeral benefits through multiple insurers, financed through required contributions from employers and employees. Employers who did not cover all of their workers were subjected to fines. It was a popular program and, by some accounts, curtailed the emigration of industrial workers who could not obtain those kinds of benefits elsewhere. Subsequently, the government added programs of accident insurance in 1884, disability insurance and old-age pensions in 1889, and unemployment insurance in 1927. White-collar workers were added in 1901; domestic, agricultural, and forestry workers in 1914; and farmers (in West Germany) in 1972. Benefits were eventually extended to the unemployed, students, the disabled, and nonworking dependents.

Over the decades, governments of different political persuasions have put their ideological imprints on the program, but Bismarck's scheme has remained fundamentally intact. There were two notable exceptions. Under the Nazi regime (1933–45), Jewish workers were excluded from coverage, and Jewish physicians were not allowed to provide care through the program. This latter development was strongly supported by non-Jewish physicians, who were the occupational group with highest representation in the Nazi Party. After the war, East Germany developed a state-run program, covering the entire population, which was dissolved after unification in 1990. In 1883, only 10% of workers were covered, but this steadily increased, reaching 51% of the population by 1925, 83% in 1960, and 88% prior to unification.

Since 2007, health insurance has been mandatory for all permanent residents of Germany, either through the public program (85%) or through private health insurance (PHI), which covers certain professional groups such as civil servants. An important exception is undocumented refugees and other immigrants, who do not receive coverage in the national program and have only limited access to medical care. Authority over the program is divided between the national government, state governments, and organizations in civil society (outside of the government). One feature of this model differs from programs that have been introduced in the United States: the government controls the prices, and the insurance companies do not make a profit from the program. During World War II, the occupying German regimes established similar programs in Belgium, France, and the Netherlands that had some influence upon subsequent reforms in those countries.[11]

France: Stepwise Development of a Program with More Control by the National Government

Bismarck's reforms had some influence in France, but in stages. The 1893 French law (discussed above), which provided health care to the destitute, was followed five years later by establishment of a workers' compensation program. In 1930, a program of health insurance for industrial and commercial workers was established with passage of the Act on Social Insurance. This law created a compulsory program of coverage up to a specified maximum income, much like the program in Germany at that time. The program covered illness, disability, maternity, old age, and death benefits. By 1939, about two-thirds of the French population had coverage through mutual benefit associations.

After World War II, France progressed toward universal coverage in a stepwise manner. In 1945, France replaced the role of the mutual benefit associations with a government program of statutory health insurance (SHI) within the government-run social security system. Initially, it covered all industrial and commercial workers' families and retirees. The program was extended to agricultural workers and farmers in 1961 and to independent professional workers in 1966. In 2000, France achieved universal coverage (*couverture maladie universelle*) by covering the unemployed and all legal immigrants, providing supplemental funding for those of low income, and including a separate program of coverage for undocumented aliens in the country.

In this system, delivery is shared by private, mostly independent physicians practicing on a fee-for-service basis, public hospitals, and nonprofit and for-profit hospitals. The system is regulated by the French government, SHI, and local communities. Except for those of low income, patients pay doctors directly, then get reimbursed. About 75% of expenses are paid by the government through SHI. The system combines elements of the German system with elements of greater involvement of the national government, as developed in the United Kingdom (see below).[12]

Adoption of Sickness Funds Elsewhere in Europe

Other European countries, including Denmark, Sweden, and Switzerland created similar programs in the 1890s, followed by England in 1911.

National Health Care Programs in the United Kingdom and Canada

Broader involvement in the health sector emerged gradually in English-speaking countries. The United Kingdom and Canada both adopted national government-sponsored programs, but not without a few perturbations.

United Kingdom: Creating a National Health Service

The European trend toward establishing a system of sickness funds was adopted in the United Kingdom in 1911, when Prime Minister David Lloyd George introduced a program of compulsory health insurance for workers in some industries. It generally covered the workers, but not other family members, and paid for visits to a doctor, but not for hospital care. For those not covered by such programs, there were mutual aid organizations and medical clubs into which people would pay when they could, then get medical care when they needed it. As for hospital care, a system had evolved in the late nineteenth century of "almoners," who assessed the ability of working-class patients to pay for their care and judged whether their hospital care should be free.

The program expanded through the 1920s and 1930s, but it did not function as an effective and comprehensive solution to the problem of accessibility of care. There was growing support for a system of free medical care prior to World War II. A report on this issue by Lord Beveridge, issued in 1942, included a national program of free care. Two years later, even as the war was still raging, the coalition war cabinet published a white paper on a National Health Service (NHS). It proposed a system of free care funded through tax revenues. After the war, the victorious Labour government of Clement Atlee moved forward with the plan.

Health Minister Aneurin Bevan wrote the act and included management by the national government as a key feature. This element elicited strenuous resistance, particularly from the British Medical Association. Notwithstanding considerable acrimony and a great deal of opposition, particularly to the fact that the government would administer the program as a government entity, it went into effect in July 1948. It is a beloved feature of British society today, although often at the center of much adversarial political discourse on the adequacy of funding and the quality of care. Bevan and a junior minister, future prime minister Harold Wilson, resigned from the cabinet in 1951 over a decision to introduce charges to patients for dentures and eyeglasses, a development that led to prescription fees. When Wilson became prime minister, he introduced legislation in 1964 to exempt the poor from these charges. A small private sector remained outside of the NHS, and some insurance companies survive to this day. Efforts to eliminate private insurance did not survive Margaret Thatcher's Conservative triumph in 1979. When devolution gave autonomy over health care to Northern Ireland, Scotland, and Wales, they abolished prescription fees, but England did not.

To fund the NHS, the UK government establishes a budget each year and allocates resources to clinician providers as well as to hospitals and other health facilities, through more than 200 "trusts," including those devoted to acute hospitals, mental health services, ambulances, and community health.[13]

Canada: Ten Provinces with Single-Payer Programs

In Canada, the Cooperative Commonwealth Federation, a Social Democratic political organization now known as the New Democratic Party, introduced a universal hospital insurance program in the province of Saskatchewan in 1947 under the leadership of provincial premier Tommy Douglas. Other Canadian provinces adopted similar programs over the next 14 years. Douglas labored long and hard to expand this to a universal health insurance program for Saskatchewan that would cover all medical services. It finally was enacted in July 1962.

The medical profession was unalterably opposed and went on strike. The strike involved about 95% of the doctors in Saskatchewan. Some sympathetic doctors came from other provinces to support the government and provide medical care during the strike. The strike finally ended with compromise on some minor issues, but the single-payer health insurance program, with no copayments or deductibles, was there to stay.[14]

I had some personal connections to the Saskatchewan strike. Two cousins of my father were physicians in Saskatchewan who participated in the strike. One of the doctors who went to Saskatchewan to support the government program and break the strike by providing medical care was Ted Tulchinsky, the deputy minister for whom I worked in the Manitoba government in the 1970s. Beyond his commitment to the health insurance program that Douglas created, Ted also married one of Douglas's daughters.

The idea of universal health insurance was popular elsewhere in Canada. The Progressive Conservative government of the day established a Royal Commission to make recommendations regarding health insurance coverage for the country as a whole. By the time the commissioner produced his report, which recommended national adoption of the Saskatchewan model, Canada had a minority Liberal government that was being supported by the New Democrats. The government went ahead with the commission's recommendation, and parliament voted in 1966 to implement the program nationally. According to Canada's constitution, however, health care was a provincial responsibility. How could they get around this? The legislation cleverly said that the federal government would pay half the cost of any province's program that met certain criteria, including universality, comprehensiveness, transferability, and the absence of user fees.

Saskatchewan and British Columbia signed up immediately when the program took effect in July 1968. Some provinces vigorously objected, but since they were paying for programs elsewhere with their federal tax dollars, all the other provinces followed within the next few years. In Quebec, this did not occur without a strike by the medical specialists in the province in October 1970, but it ended quickly. Canadians are proud of their system, in which any patient can go to any doctor: there are no networks, there is no out-of-network billing, and there are no out-of-pocket costs other than for medications and dental care.

A 2004 survey conducted by the Canadian Broadcasting Corporation asked Canadians to vote for the greatest Canadian in the nation's history. Tommy Douglas topped the list! (The top 10 also included three prime ministers, a Nobel-winning scientist, and hockey player Wayne Gretzky.)[15] In another survey in 2014, Canadians named the establishment of Medicare (the national single-payer health program) as the accomplishment that made them "most proud to be a Canadian."[16] No Canadians have illusions about the system's proximity to perfection, but almost none would care to exchange it for the situation in the United States.

US Efforts to Develop a National Strategy for Health Care Accessibility

The United States did not follow the European trend in developing sickness funds in the late nineteenth and early twentieth centuries.[17] The country had some voluntary sickness funds, covering some workers for illness, but that tradition was far less widespread than in Europe. The Progressive Era (1900–1914) witnessed some movement in that direction, but reformers could not enact a program comparable to Germany's, facing a groundswell of opposition from medical societies, opposition from the National Manufacturers Association and other business groups (including major insurers that perceived a threat to their funeral benefits business), and lack of support from the American Federation of Labor. In 1917, California's social insurance commission proposed amending the state constitution to enable establishment of a program of compulsory health insurance for the population. The state medical society was supportive but stayed neutral on the ensuing ballot initiative. However, it faced well-financed opposition from a large group of doctors and

Christian Scientists. The opposition even linked the proposal to Germany's territorial ambitions in World War I, and it was resoundingly defeated in 1918.[18]

The government was also disinclined to intervene in society with major programs such as this would be. Socialists were not much of a presence in the United States. Theodore Roosevelt, the Progressive candidate in the 1912 election (running on the Bull Moose ticket), supported social insurance, including sickness insurance, but he lost to Woodrow Wilson, who opposed it. All told, the private sickness funds in the US covered about one-third of industrial workers.[19] By the 1970s, almost every country with an advanced economy other than the US had implemented a program that at the very least was well down the road to providing some form of universal coverage. Why has the US failed to do so? It certainly has not been for lack of trying. Rather, its efforts have been met with a relentless barrage of attacks from groups deeply invested in the status quo. The political will to engage and sustain the battle for universal health insurance has been lacking at the level of the federal government. Instead, successive administrations have sought (and occasionally obtained) lesser reforms. The government likewise has been deterred from constraining costs in ways that do not disproportionately affect the poor. Even a rational public dialogue about health care spending has proved all but impossible.

The Committee on the Costs of Medical Care

In the decade following the failure of the Progressive Era initiatives, both organized labor and business interests were opposed to compulsory health insurance.[20] Interest grew in the 1920s, stimulated in part by rising hospital costs, but organized medicine, spearheaded by the American Medical Association (AMA), strenuously opposed any insurance program that the medical profession didn't control. The problem of costs did not go away, however, and the AMA acquiesced in the late 1920s in the establishment of the Committee on the Costs of Medical Care. The committee conducted a number of studies and issued a final report in 1932.[21]

As might be expected, the 48-member committee included competing factions. The majority report recommended that medical practice be organized into groups that would improve efficiency, a move the AMA opposed. Two of the committee's recommendations—public health services for the entire population and state and local agencies to study, evaluate, and coordinate services—proved less controversial. But the recommendation that medical costs be based on group payments through insurance, taxation, or both hit a wall of disdain from the AMA and conservative elements opposed to expanding government's role.

Recommendations for improved professional education were unopposed. One minority report explicitly opposed the formation of medical groups ("the corporate practice of medicine") as well as government support for the care of anyone other than the indigent, those in the armed forces, and those requiring care in government hospitals. The committee's report did not endorse compulsory insurance, although some signers of the majority report dissented on that issue.

Roosevelt and Truman

With the election of Franklin Roosevelt, many believed he would support an expanded government role in health care along with the other major programs of the New Deal. But he deferred making it an issue until after the 1938 elections, which produced a conservative majority in Congress. The issue was shelved for another decade. The labor movement, which had been far from consistent in support of such a program, cautiously put one foot forward in support of health insurance legislation in 1943. Labor leaders joined the Committee for the Nation's Health and more liberal members of the administration that year, when they drafted the Wagner-Murray-Dingell Bill. This legislation would have provided national health insurance through a social security payroll tax.

When Harry Truman succeeded Roosevelt in 1945, he endorsed this approach, which would have covered the entire population, with the government paying the premiums of those who could not otherwise afford them. Truman insisted that the plan did not constitute "socialized medicine" because people would continue to use services as they had previously. When push came to shove, however, labor leaders failed to mobilize their rank-and-file to support the legislation. By contrast, the AMA, determined to defend the medical profession's turf, boldly asserted that the Truman program would turn doctors into "slaves."[22] In addition to the AMA, the nonprofit insurers—the Blue Cross and Blue Shield Associations—also opposed the reform. The well-financed grassroots campaign succeeded in blocking the proposed legislation.[23]

The AMA was sufficiently concerned about the push for compulsory, government-sponsored insurance by the Truman administration and others that it offered support for voluntary insurance as an alternative. That position won over other influential groups, such as the American Bar Association and the American Hospital Association. In the end, Truman's reform efforts failed when he lost his majority in Congress.

Lyndon Johnson: Medicare and Medicaid

Reform finally arrived in 1965, when Lyndon Johnson signed the legislation creating Medicare (for those over 65) and Medicaid (for the poor), but not without a protracted opposition campaign by the AMA, featuring the B-movie actor Ronald Reagan as its spokesman. That campaign launched Reagan's political career.[24] He defeated Democratic incumbent Edmond "Pat" Brown to become governor of California the following year. Meanwhile, Johnson signed the legislation in the presence of Truman in the former president's home town of Independence, Missouri.

Clinton and Obama

Subsequent major reform initiatives also faced serious challenges. Apart from the elderly, most Americans were insured through their employers. The 1993 Clinton reform effort to greatly expand coverage was undone by a fiendishly clever advertising campaign funded by the health insurance industry. The ads featured "Harry and Louise," an everyman and everywoman, sitting at a kitchen table discussing the Clinton plan. They assert inaccurately that the health reform proposal would deprive them of their freedom to go to the doctor of their choice, when in reality, such "freedom" already was restricted in many health plans. (All that was missing from the ads was an image of Ronald Reagan smiling.)[25]

The Affordable Care Act (ACA) of 2010 expanded Medicaid to Americans with somewhat higher incomes than had previously qualified and required all others to obtain insurance coverage or pay fines. Beyond the Medicaid expansion, the ACA enabled middle-class Americans without employer coverage to buy into partially subsidized private plans through insurance marketplaces to be established in each state. The ACA also mandated that employers with 50 or more full-time equivalent employees offer them coverage. Support for a so-called public option, a proposed alternative to private insurance options in the new program, was vigorously opposed by Republicans and never received more than half-hearted support from the Obama administration and Democratic leadership in Congress.

The goals of the ACA were undermined by repeated court challenges to its constitutionality from Republican-led states that sought to overturn one or another (or all) of its measures, including the individual mandate to obtain insurance, the employer mandate to cover employees, and the requirement for states to participate in the Medicaid expansion. Most provisions were upheld in the courts, although the US Supreme Court allowed states to opt out of Medicaid expansion. As noted in chapter 10, 12 states still had not expanded their Medicaid program eligibility to include those with household incomes of 100% to 138% of the federal poverty level by October 2021, despite the fact that the federal government would pick up the great majority of the costs.[26] The Trump administration also eliminated the individual fine for not obtaining insurance. Those actions, along with the persistence of copayments and premiums that many cannot afford, as well as a bureaucratic system for selecting plans and obtaining coverage that is challenging to consumers, have led to the recognition that much more reform is needed. Meanwhile, some Democrats have renewed the push for single-payer insurance—

now under the banner of "Medicare for All"—or, failing that, a public option in the markets.[27]

The Role of the Insurance Corporations in US Health Reform Efforts

The health care reforms that have been enacted in the United States have left the insurance industry largely intact. The industry has successfully identified opportunities to move into public sector markets through managed care programs. Meanwhile, its defeat of a public option in the Affordable Care Act has meant that all policies in the non-Medicaid sector are issued through private insurers. The business model of health insurance corporations is to maximize revenue by minimizing risk—not the risk to the health of patients, but rather to the health of their bottom line. They accomplish this through coverage denials, marketing their products to healthier populations, and prodding allies in government to privatize the more lucrative components of care in public programs such as Medicare, Medicaid, the drug benefit in Medicare, and the medical programs of Veterans Affairs.

Insurance companies increased costs of care by having considerably higher overhead than federal Medicare. While estimates vary, Medicare administrative costs are far lower than those in the private insurance sector (2% to 5% vs. 12% to 18%).[28] Insurers would have little or no role in a one-payer system, so they fiercely resist any tendency in that direction through intense lobbying and overwhelming opposition funding for ballot initiatives that could undermine their role. In 2017 alone, insurers gave $61 million or more to political campaigns and to opposing ballot initiatives, as well as to nonprofits and trade associations promoting their interests.[29]

Workers, Their Unions, Their Employers, and Health Reform

Given how many Americans receive health insurance coverage through their jobs, a key consideration is the attitudes of employers and employees about the provision of health insurance coverage to their workforces. The organized labor movement's commitment to a national program of health insurance with compulsory participation has been mixed, at best. When progressive reformers were advocating sickness insurance on the German model for workers in the United States early in the twentieth century, Samuel Gompers, president of the American Federation of Labor, was opposed.

He argued that workers should obtain such coverage through their employers by organizing and supporting labor unions, which would negotiate for these benefits on their behalf. The sickness insurance proposal (that had coincided with the implementation of a similar program in the United Kingdom in 1911) did not gain enough traction among trade unionists, who were the group expected to benefit most from the initiative. Of note, labor unions in California and New York did support the initiative, as did women reformers, but this was not sufficient to overcome the opposition of medical practitioners, businesses, insurance companies, and legislators who considered the proposal to be a form of Bolshevism.[30]

The unions were more supportive of subsequent efforts, but after the failure to achieve universal health insurance during the Truman years, organized labor focused upon winning health care benefits in their negotiated contracts. As a result, a national program became less of a priority for them. Nonetheless, they were strongly supportive of Johnson's Medicare legislation in 1965. The American Federation of Labor and Congress of Industrial Organizations (AFL-CIO) set up a National Council of Senior Citizens in support of the legislation. Even that was more of a pragmatic than a principled position. From the perspective of organized labor, Medicare would obviate the challenge of including full health benefits for retirees in their contract negotiations. This group was active, disseminating literature, launching petition drives, and even demonstrating 14,000-strong outside of the convention hall in Atlantic City while the 1964 Democratic National Convention was under way.

Some union support for broader reform continued in the 1970s, notably through the Committee for National Health Insurance, established by Walter Reuther and the United Auto Workers, who were sensitive to the fact that corporate-provided health insurance added more to the cost of American automobiles than did the steel that went into the cars, making them less competitive in the international market.[31] The National Council of Senior Citizens (the retired union workers' organization) also continued to be supportive. When the next major effort came with the Clinton attempt at reform in the early 1990s, major union groupings like AFL-CIO and the auto workers were on board. They discouraged interest in some unions in more comprehensive reform on the model of Canada because they knew that Clinton's more limited, but ultimately doomed, effort depended upon their support, particularly in the face of opposition from business and insurance groups.

Obama's Affordable Care Act drew criticism from organized labor. Unions objected to the fact that plans they had negotiated for members and retirees were not eligible for the subsidies available to some others. They complained, too, about the burden of having to cover the adult children of members up to age 26.[32] Unions were particularly exercised that corporations were only required to cover workers employed at least 30 hours per week. One prominent labor leader suggested that Obama's reform would "shatter not only our hard-won health benefits, but destroy the foundation of the 40-hour work week that is the backbone of the American middle class."[33]

The campaign for Medicare for All, which received a boost in the 2016 and 2020 presidential campaigns of Senator Bernie Sanders, has divided the union movement, with some, such as the American Federation of Teachers and the Service Employees International Union, heavily promoting it and others, such as the International Association of Fire Fighters and Nevada's Culinary Union, opposing. In Michigan, where labor still wields some political power, several influential union leaders serve on the board of Blue Cross Blue Shield, which has a stake in the current system.[34]

Thus the union movement has supported the right of workers to receive health care, but many elements have only been willing to endorse programs they believe do not threaten union interests. They opposed government programs when they judged that obtaining coverage through union-negotiated benefits would strengthen the unions. They supported Medicare because covering retirees unburdened their negotiations for benefits for current employees. They have complained about Obamacare taxes on generous union-negotiated health benefits and have sought subsidies for the premiums associated with those benefits. The greatest impediment to union support for Medicare for All is the threat it represents to the hard-fought achievements for their membership in exchange for a new benefit funded by taxes paid by union members, whose corporations have borne the brunt of their costs up to now. Proponents reply that Medicare for All would free organized labor to negotiate for higher wages or other benefits, an argument that has not thus far carried the day.

Business owners' attitudes to health care have varied as well. On the one hand, corporations would prefer to avoid the expense of contributing to sickness funds or health insurance; on the other, health benefits are attractive to employees. For those whose employees can easily enough find work elsewhere, health care benefits make economic sense. For those mainly employing unskilled workers with few other options, such benefits are less attractive. These variable perspectives were evident in their responses to Obamacare.[35] When the ACA mandated that employers with 50 or more full-time workers (working 30 or more hours per week) provide health insurance for employees, some complied readily, while others moved to reduce headcounts, cut employee hours, or both, to avoid the legal minimum.[36]

Challenges Encountered by Canada's Universal Health Insurance Program and the United Kingdom's National Health Service

Governments have some involvement in the delivery of health care in all countries, and each has encountered challenges in implementing their programs that deserve scrutiny. How have other industrialized countries addressed problems in their implementation of national health care?

Their approaches have varied, and we can learn much by examining both their strengths and weaknesses.

Adequate Funding for Government Programs

Governments can play a number of roles: financing the care of the indigent; insuring segments of the population (such as the elderly, as in the United States); insuring the entire population, as in Canada; funding hospitals and other facilities; or running an entire health service (as in the United Kingdom). In each case, government needs to determine the appropriate level of funding and how to pay for the services, whether through payroll, income, sales, property, or value-added taxes. As always, taxing and spending present a delicate balance: You want to avoid angering taxpayers who vote, but also health care consumers, who vote as well.

Programs focused on the poor are handicapped by the fact that beneficiaries have comparably little or no voice in political discourse. They are less engaged than their better-off fellow citizens in such democratic activities as voting or writing to their representatives. And they may get little support from those citizens. People demonstrate less support for programs that don't benefit them directly in obvious ways. The lack of an effective political voice for its beneficiaries to highlight the program's shortcomings explains the ongoing difficulties Medicaid faces in the US.

There are many ways that governments can limit their medical care spending and shape clinical programs with the budget scalpel. One is to limit overall funding for a program, or, as in the case of Medicaid, to limit federal government contributions to state programs. A second approach is to limit the budgets of hospitals. (In Canada, hospitals receive global budgets to cover all operating expenses. Any new construction must be funded in other ways.) Other approaches include limiting funds for expensive services, such as intensive care units and operating rooms, and equipment (such as magnetic resonance imaging, or MRI, and computed tomography, or CT, scanners) that can be used to generate substantial charges, limiting the number of doctors entering certain specialties, and excluding expensive medications and services from eligibility for reimbursement. Not surprisingly, these cost-containing measures are not always greeted with enthusiasm by those seeking and providing care. Those concerns can influence political discourse.

Canada: The Romanow Commission

In Canada, the federal government pays a specified share of the cost for each provincial program. When universal health insurance was established in the 1960s, the federal government agreed to pay half of each provincial government's total costs. (As noted previously, the programs did not include the cost of dental care or outpatient medications.) Federal costs have risen, but the percentage share, though still substantial, has declined as a percentage of overall costs as provincial programs have grown costlier. For many years, provincial politicians, medical providers, and consumers expressed concern that the federal transfer payments were insufficient to support the provincial programs and that overall funding for the programs was inadequate. Considering all sources (including out-of-pocket expenditures for medications, dentistry, etc.), the Canadian government was paying about 35% of all health care costs in 1975. That fell to as low as 15% from 1991 to 2003.

A federal commission, led by a former premier of Saskatchewan, Roy Romanow, was established to investigate this and other issues concerning health care in Canada. The Royal Commission on the Future of Health Care in Canada, which issued its report in 2002, recommended increasing the federal share to about 25% of total governmental expenditures through a cash transfer to the provinces. It also proposed a mechanism to stabilize funding, by including an escalator clause that is set in advance for five-year periods. This recommendation was largely adopted. The funding formula has changed over time, sometimes taking account of the financial position of the different provinces, but since 2016, it has been a flat per capita transfer to all provinces. The federal government supplements the payments to certain provinces with fewer available resources. The annual increase is based on the three-year average increase in the cost of living, with a 3% minimum. The overall federal share has been between 20% and 25% in recent years.[37]

This approach allowed each province to establish funding priorities, fee schedules, hospital budgets, and the like. But the pressure on provincial budgets continues to be substantial and has resulted in some of them limiting total expenditures, for example, through various caps on fees and limits on payments to hospitals and other facilities and for procedures. The adequacy of federal contributions and the annual percentage increase in those contributions remains a major area of contention between the federal and provincial governments in Canada.[38]

Budget Allocations for the National Health Service

While no government of the United Kingdom has even hinted at being other than fully supportive of the NHS, all of them have cast a wary eye at the program's steadily rising costs. The budget of the NHS grew from about £25 billion in 1970 to about £150 billion in 2016–17 in inflation-adjusted currency. The proportion of the public services budget in the UK going to health increased from 11.2% in 1955–56 to 30.1% in 2016–17.[39]

A crucial issue in funding for the National Health Service has been the process of deciding what to spend, and the final decision rests with Parliament, which approves the budget. Insofar as the governing party makes that decision, funding reflects their priorities. Prior to 1980, there was little difference in the rate of increase in budget allocations between the parties. Since then, Conservative governments have tended to increase the budget each year by lesser amounts. As in Canada, there is much public discourse and intense disagreements between the political parties about the adequacy of funding for the NHS and what to do about it. It often is a central issue in political campaigns.[40]

Waiting Times and Program Variations

As governments have sought to optimize resources for their health care programs, they often face considerable public criticism about waiting times for appointments or procedures as risks to health and measures of the insufficiency of program funding.

Waiting Lists in Canada

One reason the Canadian government created the Romanow Commission was to investigate concerns about delays in elective surgeries. People were reportedly waiting up to several months for a hip replacement or cataract procedure. Waiting times for procedures feature prominently in critiques of the Canadian system of publicly funded medical care by advocates of a larger role for the private sector.[41] According to one report, 25% of Canadians waited four months or more for elective surgery, compared to 21% in the UK, 7% in the US, and close to 0% in Germany. Urgent or emergent procedures were dealt with far more promptly.[42]

Such findings have led to some policy changes.[43] Canada established standards for waits that were consistent with the severity and consequences of waiting.[44] The guideline specified that patients should wait no more than 4 weeks for radiation therapy for cancer, 26 weeks for hip or knee replacement, or 16 weeks for cataract surgery.[45] Subspecialties have developed guidelines for how soon patients should be seen and treated that relate to how acute the problem is. For example, people with acute gastrointestinal bleeding; acute, severe pancreatitis; or ascending cholangitis (an infection of the bile ducts) should be seen and have an endoscopic procedure, if needed, within 24 hours, while those who have difficulty swallowing that is getting worse should be seen within 2 weeks, patients with chronic hepatitis within 2 months, and those referred for screening colonoscopy can be seen within 6 months.[46] Meeting these standards continues to be a challenge.[47]

To put things in perspective, when my Canadian mother developed a stage 4 lymphoma, a situation with a mortality rate of about 50% at the time, she never had to wait for a diagnostic procedure or for treatment. She was able to see the most experienced oncologist in Manitoba, where she lived. The principal of "portability" in the Canada Health Act means that she could have been referred to another province for similar care, as appropriate, at no cost to her.[48] She never had to pay a penny for surgery, physician visits, hospital care, or chemotherapy. Finally, she received home care services daily, also at no charge, for the remaining 11 years of her life. That does not happen in the United States. So, while Canada still has lots to do to ensure that everyone gets the best care possible in a timely manner, my mother's provincial health care system certainly delivered the goods when she had a serious health problem.

Waiting Lists in the United Kingdom

In the UK, the National Health Service experiences chronically long waiting lists for nonemergent services. The UK government also has targets: that 85% of cancer patients start treatment within 62 days of an urgent referral, and that 92% of patients receive routine hospital care (likely elective surgeries) within 18 weeks. As of 2019, these standards were not quite being met, with 77% of those with cancer and 86% of people needing routine hospital care getting treated within the recommended window. This has been a matter of intense political contention, because the cure for longer-than-acceptable waiting times is widely regarded as providing more funding for the NHS.[49]

Provincial Inequities in Canada

Some Canadian provinces are wealthier than others, for example, because of greater tax revenues related to extraction industries. As a result, they can afford to spend more on their health care systems, thereby improving access, quality, and waiting times. The federal government has attempted to level the playing field with greater financial support to the less advantaged provinces.[50]

Getting Right the Number of Specialists to Be Trained

One strategy for controlling costs is to limit the numbers of physicians entering particular procedural specialties that generate high expenditures. While this makes sense from the perspective of containing costs as a way to reduce low-value or unnecessary care, estimating the needed numbers of practitioners can be challenging. In some instances, these constraints may contribute to waiting times for procedures. In Canada, for example, waiting times for elective orthopedic procedures increased from a median of 19.5 weeks in 1993 to 32.2 weeks in 2003. By one estimate, there was a need for 400 more orthopedic surgeons in addition to the 1,126 practicing in Canada in 2003.[51] Of course, estimates of need by members of a specialty are subject to professional biases. The increase would need to be even greater were the goal being to achieve the numbers of orthopedists thought to be optimal in the United States, although the mix of specialties in the US is associated with costs to the system that are recognized as unsustainable.[52]

Ensuring Adequate Funding for Government Programs

We have seen that governments are often reluctant to spend all that is needed to optimize health. Would it be appropriate for external experts and others to have substantial roles in formulating policy about how much to spend for public health care programs? If the government is responsible for funding the programs, they cannot help but be involved. Arguably, an enforceable recommendation, imposed on them by an independent group, that they pay any amount, even up to the point of allowing health care to consume their entire budget, could make other important programs lose all or much of their funding. But if government officials and legislators *alone* establish the levels at which to fund these programs, they are much more likely to underfund programs and to be swayed by constituencies whose priorities do not include optimizing health for the population as a whole.

Ideally, appropriations would be approved by government after being specified in detail by an outside entity that is not beholden either to the government or the various constituencies (taxpayers, scientists, practicing doctors, clinical corporations, manufacturers, and disease advocacy groups) that dot the landscape and are ready to pounce. Such a group would include people who understand financing, science, and clinical operations, as well as other budgeting needs outside of health. Would such a process ever be entirely objective? That is unlikely. But such an approach might, on the model of Canada's Romanow Commission, lead to more even-handed consideration of evidence, need, competing needs, and capacity.

What Kind of Country?

It seems self-evident that any nation should have the goal of achieving, as far as possible, a comparable standard of physical, emotional, and social health for all citizens. Many states with the greatest burden of important chronic diseases have the least generous Medicaid programs, in part because of political ideology, but also because of the states' financial circumstances. The same states also have the lowest life expectancy at birth (75 to 77.2 years in Alabama, Arkansas, Georgia, Kentucky, Mississippi, Oklahoma, South Carolina, and Tennessee, compared to 80 years or more in California, Colorado, Kansas, Hawaii, Minnesota, New York, and most of the New England states).[53] African Americans migrated to escape racism in the past century. While we might expect similar migration between states to obtain better health benefits, one study of immigrant children did not find evidence of such migration.[54]

The World Health Organization's 1946 constitution envisages "the highest attainable standard of health as a fundamental right of every human being." More recently, WHO stated, "The right to health must be enjoyed without discrimination on the grounds of race, age, ethnicity or any other status. Non-discrimination and equality require states to take steps to redress any discriminatory law, practice or policy."[55] Government policies alone don't explain the inequitable system for health care in the

United States. Why should government have to solve these problems? It is clear that none of the other major actors in the system are particularly motivated to address them in a meaningful way.

This was brought home to me when an incoming dean in my former medical school at the University of California, Los Angeles, announced at his first faculty meeting, "We must pay more attention to our community." I mistakenly thought that he was talking about the disadvantaged who received poor care. Alas, he was instead referring to the wealthy people in Los Angeles who could donate funds to the medical school!

The reality is that only a government so disposed has any inclination to ensure care for the most disadvantaged. When I asked a prominent health care leader, who has run the public health care systems in three major cities, whether it is possible for systems that are separate to be equal, he responded that they could not. Care for the disadvantaged will improve only when the population as a whole share the same risk of receiving the same inadequate health care. The Canadian and British examples demonstrate that when the entire population is affected by deficiencies in health care, politicians are more responsive to the need for change, even if not always to the degree required to solve the problems.

Beyond that, equitable health care would require that more resources be directed toward those most in need. For example, COVID-19 testing and vaccination programs in the United States should have anticipated the need to prioritize the poor and minority communities, who, as is generally the case with epidemics, were at greatest risk. Testing among these populations at the peak of the epidemic in New York City occurred at a significantly lower rate than in advantaged communities in New York.[56] Vaccinations followed a similar pattern nationwide.[57] The inadequate funding of public health programs and the broken health insurance system made it impossible to reach out systematically to people at risk, to make sure that persons in multigeneration housing were able to quarantine, or to assure people concerned about infection that they could seek care without worrying that they would accrue medical expenses that they could not afford. National health care programs are far better positioned to take all of the measures that are needed to ensure that all people have every opportunity to benefit from measures to prevent and treat potentially lethal illnesses like COVID-19.[58]

The American health care system is an unqualified disaster. That is not to idealize programs in other countries. Government-sponsored health care coverage does not ensure equitable access, let alone equitable care. In Canada, disparities in access to a regular doctor are not as extensive overall as those reported in the United States. In Canada's substantial aboriginal population, however, and among longer-term Latin American immigrants, access is a problem.[59] One study found that 16% of Canadians and 7% of persons in the United Kingdom reported cost-related access barriers. This was substantially less than in the United States, but still a more than negligible problem.[60] Another study of mental health services in Canada found that lower-income Canadians were significantly more likely than others to report that such services were inaccessible or unavailable.[61] These problems, along with long waits for elective surgery and lack of pharmaceutical coverage, engender active policy discussions of ways to address these needs.[62]

So, no government can wave a wand and obliterate health and health care disparities, but if governments invest sufficiently and create systems to prioritize the well-being of the people *as a whole* (all of whom are potentially at risk for deficient care), they can address systemic problems while diminishing disparities. No one else has the incentive or the resources to accomplish that.

Notes

1. Saul A. Miller, *White Paper on Health Policy* (Winnipeg: Government of Manitoba, July 1972).

2. "Rights and Assistance in the French Revolution," in *Health and Citizenship: Political Cultures of Health in Modern Europe*, ed. Frank Huisman and Harry Oosterhuis (London: Routledge, 2015), 49–56.

3. These sections on public health in Europe and the United States draw extensively upon "Public Health and the Modern State: France, Sweden, and Germany," and "Localization and Health Salvation in the United States," in Dorothy Porter, *Health, Civilization and the State: A History of Public Health from Ancient to Modern Times* (New York: Taylor & Francis e-Library, 2005), 96–109 and 147–62.

4. Porter, *Health*, 98–103.

5. Porter, *Health*, 96–98.

6. Porter, *Health*, 104–9.

7. Richard Brown, "Looking at History: Public Health 1832–1854," April 30, 2008, http://richardjohnbr.blogspot.com/2008/04/public-health-1832-1854.html; William Cunningham Glen and Alexander Glen, *The Public Health Act, 1875, and the Law Relating to Public Health, Local Government, and Urban and Rural Sanitary Authorities* (London: Butterworths, Knight, 1876).

8. John Henry Griscom, *The Sanitary Condition of the Laboring Population of New York with Suggestions for Its Improvement* (New York: Harper & Bros., 1845).

9. Lemuel Shattuck, Nathaniel P. Banes, and Jeniel Abbott, *Report of a General Plan for the Promotion of Public and Personal Health* (Boston: Dutton & Wentworth, 1850).

10. Warren Winkelstein, "Lemuel Shattuck: Architect of American Public Health," *Epidemiology* 19, no. 4 (July 2008): 634, https://doi.org/10.1097/EDE .0b013e31817307f2.

11. Reinhard Busse and Miriam Blümel, "Germany: Health System Review," *Health Systems in Transition* 16, no. 2 (2014): xxiii–xxvii, 17–41, PMID 25115137; Mimi Chung, "Health Care Reform: Learning from Other Major Health Care Systems," *Princeton Public Health Review*, December 2, 2017, https://pphr.princeton.edu/2017/12 /02/unhealthy-health-care-a-cursory-overview-of-major-health-care-systems/; Lorraine Boissoneault, "Bismarck Tried to End Socialism's Grip—by Offering Government Health Care," *Smithsonian Magazine*, July 14, 2017, https://www .smithsonianmag.com/history/bismarck-tried-end-socialisms-grip-offering -government-healthcare-180964064/; Roosa Tikkanen et al., "International Health Care System Profiles: Germany," Commonwealth Fund, June 5, 2020, https://www .commonwealthfund.org/international-health-policy-center/countries/germany; Reinhard Busse et al., "Statutory Health Insurance in Germany: A Health System Shaped by 135 Years of Solidarity, Self-Governance, and Competition," *Lancet* 390, no. 10097 (August 26, 2017): 882–97, https://doi.org/10.1016/S0140-6736(17)31280-1.

12. Philip Nord, "The Welfare State in France, 1870–1914," *French Historical Studies* 18, no. 3 (Spring 1994): 821–38, https://doi.org/10.2307/286694; Victor G. Rodwin, "The Health Care System under French National Health Insurance: Lessons for Health Reform in the United States," *American Journal of Public Health* 93, no. 1 (January 2003): 31–37, https://doi.org/10.2105/ajph.93.1.31; Roosa Tikkanen et al., "International Health Care System Profiles: France," Commonwealth Fund, June 5, 2020, https://www.commonwealthfund.org/international-health-policy-center /countries/france; Karine Chevreul et al., "France: Health System Review," *Health Systems in Transition* 17, no. 3 (2015): 1–218, v–xxvii, PMID 26766545.

13. "Authorities and Trusts," National Health Service, accessed July 12, 2020, https://www.nhs.uk/servicedirectories/pages/nhstrustlisting.aspx; "The Formation of National Health Service," University of Warwick, accessed June 2, 2020, https:// warwick.ac.uk/services/library/mrc/archives_online/digital/health/nhs/; Roosa Tikkanen et al., "International Health Care System Profiles: England," Common- wealth Fund, June 5, 2020, https://www.commonwealthfund.org/international -health-policy-center/countries/england; George Campbell Gosling, "Paying for

Healthcare: Life in Britain before the 'Free' NHS," History Extra, August 9, 2018, https://www.historyextra.com/period/20th-century/nhs-history-pay-healthcare-free/.

14. Robin F. Badgley and Samuel Wolfe, *Doctors' Strike: Medical Care and Conflict in Saskatchewan* (New York: Atherton Press, 1967).

15. "Tommy Douglas Crowned 'Greatest Canadian,'" CBC News, November 29, 2004, https://www.cbc.ca/news/entertainment/tommy-douglas-crowned-greatest-canadian-1.510403.

16. "Poll: Canadians Are Most Proud of Universal Medicare," CTV News, November 25, 2012, https://www.ctvnews.ca/canada/poll-canadians-are-most-proud-of-universal-medicare-1.1052929.

17. Much of the discussion about efforts to reform American health care in the first half of the twentieth century draws on Paul Starr's discussion in Paul Starr, *The Social Transformation of American Medicine* (New York: Basic Books, 1982), 240–89.

18. Starr, *Social Transformation*, 253; Artur Viseltear, "Compulsory Health Insurance in California, 1915–1918," *Journal of the History of Medicine and the Allied Sciences* 24, no. 2 (April 1969): 151–82, https://doi.org/10.1093/jhmas/XXIV.2.151.

19. John Murray, *Origins of American Health Insurance: A History of Industrial Sickness Funds* (New Haven, CT: Yale University Press, 2007).

20. The perspective of organized labor is discussed toward the end of this chapter.

21. Isidore S. Falk, C. Rufus Rorem, and Martha D. Ring, *The Costs of Medical Care: A Summary of Investigations on the Economic Aspects of the Prevention and Care of Illness* (Chicago: University of Chicago Press, 1933).

22. Starr, *Social Transformation*, 282.

23. Beatrix Hoffman, "Health Care Reform and Social Movements in the United States," *American Journal of Public Health* 93, no. 1 (January 2003): 75–85, https://doi.org/10.2105/ajph.93.1.75.

24. Max J. Skidmore, "Ronald Reagan and 'Operation Coffeecup': A Hidden Episode in American Political History," *Journal of American Culture* 12, no. 3 (Fall 1989): 89–96, https://doi.org/10.1111/j.1542-734X.1989.1203_89.x.

25. Darrell M. West, Diane Heith, and Chris Goodwin, "Harry and Louise Go to Washington: Political Advertising and Health Care Reform," *Journal of Health Politics, Policy and Law* 21, no. 1 (Spring 1996): 35–68, https://doi.org/10.1215/03616878-21-1-35.

26. "Status of State Medicaid Expansion Decisions: Interactive Map," Kaiser Family Foundation Medicaid, October 8, 2021, https://www.kff.org/medicaid/issue-brief/status-of-state-medicaid-expansion-decisions-interactive-map/.

27. Linda J. Blumberg et al., "Comparing Health Insurance Reform Options: From 'Building on the ACA' to Single Payer," Commonwealth Fund, October 16, 2019, https://www.commonwealthfund.org/publications/issue-briefs/2019/oct/comparing-health-insurance-reform-options-building-on-aca-to-single-payer; Robert Doherty et al., "Envisioning a Better U.S. Health Care System for All: A Call to Action by the American College of Physicians," *Annals of Internal Medicine* 172, no. 2 Supplement (January 2020): S3–S6, https://doi.org/10.7326/M19-2411; Steffie Woolhandler and David U. Himmelstein, "The American College of Physicians'

Endorsement of Single-Payer Reform: A Sea Change for the Medical Profession," *Annals of Internal Medicine* 172, no. 2 Supplement (January 21, 2020): S60–S61, https://doi.org/10.7326/M19-3775.

28. Glenn Kessler, "Medicare, Private Insurance and Administrative Costs: A Democratic Talking Point," *Washington Post*, September 19, 2017, https://www.washingtonpost.com/news/fact-checker/wp/2017/09/19/medicare-private-insurance-and-administrative-costs-a-democratic-talking-point/?utm_term=.9709a72b2cc1.

29. Frank Bass, "Health-Care Corporations Flooded Political Campaigns with Cash in 2017," Maplight News Archive, April 10, 2019, https://maplight.org/story/health-care-corporations-flooded-political-campaigns-with-cash-in-2017/.

30. Hoffman, "Health Care Reform"; Ronald Numbers, *Almost Persuaded: American Physicians and Compulsory Health Insurance, 1912–1920* (Baltimore: Johns Hopkins University Press, 1978); Beatrix Hoffman, *The Wages of Sickness: The Politics of Health Insurance in Progressive America* (Chapel Hill: University of North Carolina Press, 2001), 68–91.

31. Igor Volsky, "The Auto Makers and the Health Crisis," Think Progress, November 18, 2008, https://archive.thinkprogress.org/the-auto-makers-and-the-health-care-crisis-55282007c3de/.

32. Steven Mufson and Tom Hamburger, "Labor Union Officials Say Obama Betrayed Them in Health-Care Rollout," *Washington Post*, January 31, 2014, https://www.washingtonpost.com/business/economy/labor-union-officials-say-obama-betrayed-them-in-health-care-rollout/2014/01/31/2cda6afc-8789-11e3-833c-33098f9e5267_story.html.

33. James Hoffa, quoted in Avik Roy, "Labor Unions: Obamacare Will 'Shatter' Our Health Care Benefits, Cause 'Nightmare Scenarios,'" *Forbes*, July 15, 2013, https://www.forbes.com/sites/theapothecary/2013/07/15/labor-leaders-obamacare-will-shatter-their-health-benefits-cause-nightmare-scenarios/#135b49393da1.

34. Ian Kullgren and Alice Miranda Ollstein, "Labor's Civil War over 'Medicare for All' Threatens Its 2020 Clout," Politico, February 19, 2020, https://www.politico.com/news/2020/02/18/medicare-for-all-labor-union-115873; Natalie Shure, "Why Are These Labor Unions Opposing Medicare for All?," *In These Times*, December 17, 2018, https://inthesetimes.com/working/entry/21642/labor_unions_new_york_medicare_for_all_bernie_sanders.

35. Paul Starr, *Remedy and Reaction: The Peculiar American Struggle over Health Care Reform* (New Haven, CT: Yale University Press, 2013), 114–17, 219–20, 248–49.

36. Jacob Passy, "Businesses Eliminated Hundreds of Thousands of Full-Time Jobs to Avoid Obamacare Mandate," Marketwatch, November 24, 2017, https://www.marketwatch.com/story/businesses-eliminated-hundreds-of-thousands-of-full-time-jobs-to-avoid-obamacare-mandate-2017-11-24; Karen McVeigh, "US Employers Slashing Worker Hours to Avoid Obamacare Insurance Mandate," *The Guardian*, September 30, 2013, https://www.theguardian.com/world/2013/sep/30/us-employers-slash-hours-avoid-obamacare.

37. Sonya Norris, "Federal Funding for Health Care," Canada Library of Parliament, July 18, 2018, https://lop.parl.ca/sites/PublicWebsite/default/en_CA

/ResearchPublications/201845E; "Major Federal Transfers," Department of Finance Canada, accessed April 23, 2020, https://www.canada.ca/en/department-finance /programs/federal-transfers/major-federal-transfers.html; Roy J. Romanow and Commission on the Future of Health Care in Canada, *Building on Values: The Future of Health Care in Canada: Final Report* (Saskatoon, SK: Privy Council of Canada, 2002).

38. A detailed discussion of this history can be found in C. David Naylor, Andrew Boozary, and Owen Adams, "Canadian Federal-Provincial/Territorial Funding of Universal Health Care: Fraught History, Uncertain Future," *Canadian Medical Association Journal* 192, no. 45 (November 9, 2020): e1408–12, https://doi.org/10.1503 /cmaj.200143.

39. Nick Triggle, "10 Charts That Show Why the NHS Is in Trouble," BBC News, May 24, 2018, https://www.bbc.com/news/health-42572110.

40. From 1955 to 1979, a period during which there were both Conservative and Labour governments, the average annual increase in funding was about 4.3%. During the rule of the Conservative governments of Margaret Thatcher and John Major, the annual budget increase was about 3.3%. The Labour governments from 1997 to 2010 increased the budgets by an average of 6% per year. The Conservative-led governments after that dropped the increases to 1% to 2%. Thus, when the decision about funding is entirely in the hands of politicians, the budget decisions often reflect the perspectives and priorities of the political parties. Triggle, "10 Charts." In the 2019 election, the winning Conservatives proposed increasing the budget by 2.3% per year for five years. The Labour Party considered that inadequate to address the problem and proposed increasing the budget by 3.9% per year. Nick Triggle, "Hospital Waiting Times at Worst-Ever Level," BBC News, November 14, 2019, https://www.bbc.com/news/health-50397856.

41. Peter St. Onge and Patrick Déry, "Waiting for Health-Care Reform: Patients Are Paying the Price for Our Public Health-Care Monopoly," *Financial Post*, December 18, 2019, https://business.financialpost.com/opinion/waiting-for-health-care -reform-patients-are-paying-the-price-for-our-public-health-care-monopoly.

42. Cathy Schoen et al., *The Commonwealth Fund 2010 International Health Policy Survey in Eleven Countries* (New York: Commonwealth Fund, 2010), http://www .commonwealthfund.org/Surveys/2010/Nov/2010-International-Survey.aspx.

43. Canadian Institute of Health Information, *National Health Expenditure Trends*, 1975 to 2019 (Ottawa: Canadian Institute for Health Information, 2019), https://www .cihi.ca/sites/default/files/document/nhex-trends-narrative-report-2019-en-web.pdf.

44. "Patient Wait Times Guarantees," Government of Canada, accessed October 25, 2021, https://www.canada.ca/en/health-canada/services/quality-care/wait -times/patient-wait-times-guarantees.html.

45. Sonya Norris, "The Wait Times Issue and the Patient Wait Times Guarantee," Government Canada, revised July 24, 2007, https://publications.gc.ca/collections /collection_2007/lop-bdp/prb/prb0582-e.pdf.

46. William G. Patterson et al., "Canadian Consensus on Medically Acceptable Wait Times for Digestive Health Care," *Canadian Journal of Gastroenterology* 20, no. 6 (June 2006): 411–23, https://doi.org/10.1155/2006/343686.

47. "Explore Wait Times for Priority Procedures across Canada," Canadian Institute for Health Information, accessed October 16, 2021, https://www.cihi.ca/en/explore-wait-times-for-priority-procedures-across-canada.

48. "17.4 Portability," in Standing Senate Committee on Social Affairs, Science and Technology, *The Health of Canadians—The Federal Role, Final Report, Volume Six, Part VIII: The Canada Health Act* (Ottawa: Government of Canada, 2002), https://sencanada.ca/content/sen/committee/372/soci/rep/repocto2vol6part7-e.htm.

49. Triggle, "Hospital Waiting Times."

50. Jenny Yang, "Government Sector Health Spending per Capita in Canada by Province in 2019," Statista, September 8, 2021, https://www.statista.com/statistics/436343/governmental-health-spending-per-capita-canada-by-province/.

51. Pauline Comeau, "Crisis in Orthopedic Care: Surgeon and Resource Shortage," *Canadian Medical Association Journal* 171, no. 3 (August 3, 2004): 223, https://doi.org/10.1503/cmaj.1041073.

52. Deborah Shipton, Elizabeth M. Bradley, and Nizar N. Mahomed, "Critical Shortage of Orthopaedic Services in Ontario, Canada," *Journal of Bone and Joint Surgery, American* 85, no. 9 (September 2003): 1710–15, https://doi.org/10.2106/00004623-200309000-00009.

53. "Life Expectancy by State 2020," World Population Review, accessed April 27, 2020, https://worldpopulationreview.com/states/life-expectancy-by-state/.

54. Vasil I. Yasenov et al., "Public Health Insurance Expansion for Immigrant Children and Interstate Migration of Low-Income Immigrants," *JAMA Pediatrics* 174, no. 1 (January 1, 2020): 22–28, https://doi.org/10.1001/jamapediatrics.2019.5477.

55. "Human Rights and Health," World Health Organization, December 29, 2017, https://www.who.int/news-room/fact-sheets/detail/human-rights-and-health.

56. Michelle Young, "Interactive Map of the Coronavirus Cases in NYC by Zip Code," Untapped New York, April 21, 2020, https://untappedcities.com/2020/04/28/interactive-map-coronavirus-cases-nyc-zip-code/. For example, as of April 20, 2020, zip code 10128 on the affluent Upper East Side of New York had 9.05 cases per 1,000, and 3.05 people had been tested for every person diagnosed; in zip code 11372 in Queens, they had 32.05 cases per 1,000 residents, and only 1.60 tests for every person diagnosed. The pattern was consistent throughout the city, with clear stratification by socioeconomic status in access to the tests.

57. Jennifer Tolbert et al., "Vaccination Is Local: COVID-19 Vaccination Rates Vary by County and Key Characteristics," KFF Coronavirus (COVID-19), May 12, 2021, https://www.kff.org/coronavirus-covid-19/issue-brief/vaccination-is-local-covid-19-vaccination-rates-vary-by-county-and-key-characteristics/.

58. Zeynep Tufekci, "The Unvaccinated May Not Be Who You Think," *New York Times*, October 15, 2021, https://www.nytimes.com/2021/10/15/opinion/covid-vaccines-unvaccinated.html.

59. Arjumand A. Siddiqi et al., "Racial Disparities in Access to Care under Conditions of Universal Coverage," *American Journal of Preventive Medicine* 50, no. 2 (February 2016): 220–25, https://doi.org/10.1016/j.amepre.2014.08.004.

60. Danielle Martin et al., "Canada's Universal Health-Care System: Achieving Its Potential," *Lancet* 391, no. 10131 (April 2018): 1718–35, https://doi.org/10.1016/S0140-6736(18)30181-8.

61. Amanda K. Slaunwhite, "The Role of Gender and Income in Predicting Barriers to Mental Health Care in Canada," *Community Mental Health Journal* 51, no. 5 (July 2015): 621–27, https://doi.org/10.1007/s10597-014-9814-8.

62. Martin, "Canada's Universal Health-Care System."

| Dialogue #9 |

Student: I was always puzzled that it took hundreds of years to build some of those old cathedrals in Europe. In the United States, we build structures more quickly than that, but it is 100 years and counting for trying to create a comprehensive system for health care.

Professor: This bit of American exceptionalism is not one we can be proud of.

Student: Are we ever going to be able to fix health care? Will the insurance industry ever get out of the way?

Professor: They probably won't disarm unilaterally.

Student: Your point is well-taken. Even with government programs, a lot of things can go wrong.

Professor: They sure can.

Student: I think that we've done a decent job of covering the major topics. I know there is so much more that could be said about each of them, but let's move on to the solution.

Professor: There's more to do.

Student: Professor, haven't we done enough? This is project may outlive me!

Professor: We've identified some issues that pop up again and again. We need to weave them together. We should probably discuss a few of them. Can you think of one that seems important to you?

Student: Hmm. How about money? It came up a lot. Getting things. Everyone is trying to get something out of the health care system.

Professor: Nice insight. Perhaps you are talking about commodities? That is indeed a key theme. As you look into it, think about health as well as health care. There might be some parallel issues. I'll send you links to a few relevant papers.

12

Rectitude or Revenue?

American Health Care in the Marketplace

Is the physician . . . a healer of the sick or a maker of money? I am speaking of the true physician.
—Plato, quoting Socrates, in *The Republic*, Book I

"Sales."

I never really have gotten over that comment by the executive from Henry Ford Hospital years ago, when he used the term to refer to patient visits and admissions. "Have we sunk so low as that?" I ask myself. Then I think of the dermatologist who wasn't going to see me because I owed $4. And the diabetic patients in New England who cut down on their insulin because they couldn't afford the $1 "copayment."

Copayment—what a strange word. Sure, there needs to be a mechanism for reimbursing clinicians for their time, effort, and expenses. But making the potential recipients of care pay to be seen when they might not be able to afford it, or may suffer grave consequences to their health or financial circumstances? Calling for "skin in the game" when the game is survival? Putting people at risk for medical bankruptcies? Does this make sense in a country that purports to value life?

Commodities and Health Care

Has health care become a commodity? "Commodity" is defined by *Webster's Third New International Dictionary* as "something used or valued especially when regarded as an article of commerce." Commodities are "economic goods," things bought and sold in a market.[1] In modern parlance, a commodity is generally recognized as a good that is produced for exchange in the market, either for other goods or for money. Humans have been in the commodities trading business for at least 6,000 years, since the residents of Sumer (in ancient Mesopotamia) used clay tokens to trade for goats.

It is simple enough to think of corn, oil, beef, cars, and clothing in this way. Can the same be said of health care or health? Can provision of treatment to a sick individual be regarded in the same way as a pound of butter? Some health care is clearly neither an item produced nor a service provided for the marketplace. Consider soldiers injured on a battlefield. No one would suggest that they be required to present a credit card or insurance card to get their wounds treated. Public health officials who monitor air quality are salaried and don't issue reports to individuals for a fee. Granted, these are exceptions, but what about office- or hospital-based medical care? After all, don't doctors and hospitals need to get paid for their time and effort?

They do, but it is not inevitable that their compensation needs to be determined in the marketplace of commodities. When clinical decisions have implications for revenue accruing to individuals or organizations making those decisions, health care enters the marketplace of commodified goods and services. Recall my gastroenterology colleague, Art Schwabe, who lamented that younger practitioners barely take time to evaluate patients before ordering procedures that generate more revenue than "evaluation and management." Recall the cardiologists, of whom the house staff joked that they would put a catheter in the heart of anyone with a heartbeat. Their decisions may or may not have been defensible clinically, but they were unquestionably beneficial to them financially.

Practicing physicians need to be fairly compensated. In the United States, this typically takes the form of fees for service or salaries consistent with the amount of revenue they are expected to generate. In either case, doctors' compensation varies widely across specialties, differences not explained by years of training. Although no physicians are destitute, these pay differentials have implications.

When my family took a summer road trip to visit baseball stadiums on the East Coast, we faced a dilemma: Boston's Fenway Park was sold out for every game. Fortunately, JudyAnn, a friend and general internist colleague at Harvard, told me that she had a share of two season tickets. Since there were four of us, I asked her if she had a lead on another pair. She did. When I reimbursed her, she pointed out that one pair of seats was much better than the other. The really good seats came from a surgeon, while the other pair were the ones she shared with other generalist clinicians.

Does the world work this way because surgeons' services have greater value than those of generalists? That depends. What do we mean by "value"? And how does that relate to price? Anyone with something to sell has to recoup the costs incurred along the way. In the case of medical care, this includes the time and effort of the personnel (including the physician), and a number of other expenses (see below). The sum of these inputs comprises the cost of the health care service to those who render care. Is that the same as its value? How does that relate to the price that is charged?

Commodities, Value, and the Marketplace

In John Huston's classic film *The Treasure of the Sierra Madre*, based on B. Traven's novel, three desperately poor men prospect for gold. The oldest man, Howard, muses about why gold sells for such a high price.

"A thousand men, say, go searching for gold. After six months one of 'em is lucky—one out of a thousand. His find represents not only his own labor but that of nine hundred and ninety-nine others to boot. Six thousand months or fifty years of scrabbling over mountains, going hungry and thirsty. An ounce of gold, mister, is worth what it is because of the human labor that went into the finding and getting of it . . . There's no other explanation. In itself, gold ain't good for anything much except to make jewelry and gold teeth."[2]

"Free-market" economists don't believe that a commodity's price needs to reflect the cost of producing it or its usefulness to the buyer. They regard it as driven primarily by supply and demand. But real markets are far from free: the "price point" is often set without respect to actual costs, and demand can be manipulated through advertising that inflates perceptions of usefulness. Other economists who reject free market ideology recognize the salience of supply and demand to prices, for example, in the relationship of higher interest rates to the preference for greater liquidity of investments.[3] In spite of these complexities, I find it clarifying to think about three components of price in the context of medical care.

First, presuming that an item is potentially useful, *what does it cost to produce and distribute?* In health care, this involves not only the time and effort to provide a service, but also the costs of producing and distributing supplies or medications, paying for office or hospital space and equipment, and training clinicians. Second, *what price can the seller charge?* In an unregulated market, this price bears only a passing relationship to costs. It can also easily be manipulated: the seller can make exaggerated claims for the product's usefulness or can drive up price by limiting supply (and competition from other producers). Third, *when there is a nontrivial difference between the cost of all inputs and the price obtained, the transaction generates surplus or profit.*[4]

Not everyone wants to describe that surplus as "profit." That would seem crass for clinicians and would represent tax problems for so-called nonprofit hospitals that generate hundreds of millions of dollars of such revenue yearly. Conversely, manufacturers of health care products and those who own medical office space have no such reluctance to talking about profits shamelessly. All are interested in maximizing their revenue, as are most actors in our economy.

Extraction of Surplus in US Health Care

In the United States, many providers charge substantially more for a service or a medication than their costs would dictate. In short, they generate large profits.[5] Take a hospital with an average of 500 inpatients per day and an annual surplus of $365 million. Its operating profit is $1 million per day, or $2,000 per day per patient. Maybe that's justified, for example, because of a need to periodically update the facilities. But many would disagree, especially when such hospitals obscure the distinction between revenue that is needed to maintain satisfactory facilities and revenue that exceeds such needs and contributes to inequity in health care, particularly when hospitals game the system to avoid caring for Medicaid patients, for whom reimbursement is lower. The push to generate more surplus can amplify social inequality beyond health care, particularly if the rate of return on capital (extraction of surplus) exceeds the rate of growth in the economy.[6]

What is difficult to refute, however, is that the price charged for medical care is neither the embodiment of its intrinsic value to the patient or society nor necessarily of the actual cost of providing that care. If it were, then medical care in the United States, which produces worse outcomes, would not cost much more than similar care in other countries. Let's review briefly the evidence in the preceding chapters about how this phenomenon manifests in different areas of American health care.

Practicing Clinicians: What Kind of Value?

Back to the disparities in specialty income in the United States: If challenged, highly paid specialists would say that they provide something more valuable than what generalists, psychiatrists, or pediatricians do. But as we saw with the Relative Value Scale Update Committee, which advises on prices across specialties, specialists get paid more because they have been able to work the system to pay them more.

I have made clear my belief that spending an hour helping a patient come to terms with a diagnosis, treating them empathically, and providing them with the information they need to navigate the road ahead, is no less valuable than spending an hour administering anesthesia, cutting out a tumor, or infusing drugs to treat the tumor.

Because these activities are not treated as equivalent, the system is tilted severely toward doctors wanting to do more and more procedures for which they can charge more and more money. When medical work is piecework, it is the act of producing and selling a commodity. The incentive to "sell" as many of the expensive procedures as possible is substantial. A clinical decision is partly an economic one, and that part is often in conflict with other essential dimensions of the role of the physician, as I discuss below.

Health Care Systems: Commodification of Care and of Clinicians

Hospitals and health systems are also in the business of buying and selling products in the marketplace. While the clinician is a relatively small-business person, the health system chief executive is a corporate tycoon. Yes, he or she is interested in sales, but also in getting the best price for the transaction (from the corporation's perspective). As a result, health systems prefer contracts with private insurers that pay more than public insurance. They want practitioners who do a lot of procedures for which they can charge high prices. They advertise to stimulate demand and increase both sales and prices. They deny service whenever they can to large swaths of the population that need care, but don't or can't pay top dollar.

Health care systems notoriously lack transparency about pricing. They generally set their "sticker" prices to be much higher than any insurer will pay. For private insurance plans for which they are in-network providers, they contract for a specified level of reimbursement for each service that is less than the sticker price. In the case of Medicare and Medicaid, the government sets the payment level. Insurers specify how much of a provider's nominal price is an allowable charge, and what proportion is to be paid by insurance and by the patient. An insurer may specify that $100 of a provider's $400 bill is an allowable charge, of which the insurer will pay $80 and authorize the provider to charge the remaining $20 to the patient.

Those lacking insurance or who are out-of-network are less fortunate: they are confronted with a bill for $400. Indeed, providers set the price that high in order to collect the most that they can from such individuals. For patients who are affluent or who understand how to work the system, that may not be a serious problem. My neighbor, who was savvy, knew that she could request and get 30% knocked off the quoted price when seeing an out-of-network provider. Financially disadvantaged patients often lack both health insurance and negotiating skills. When confronted with this sort of situation, they don't know that they can seek relief. Even if they obtain some price reduction, they often cannot pay the fee, which remains much greater than what Medicare or private insurance companies pay. The nature of the medical marketplace allows clinical corporations to charge whatever they can get away with, and not necessarily what the intrinsic value is to the person receiving the service.

Health systems hire workforces of clinicians to feed their money machines. Some (the proceduralists) they pay well, others (the primary care doctors) they pay just enough to ensure that they will continue to channel people into the system in search of procedures. In this sense, the physicians are also, from the perspective of the health system, commodities.

Like many other medical centers, UCLA hired high-priced consultants some years ago to advise it on improving its financial position. The consultants were known for their "slash and burn" approach, so it came as no surprise when they concluded that UCLA was overpaying its generalist physicians. They proposed getting rid of most of them. The medical school did just that, notwithstanding intense protests from the chair of my department of internal medicine, who argued that generalists were essential to the system—after all, they referred patients for hospitalizations and specialists' procedures. Soon after many of the generalists' contracts were not renewed, health system leadership realized that they faced a looming disaster of diminishing hospital admissions and procedural revenue. The institution reversed course and hired generalists again. All parties involved viewed the situation in financial terms. As Plato would put it, "maker of money" was more important than "healer of the sick."

Even referring to generalists as "providers" expresses a view of them as being interchangeable workers on a health care product assembly line.[7] Like all grand enterprises in the marketplace, health systems are devoted to maximizing market share and surplus. They don't see public health as their responsibility, notwithstanding eloquent affirmations of their commitment to the health of their communities. Instead, they view as their constituency the subset of "covered lives" within society from which they seek to extract revenue. The so-called nonprofit voluntary hospitals are in the business of optimizing patient mix and making lucrative sales in order to generate and retain surplus revenue, whether or not you call it profit.

Medical Schools: Reinforcing the Status Quo

Medical schools are mostly populated by physicians who accept their employers' values and priorities and train the system's future clinicians. In so doing, the schools and their faculties help reproduce the commodified nature of American medicine. They maximize their revenue generation by deploying subspecialty trainees in their practices, thus expanding the overspecialized workforce that sells expensive products and procedures the public may not need. They mostly select students who aspire to the socioeconomic rewards that accrue to physicians and who accept the tenets of a system that provides them. When schools do admit more idealistic students, their sprinkling of humanistic courses is insufficient to counteract the negative socialization that occurs during training.

Insurers: Serving Their Shareholders' Interests

The insurance industry is pretty much shameless in its pursuit of profit. It vigorously opposes any health reform that might threaten its business model. Companies deny coverage and payment whenever possible. As for-profit entities, they are responsible first and foremost to their investors, not their clients. The system produces administrative overhead without parallel in the advanced, industrialized world. Only certain health maintenance organizations, such as Kaiser Permanente, and public sector "safety net" clinics and hospitals are not singularly devoted to the pursuit of surplus revenue.[8]

Medical Research and the Marketplace

Research enterprises, including those in the medical schools, also deal in commodities. Academic prestige is linked to research dollars from the National Institutes of Health. For the individual investigator, generating substantial research dollars typically heralds career advancement. Grants received are a measure of a researcher's "productivity"; dollar amounts of the grants are another. The prestige of such grants attracts philanthropic dollars as well. Finally, and certainly not least, under current law, scientists and their institutions can share in the profits and royalties from inventions. A potential inventor thus becomes a particularly attractive faculty hire. Researchers in sociomedical sciences and humanities, by comparison, are seen as dead weights, attracting far fewer research dollars and no lucrative patents.

Manufacturers and Other Corporations: For the Good of the Firm

Other corporate interests seek to maximize their take of the goodies: pharmaceutical companies and major equipment manufacturers do very well—and they have lobbyists and marketing divisions working for them to make sure they do even better—setting prices, fighting government price controls, stimulating demand, and so on. They employ economists to calculate optimal "price points" to maximize profit, even when it means that some people will die because they cannot afford expensive products. Equity firms are particularly notorious for squeezing every last penny from the enterprises on which they feed.

Patients in the World of Commodified Health Care

Which brings us to the patients. In health care, they encounter a commodified world in which their relationships are at least as much economic as clinical. They have to buy insurance, sort through impenetrable policies with deductibles, copayments, and provider networks whose implications are not clear to them until they need care. They have to hope that their diagnoses and needed procedures are covered services. They need to pay their medical bills or risk getting sued if they do not. They even can face loss of their life savings.

Pharmaceutical ads encourage patients to ask their doctors for expensive new medicines when less expensive treatments will do. Doctors and health systems sell procedures (product lines), as well as some of the most expensive medications, directly to the patients. Workers find themselves locked into unrewarding and unsatisfying jobs in order to maintain their insurance coverage. Too often, health systems and providers treat the patients themselves as commodities (known as "covered lives"). There is some evidence, for example, that physicians have received kickbacks for referring patients to specialists, even though that practice violates federal law.[9]

Health and Life as Commodities

When health care is treated as an array of commodities, patients may decide they want their fair share. After all, they have paid for them: through premiums, deductibles, copayments, job lock, worry, poor access, and time spent appealing claims or figuring out their coverage. Under these circumstances, is it any wonder that patients want the scan, seek the visit, request the many laboratory tests, demand the procedure?

Many want more medical goods, including measures to prolong of life, even when the prospects for meaningful recovery are negligible:

"Keep my mother intubated in the ICU."

"Put a feeding tube in my uncle with advanced dementia."

"Don't talk to me about the cost to society, the cost of health insurance for others, or the availability of this bed for others."

When the pursuit of more medical care becomes a pursuit of more days of life, even at the expense of others' health care needs, the commodification of medical care goes hand in hand with the commodification of life, a phenomenon certainly not limited to the domain of health.[10] It is not just patients and their families who commodify their lives. Other actors in health care commodify them as well when they decide in favor of their own financial interests rather than patients' lives and fail to fund life-saving treatments adequately, deny or delay insurance approval for vital care, and fail to give follow-up care to those lacking "good" insurance. The very pursuit of "covered lives" speaks to the devaluing of "uncovered lives" or even of "less well-covered lives."

Ethical Consequences of Commodification of Health Care and Health

Our society teems with commodities. Isn't it inevitable that health care and health are commodities in our capitalist society as well? Isn't that for the good? Why not allow the workings of the marketplace to sort out such matters as the cost and quality of care, and how it is priced and distributed? In this model, patients are regarded as consumers, as they would be of any commodity, and the sellers of medical care presumably compete to reduce waste and conserve societal resources.

Classical economic theory holds that the market maximizes efficiency and productivity. As Notre Dame University economist Stephen Worland noted, however, even Adam Smith, the father of modern economics and market capitalism, didn't believe that everything could be left to the marketplace; some form of government intervention was necessary.[11] That view is not shared by conservative economists such as the influential Milton Friedman, who favored an unrestrained market. Critics of Friedman's perspective who are concerned about health care contend that an unregulated market would empower doctors to avoid patients who are time-consuming and expensive to care for, and that putting clinicians at financial risk for the consequences of caring for such patients would promote behaviors that lead to a loss of professionalism (such as disenrolling certain patients or making it difficult for others to enter the practice).[12] But how rational can a market be, whether regulated or not, if many people are not receiving the care they need? When the governing ethos is "your money or your life," the consequences are bound to be dire for some, perhaps many.

Physician-ethicist Edmund Pellegrino identifies other problems with a shift from a professional to a market ethic. He contrasts marketplace transactions, in which the relationship between buyer and seller "does not extend beyond the sale or consumption of that commodity," with the medical relationship, in which "confidence and trust are crucial as is a continuing relationship, at least in general medicine."[13] If health care is treated as a commodity, "one health care is like any other, just like any bag of beans of the same weight and quality is like any other bag of beans."[14] By the same logic, any physician can be substituted for another, any patient for the next, and both are interchangeable profit or loss centers. Continuity of their relationship is, at best, a secondary concern when the primary goal of the transaction is generation of surplus revenue.

But health care involves education, prevention, and treatment or other services for someone in need: it centers on a "personal relationship between a health professional and the person seeking help."[15] Physicians "enter implicitly into a covenant with society to use their knowledge for the benefit of the sick."[16] They are stewards of this knowledge, not its proprietors, like merchants who own the goods they sell. They are entitled to compensation for their time and effort. But they are healers first, not merchants. Accordingly, commodities may be used in care, but the care itself should not become a commodity.[17]

Pellegrino is expressing a view of the way it should be, not the way it is. For many doctors who spend most or all of their time doing procedures, there is no ongoing relationship beyond the transaction. For health systems, the intimate relationships are with the rich and powerful, with the insurance companies and pharmacy benefit managers, and not even with most physicians. For patients, clinical encounters often are impersonal and involve financial risk and indebtedness. When care is commodified, intimacy is lost, and relationships between patients and doctors or health systems become little more than commercial transactions.

Pellegrino sees the clinician's divided loyalty as ethically consequential; profit-making is legitimized, and inequities are "unfortunate but not unjust," although altruism remains a possibility.[18] In commodified care, the business ethic of *non-malfeasance* (don't do something wrong or bad) would not preclude self-interest, striving for a competitive edge, or unequal treatment based on unequal ability to pay. In an ethical universe, *beneficence* (doing good) would orient care to patients' interests, not those of clinicians or health systems.[19]

Do Market Principles Apply in Health Care?

The eminent economist Kenneth Arrow has demonstrated that health care cannot meet the conditions of a perfect self-functioning market. Because of the patient's inherent uncertainty about "the quality of the commodity he is purchasing," we cannot be confident that the injury to some (caused by change to an unconstrained market) "is not enough to offset the benefit" to others.[20] Pioneering bioethicist Daniel Callahan makes much the same point, observing that the formal goals of medicine are "explicitly altruistic," whereas the market is "explicitly oriented to the maximization of choice and efficiency, aiming at satisfying individual self-interest." He also comments that "it is hard to find evidence anywhere that a turn to the market improves or even sustains earlier levels of access to care."[21]

Many of the reforms advocated in recent years have striven to apply market principles by rewarding efficiency and promoting competition on quality.[22] But the freewheeling American health system could not be less efficient. As for competing on quality, health systems rarely go beyond attempting to improve performance on some quality metrics for which reporting is required, such as glucose control in diabetics. They tend to publicize only their good results, if they have some, or make unsubstantiated claims about their care to attract even more market share.

Reform efforts in American health care rarely stray far from an abiding faith in the market and the commodification it depends on. Consider the Affordable Care Act. Its health care exchanges provided rewards for meeting certain measures of quality and created Accountable Care Organizations that imposed financial risk on providers who failed to reduce costs and gave rewards to those who succeeded. Because large systems are better positioned to assume these risks, these initiatives may well result in an even more consolidated health system that ultimately may be even more expensive, whether or not they achieve some short-term cost savings.[23]

If health care is a fundamental human need (since everyone gets sick at some point), Pellegrino argues that there should be just distribution of care, and it should not be based on a social lottery. Only government, not the market, will place the public good ahead of private interests.[24] If we agree that we have an obligation to help the sick through just distribution of care, and that health care is both a common good and an individual one, we can conclude that it is something that a good society owes to all its members.[25]

That is clear enough, but how can we get to that point? Simply believing will not make it so. Will society, particularly all of those participating in health care, be motivated to take the path that could make "all the difference?" If not, participants in health care may well discover that they fail not only to meet the ethical imperatives of their disciplines, but also to live lives that command respect. In *The Treasure of the Sierra Madre*, prospectors were transformed by their pursuit of gold and its acquisition. As the novelist Traven described it in the novel, "with every ounce more of gold possessed by them, they left the proletarian class and neared that of the property-holders, the well-to-do middle class . . . Since they now owned certain riches, their worries about how to protect them had started . . . They had reached the first step by which man becomes the slave of his property."[26] In this context, it is worthwhile to reflect on Plato/Aristotle's answer to the question posed at the beginning of this chapter about the material pursuits of physicians: "no physician, insofar as he is a physician, considers his own good in what he prescribes, but the good of his patient; for the true physician is a ruler having the human body as his subject, and is not a mere money-maker."[27]

Notes

1. *Webster's Third New International Dictionary of the English Language, Unabridged* (Springfield, MA: Miriam-Webster, 1986), 458.

2. Robert Rossen, "The Treasure of the Sierra Madre," Screenplay by Robert Rossen from the Novel by B. Traven, First Temporary White Draft, January 1, 1947, SimplyScripts—Complete Listing of Movie Scripts on the 'Net, accessed June 14, 2020, http://www.awesomefilm.com/script/treasureofthesierramadre.pdf.

3. Franco Modigliani, "Liquidity Preference and the Theory of Interest and Money," *Econometrica* 12, no. 1 (January 1944): 45–88, https://doi.org/10.2307/1905567.

4. Karl Marx, *Capital: A Critique of Political Economy*, vol. 1, trans. Ben Fowkes (New York: Penguin, 1990), 126–41.

5. Elisabeth Rosenthal, *An American Sickness: How Health Care Became Big Business and How You Can Take It Back* (New York: Penguin Books, 2017), 1–7.

6. Thomas Piketty, *Capital in the Twenty-First Century* (Cambridge, MA: Belknap Press of Harvard University Press, 2014), 20–27.

7. Bruce Y. Lee, "Time to Stop Labeling Physicians as Providers," *Forbes*, May 5, 2019, https://www.forbes.com/sites/brucelee/2019/05/05/time-to-stop-labeling-physicians-as-providers/#4dc31128118e.

8. Ryan Crowley et al., "Financial Profit in Medicine: A Position Paper from the American College of Physicians," *Annals of Internal Medicine* 174, no. 10 (October 2021): 1447–49, https://doi.org/10.7326/M21-1178.

9. Sandeep Jauhar, "Referral System Turns Patients into Commodities," *New York Times*, May 25, 2009, https://www.nytimes.com/2009/05/26/health/26essa.html; Laurie Zoloth-Dorfman and Susan Rubin, "The Patient as Commodity: Managed Care and the Question of Ethics," *Journal of Clinical Ethics* 6, no. 4 (Winter 1995): 339–57, PMID 8750596.

10. Mammo Muchie and Li Xing, *Globalization, Inequality, and the Commodification of Life and Well-Being* (London: Adonis & Abbey, 2006).

11. Stephen T. Worland, "Adam Smith, Economic Justice, and the Founding Father," in *New Directions in Economic Justice*, ed. Roger Skurski (South Bend, IN: University of Notre Dame Press, 1983), 7.

12. Edmund D. Pellegrino, "The Commodification of Medical and Health Care: The Moral Consequences of a Paradigm Shift from a Professional to a Market Ethic," *Journal of Medicine and Philosophy* 24, no. 3 (January 1999): 243–66, https://doi.org/10.1076/jmep.24.3.243.2523; John H. McArthur and Francis D. Moore, "The Two Cultures and the Health Care Revolution: Commerce and Professionalism in Medical

Care," JAMA 277, no. 12 (March 26, 1997): 985–89, https://doi.org/10.1001/jama.1997
.03540360053031.

13. Pellegrino, "Commodification," 249.

14. Pellegrino, "Commodification," 247.

15. Pellegrino, "Commodification," 247.

16. Pellegrino, "Commodification," 251.

17. Pellegrino, "Commodification," 247.

18. Pellegrino, "Commodification," 252.

19. Pellegrino, "Commodification," 254.

20. Kenneth J. Arrow, "Uncertainty and the Welfare Economics of Medical Care," *American Economic Review* 53, no. 5 (1963): 941–73, http://www.jstor.org/stable /1812044.

21. Daniel Callahan, "Medicine and the Market: A Research Agenda," *Journal of Medicine and Philosophy* 24, no. 3 (January 1999): 224–42, https://doi.org/10.1076 /jmep.24.3.224.2527.

22. James C. Robinson, "Hospital Quality Competition and the Economics of Imperfect Information," *Milbank Quarterly* 66, no. 3 (September 1988): 465–81, https://doi.org/10.2307/3349965.

23. Jenny Gold, "Urgent Care: What's in an Accountable Care Organization?," Kaiser Health News, September 14, 2015, https://khn.org/news/aco-accountable-care -organization-faq/.

24. Pellegrino, "Commodification," 258.

25. Pellegrino, "Commodification," 259.

26. B. Traven, *The Treasure of the Sierra Madre* (New York: Penguin, 1956), 86–87.

27. Plato, quoting Socrates, *The Republic*, Book I (London: Global Classics, 2017), 22.

Dialogue #10

Professor (looking up from the document): Commodification of health care appears to be an important problem. Are Americans prepared to do something about it? There's an old joke: It only takes one psychiatrist to change a light bulb, but the light bulb really has to want to change.

Student: I am struggling with that question. Commodification is easy to diagnose and difficult to treat. I'm afraid there are additional disorders (some doctors would call them "comorbidities") that make it even harder. The fact that human life is treated like a commodity is even more bothersome.

Professor: It's a complicated problem. But what else, beyond economics, is preventing us from making the system more effective, just, and equitable?

Student: I thought you'd ask that. Yes, there are factors affecting the behavior of doctors and patients. But why not go ahead and figure out what to do about commodification, instead of worrying about other things that may or may not get in the way, and may be even harder to change?

Professor: True. On the one hand, if they are minor perturbations, perhaps we can ignore them. On the other hand, can we be sure that they are not major roadblocks to change?

Student: I suppose that we can't be sure unless we look at issues in all the relevant groups, including patients and their doctors, medical students and their teachers, scientists and their employers, health systems and their administrators, governments and their constituencies.

Professor: I agree. There seem to be distinct issues involving each group. We should also figure out what they have in common. And what their implications might be.

Student: That's a tall order.

13

Atomization and Its Discontents

The Consciousness and Connectedness of Participants in Health Care

No man is an island, entire of itself; every man
is a piece of the continent, a part of the main . . .
any man's death diminishes me,
because I am involved in mankind.
—John Donne, "Devotions on Emergent Occasions, Meditation XVII"

There is little doubt that we need to transform the world of American health care—to radically reorder priorities, approaches, practice styles, and patterns of care rendered and received. Such change won't be possible if we don't address the expectations, perceived needs, values, and capacities of everyone involved. That not only includes the clinicians and health care systems that deliver care, governments that organize care, and corporations that produce a range of products. It also means considering how to accomplish this in relation to the recipients of care. How realistic is that?

A Potential Framework

Attacking that question requires some insight into how Americans think about their lives, their society, and their roles and responsibilities within that society. A useful guide is sociologist Robert Bellah's wonderful book, *Habits of the Heart: Individualism and Commitment in American Life*.[1] Bellah and his colleagues interviewed hundreds of Americans about what they found fulfilling in their lives as well as what they saw as lacking. The research team concluded that many people struggle with the conflict between a tradition of individualistic interests (self-interest) and the meaning that comes from commitment to something larger. "It is easier," they write, "to think about how to get what we want than to know exactly what we should want."[2] In this context, the researchers probe "the nature of success, the meaning of freedom, and the requirements of justice." They find that Americans' language (for organizing their thinking and discourse) is one of autonomy, a deeply ingrained American ideal. They argue, however, in postindustrial society, American individualism has become an autonomy that is dissociated from meaningful societal integration.[3]

In this circumstance, connections to community and commitments to a moral and just society are hard to come by. At the center of life "is the autonomous individual, presumably able to choose the roles he will play and the commitments he will make, not on the basis of higher truths but according to the criterion of life-effectiveness as the individual judges it."[4] The individual is free to do many things and exercises that freedom with little consideration for the impact of his or her decisions on society.

Such attitudes become commonplace when "what has dropped out are the old normative expectations of what makes life worth living,"[5] for example, by making life better for others. The people they studied find themselves in a society in which "the virtual meaning of life lies in the acquisition of ever-increasing status, income, and authority, from which genuine freedom is supposed to come," in a world "damaged by the destruction of the subtle ties that bind human beings together, leaving them frightened and alone."[6]

Bellah and his colleagues characterize this situation as a "culture of separation." They observe that some people seek respite and meaning in intense, loving relationships, but this a strategy that does not solve the problem of isolation in a meaningful way. It can even make things worse. Many abandon any notion of finding meaning in relation to society as a whole and particularly in the idea of a common good, which the authors call "the uncompleted American quest."[7]

The authors find inspiration for that quest in earlier American history. John Winthrop, the first governor of the Massachusetts Bay Colony, spoke of "our community as members of the same body."[8] In Federalist Paper 71, James Madison asserted that "the people commonly intend the PUBLIC GOOD."[9] Bellah and his colleagues are not directly prescriptive, but they do insist that "individuals need the nurture of groups that carry a moral tradition reinforcing their aspirations,"[10] "to link interests with a conception of the common good."[11]

Thus the business owner who provides generously for his or her family while paying the employees less than a living wage has abandoned this quest. So too have office workers, who support policies that lower their taxes but deprive others of needed services, and homeowners who oppose housing disadvantaged families in their neighborhoods, thereby contributing to racial and socioeconomic segregation. Such individuals may regard themselves as good and ethical people. They may even contribute to charities or volunteer at food banks, have friends and admirers, and feel successful in life. But they are unlikely to have the same kind of sense of meaning and fulfillment as those who truly are committed to the common good and connected through their actions to efforts to create a world that is more just.

Medical Students and Their Educators

How does this apply to American health care? Let's start with the medical students. They are citizens of our society, mostly from the upper-middle to upper class. Their postures with respect to individualism, community, and commitment certainly vary considerably, but like so many others in our society, most did not grow up in environments in which the common good was the dominating ethos or even an expression often mentioned. Those from economically advantaged backgrounds may have had little or no experience with the struggles that many others face. Taken alone, that might not be a problem. Some are capable of learning to see the world differently and do so. But many other students, including some from working-class families, may be pursuing medical careers, at least in part, to acquire or maintain economic security and to attain the social standing accorded to physicians. As Bellah and his colleagues observe, "when education becomes an instrument for individual careerism, it cannot provide either personal meaning or civic culture," meaning the well-being of the community as a whole.[12]

Medical school admissions can be intensely competitive, a Hobbesian world of unrestrained competition, in which conflict is perpetual and getting ahead is all that matters.[13] What's involved is neither physical competition nor mortal combat. It is college grades and test scores. Almost every student who gets into medical school does so on this basis. We might be tempted to conclude, therefore, that admissions criteria are objective measures of "merit" and are thus consistent with ideas of fairness and justice. This idea has come under considerable criticism of late. As Daniel Markovits, a Yale University law professor, notes, success on college admissions tests is strongly correlated with the resources that families are able to devote to helping their children.[14]

The inherent inequity of that approach, from the applicant's perspective, is one problem. At least as important is the consequence for the patient. Evidence suggests that shared racial, ethnic, and language backgrounds between patient and provider are associated with greater patient satisfaction and superior health care.[15]

The idea that much more than academic performance matters in the selection of future physicians was brought home to me when I was applying to medical school. I went to one of my professors, Willy Moser, a gifted teacher of mathematics, for a letter of recommendation, having done well in his course. He surprised me when he said, "I'll be happy to write you a letter. Anyone can be a doctor." I thought that he was jesting, but I later recognized the wisdom of his remark. The technical knowledge that one needs to acquire in medical school is substantial, but not over-whelming. Attributes beyond ability to memorize scientific information and spew it out on tests matter much more.

It would be great if more students had backgrounds in the social sciences and humanities, but that is not the greatest deficiency. The main problem is the destructive effect of selecting students based on grades and test scores. Successful applicants are those who focus on optimizing their performance on those critical measures, diverting from that mission only to fill out their résumés with activities that can make medical schools feel good about whom they admit. The résumé attests to well-roundedness, to wonderfulness, but it is almost always illusion. Once the students are in the doors of a medical school, those traits and interests dissipate rapidly for far too many. Students who might bring other qualities to the table usually don't play that game as well and are only infrequently admitted. Doctors who maintain their idealism throughout their careers, like the ones I described in chapter 3, should be the norm, not the exceptions.

What qualities *should* drive selection of students? Ideally, those that increase the likelihood that future physicians will have both the capacity and the inclination to meet the needs of patients and the larger society, and to contribute to addressing problems in the health care system, even when those needs run contrary to the physician's immediate self-interest.

Among these qualities I would include empathy, altruism, ability to deal with ambiguity in socially constructive ways, sufficient psychological maturity to be able to handle emotional intensity, commitment to redistributive justice, familiarity with groups traditionally underserved by the health care system, and unswerving commitment to the well-being of others, even at some sacrifice to oneself. Grade point average, knowledge of genetics and biochemistry, and Medical College Admission Test (MCAT) scores don't even make my list, which appears below.

There are students for whom science courses are challenging. They are often the same students who lack the kind of family support that many upper-middle-class students have, and they may be distracted from their studies by challenges at home. None of this should be disqualifying. It simply calls for programs to support such students so that they can succeed in bringing their other fine qualities to the work of medicine. Can such a reordering of admissions requirements and selection criteria be effective? Making it work wouldn't be easy. Some students would try to game the system. Nonetheless, if we made this an explicit goal—perhaps the central goal—of the selection process, it might make a difference. Members of communities that currently are underserved are well positioned to judge which candidates are best equipped to meet their communities' needs. Involving them in the selection process might improve it.

Schools already pay lip service to these qualities but only infrequently do they give them real weight in the selection process. Consequently, too many incoming students share values that prioritize acquisition and competing successfully to address their perceived personal needs. Products of their society and culture, they often lack the disposition and experiences that might lead them to pursue an alternate path. Some students do arrive with idealistic concerns about making the world a better place. For many, these qualities are fragile and need to be nurtured. That task falls to the medical schools.

To be sure, many medical schools provide instruction on morals, ethics, and social responsibility. Such instruction generally takes the form of lectures, not the best forum for learning about values. Lectures offer the student little time to reflect or pursue a topic in depth—to analyze it from multiple perspectives, examine conflicting interpretations, struggle with its meaning, and consider possible answers. A student preparing for an exam in neuroscience is unlikely to absorb or retain subtle points from a lecture on moral philosophy that was watched online, perhaps at double speed while multitasking. That situation brings to mind the quip attributed to Woody Allen: "I took a speed-reading course and read *War and Peace* in twenty minutes. It involves Russia." Nor do the medical schools do enough to nudge their charges toward psychological insights and psychological health that would allow them to engage more fully with their patients. They also don't immerse the students meaningfully in the diverse subcultures that they might serve.

Some clinicians and clinical experiences can inspire by exemplifying humane values, but others do not. Far too often, the clinical environment is toxic. Too many students learn to model their own behavior and values on those of the more senior trainees and professors—values at odds with the idealistic words recited at the white coat ceremonies. To be fair, there are exceptions. In some instances, students choose to model their behavior in reaction to what they observe. One professor of behavioral medicine told me that many of his students spoke of the crucial importance of negative role modeling: Never wanting to act like a certain doctor can be more powerful than wanting to be like another! Alas, such independence of mind, while admirable, is relatively uncommon.[16]

The structure and content of medical learning, both preclinical and clinical, are frequently anti-intellectual. There is a great deal of rote and formulaic learning and little opportunity to reflect on life, values, society, and how we could make the biggest difference in the world.[17]

I was fortunate to encounter a few professors who encouraged me to think about those things, and then to stumble into a graduate program in history, where I could dwell in a world shaped by those concepts and think about how they applied to medicine. Unfortunately, that experience is uncommon. Some students do emerge with decent values and perspectives, but that is in spite of the nature of their formal medical education and training. They should have an opportunity to be immersed deeply in studying such issues.

What might a transformed educational environment look like? Change is never easy. Getting it right will require trial and error, rigorous evaluation, and continuous improvements. Here are some modest proposals:

- Eliminate the prerequisite premedical courses in the sciences and mathematics. Students can take all the science courses they need in medical school. Add extensive premedical course requirements in the humanities and social sciences.[18]
- Develop mechanisms to identify applicants who are driven fundamentally by altruism rather than potential income and professional prestige.
- Use available strategies for assessing empathic capacity, psychological openness, and moral and ethical outlook in the selection of medical students.
- Involve members of underserved communities in the selection process.
- Introduce premedical requirements that would provide meaningful evidence of sustained commitment to societal well-being. Volunteer-

ing in a health care setting would not suffice. Sustained, substantive involvement with an organization or program over time would be more meaningful.

- Up to half of the curriculum in the first two years should be devoted to ethics, morality, and communications skills. This should be integrated with early clinical experiences, such as following a patient with chronic medical and social problems. The scientific and clinical half of the curriculum should consistently reinforce the ideal of social responsibility.
- The curriculum should embrace psychological openness. Toward that end, students should be encouraged to undertake some form of psychotherapy.
- Rebalance the curriculum in the classroom and in clinical conferences to give much more weight to social context and causes of illness, and less to biological reductionism.
- In the subsequent years, the medical school curriculum should include courses that reinforce ethics, morality, and social responsibility, and postgraduate trainees should have seminars in which they can reflect on experiences in clinical and other educational settings in relation to their ideals.
- Residency recommendations should be based primarily on the metrics that reflect the above curricular content.

Medical Practitioners

As we have seen, the physicians who are products of this medical education system were not chosen for their roles because of their ability to empathize and connect emotionally, nor does their training prepare them for that. When asked to choose between being an emotional resource for others in times of great crisis or chronic need, or being someone who does procedures and has little if any emotional connection, the choice that doctors often make is predictable. In fairness, we should note that many proceduralists come to love what they do, apart from the financial rewards.

In the absence of strong moral and ethical grounding and guidance, and in the context of discomfort with ambiguity or uncertainty, it becomes easier for physicians to nudge, prod, or cajole patients toward procedures that they may not need, inducing demand or acquiescence in a thousand ways. For too many, it is almost unheard of to discourage a procedure unless it poses a danger to the patient. Many clinicians not only benefit financially from practicing this way—they also feel fully justified in doing so.

My friend Norman, a surgical subspecialist who also studies health care delivery, told me that people in his field deserve to earn much more than generalists because what they do is so demanding and stressful. This sense of entitlement (and failure to recognize the comparable demands of what generalists do) is, sadly, quite common. Norman is otherwise reasonable, collegial, and liberal-minded. Many trainees in the procedural fields develop an arrogance about their impending status, going so far as to refer to internal medicine doctors as "fleas." The professional organizations of many medical subspecialties advocate vigorously for the way things are. They fight tenaciously against any redistribution of income toward the cognitive fields. Establishing guidelines or clinical policies that could have the effect of trimming their incomes from activities of questionable benefit is rarely their notion of "choosing wisely." Yes, these attitudes and behaviors have an economic underpinning, but they also are fully justified by their worldview and mesh all too well with the disinclination of many procedural doctors to connect more than superficially with their patients.

When I was a student, many fine surgeons attended closely to their patients before and after their procedures. Nowadays, such close follow-up is rarer. After an operation, the surgical team checks on the wound and other issues related to the area of the operation. If there are other problems, they call for a generalist or another specialist to deal with them. Patients with broken hips often reside on internal medicine wards before and after their operations. Some oncologists do a great job of discussing prognosis with their patients and limiting care, when appropriate; others, not so much.

The failure to connect, to have difficult conversations, to deal with ambiguity, to offer a shoulder to cry on, rather than giving patients futile treatments, performing avoidable procedures on them, or transferring them to other teams of doctors, is not only a matter of convenience and economics. It also can be a consequence of emotional, moral, and intellectual limitations in the physicians' capacity to respond to such challenges in different ways, as well as lack of exposure to clinicians modeling this kind of communication. Sending an intern to discuss the fact that there is nothing more to be done is clinically negligent. Showing a trainee that passing a box of tissues to a patient bursting with emotion is a kind, empathic act can be empowering. Doctors lacking capacity for empathy are ill equipped to teach their students to connect at a meaningful level with patients.

The valuing of revenue generation over relationships also reflects expectations that society condones. I recall many of my classmates in medical school seeming to move toward the values and lifestyle expectations of practicing physicians as we progressed through our training and spent time with them. My friend Henry (whom we encountered in chap. 3 ordering unneeded breathing tests) once referred mirthfully to a *New Yorker* cartoon with the caption, "Money is life's report card." He implied that that was not his perspective, notwithstanding his actions. Well, just as the report card is not the measure of a person's worth (as a potential physician or in most other ways), neither is money. The Hobbesian push for ever more, notwithstanding the implications for others, dominates perceptions for what is culturally and professionally acceptable. And the culture barely notices the individual who sits with someone in despair and provides comfort to them.

Can anything change physicians' behavior and their perceptions of their roles and capabilities? Perhaps. Much depends on who is selected into the medical profession, and what happens in their training, but some measures aimed at practitioners might be worth a shot. Doctors regularly have to do a certain amount of "continuing medical education," much of which has no effect on learning or knowledge retention, particularly when in the form of didactic sessions.[19] Intense programs with different structures could be designed to address values, ethics, self-perceived capabilities, and how doctors might overcome barriers to behaving differently. Here are a few ideas drawn from my experiences as a clinician, educator, and researcher:

- Balint-like groups (see chap. 4), moderated by a trained psychologist, a social worker, or both, in which physicians in one specialty or across specialties meet regularly to discuss challenges in the doctor-patient relationship, might empower some clinicians to take these on more directly.
- Required small-group sessions may provide opportunities to improve communication skills and overcome other barriers. Recertification requirements for medical specialists could include participating in simulated interviews involving difficult conversations.
- Ongoing seminars on ethics, moral responsibilities of the profession, and social responsibility that are integrated with discussions of clinicians' actual caregiving experiences.
- Regular sessions in which physicians, especially those who perform procedures, and the administrators of health care systems critically appraise their practice patterns and discuss how to reduce the use of clinical services that are unlikely to contribute meaningfully to outcomes, including those that contribute substantially to their incomes. This program will be particularly difficult to pull off. Getting doctors who implant pacemakers, do deep brain stimulation, or biopsy prostate glands even to attend such sessions, much less reduce the use of procedures that generate much of their income, is a daunting challenge. Many have contracts from their institutions that specify the expected revenue and/or relative value units to be generated from their work to support their salaries. As for the administrators, the goal of such sessions is likely to be inconsistent with the business model in most US health care systems, if it were to be applied to their fee-for-service clients.

Two additional strategies that might affect the behavior of some physicians:

- Providing incentives for interested physicians to seek insight-oriented psychotherapy or cognitive-behavioral therapy that could help them better understand and relate to patients, their needs, and their values.
- Paying doctors for their time, not for their acts. Being a physician is intrinsically rewarding. Society grants the practitioner moral prestige. The financial incentive to perform more procedures and spend less time with patients distracts clinicians from their moral purpose. Without a change in the incentive structure, interventions aimed at values, ethics, and capabilities may have little if any impact.

Executives and Managers of Health Care Systems

What about the managers and executives of health systems? Many are physicians with some managerial training. Others are graduates of health care management programs or traditional management schools. They tend to be trained in the technical requirements of their jobs: managing the workplace, improving quality, assembling and analyzing data. They learn how to run a big business successfully. They even may be exposed to some instruction in corporate social responsibility. They talk a good game:

"Population health."

"Access."

"Serve our community."

"High-value care."

But they, too, are caught in a web of self-deceit, of false consciousness: They see themselves as forces for good in the world, but their actions often say otherwise. And the financial rewards at the higher levels of management are enormous.

What is missing is a moral core in the form of other-directed values, modesty of their perceived needs and of their lifestyle expectations, ingrained altruism, and commitment to the betterment of society. Managers see it as their job to negotiate favorable contracts, promote a financially advantageous patient mix, and bring on "product lines" that will enhance their bottom line. Their "population" is those with generously "covered lives." Their "community" is not people who live in a large, populated area where the health system is located, but rather those whom they can attract to their systems and potential donors to their hospitals. They invest in "bricks-and-mortar" and place clinicians in settings where they will attract the right kinds of clients for their systems.

None of this is malevolent. It is the way that business is done. Sending the collection agency after the unpaid bill, suing the person who hasn't paid—these, too, are part of the job. Managers commit to fixing the holes in the hearts of their patients, but they ignore the holes in their own hearts. Is this inevitable? Sociologist Bellah and colleagues seem to believe that managers could be transformed, partly through better education, in order to change so-called corporate responsibility from "a kind of public relations whipped cream decorating the corporate pudding, to the constitutive structural element of the corporation itself." They call for:

> a fundamental alteration of the role and training of the manager. Management would become a profession in the older sense of the word, involving not merely standards of technical competence but standards of public obligation that could at moments of conflict override obligations to the corporate employer. Such a conception of the professional manager would require a deep change in the ethos of schools of business administration, where "business ethics" would have to become central in the process of professional formation. If the rewards of success in business management were not so inordinate, then choice of this profession could arise from more public-spirited motives.[20]

Not paying hospital executives for their "winnings" might make room for some of these value-oriented efforts to take hold.

Insurers, Investors, Manufacturers, and Other Corporate Interests

Occasionally, we hear about a ravenous chief executive officer who jacks up prices of a pharmaceutical company's products, or an investor who makes a fast billion by juicing a clinical practice or network to maximize revenue and inflate market value. Most corporate titans are not different from health system CEOs. They operationalize their fiduciary responsibility to investors as an obligation to maximize profits. Carefully selecting insurees, inducing demand, extending patents, optimizing "price point," and opposing efforts to rein them in are all part of the job. As with health system executives, changing their behavior would require a reordering of values, morals, ethics, and rewards.

Medical Scientists and Their Organizations

The professional circumstances of biomedical scientists have transformed radically in recent decades. Early in the twentieth century, there were not nearly as many of them. Funding was sparse. Most were professors who had laboratories and some staff, and that was it. There were relatively few people in training who aspired to similar positions. Science today is a highly competitive enterprise. Anyone entering the field has to be concerned about their career. To gain and retain employment in the field, you must be productive and focused on your career. There's little time to acquire a broad education or think much about the world.

Those training the scientists do so, in part, to be generative—to produce scientific progeny—but also to increase the efficiency of their research factories. I knew of one famous scientist who once a week would go into the lab, where there were many predoctoral students sharing benches. Each bench was supervised by a postdoctoral scholar (generally, someone spending a couple of more years to get the résumé in shape to compete for desirable positions in academia or elsewhere). The professor would walk down the row of benches, having a detailed discussion with each postdoc (with the predocs listening in) as he moved through the room. Were questions of ethics and public responsibility discussed? At moments, perhaps. But they would have been drowned out by the relentless hum of scientific production.

Students enter science with a love for the field. Successful scientists are passionate about their work. Many can imagine nothing more exciting.

They believe in their work. Seeking recognition for their contributions and perhaps aspiring to prominence or leadership in the scientific world, many are too caught up in their work to judge objectively the merits of their field of research either as a scientific priority or in relation to its social significance and implications.

Scientists form organizations to advance their interests, much like the medical specialty and subspecialty societies. One can claim (as do I) that the priorities and goals of these organizations are misplaced, that they sometimes run contrary to the public interest in the ways they influence funding and public discourse. But given the life courses, professional experiences, and predilections of people in science, their organizations hardly can be expected to behave otherwise.

Can the consciousness of scientists be geared more to serving societal needs? That is an extremely challenging goal. It would require a curriculum for trainees in which moral and ethical principles and social responsibility were prominent. Crucially, scientists, their employers, and funders would need to restructure the opportunities and rewards in scientific practice to be more compatible with the kind of ethos of science about which Robert Merton wrote (see chap. 8). If that does not happen, any lessons acquired in training are likely to be washed away in the pursuit of employment, grants, and patents. Some approaches suggested earlier for medical students and practicing physicians may be worth considering.

Patients and Their Families

Patients are a heterogeneous group. What inner needs, agendas, and expectations do they bring to medical care? More often than not, a medical encounter is a clinical transaction. Someone needs an immunization or a mammogram, or has a urinary tract infection or a pain the back. They would like a diagnosis or the appropriate treatment. In other cases the challenge is less straightforward. When a person is seriously ill, there often is more at stake. When that person's distress is existential rather than physical, there is also much to understand.

The lived experience of patients may prompt visits to physicians for problems, needs, and challenges to which medical training pays little, if any, attention. Think of my patient Ruth, who was living a "life without connections." She was isolated, with no real friends. Her son was a source of disruption. She had no community as a source of succor. She felt lost and anxious in her loneliness. Family, far from being a haven or a protected space, was a source of additional distress.[21] In the absence of any such connections, she looked to her doctor for what she was missing, but her needs were limitless, and the physician's capacity to respond was finite.

Think of Georg, the young scholar crippled by his sense that he never could match his father's level of success even though he had accomplished a great deal. He was caught on the treadmill of a society where there is no upper bound for success, which can leave those who pursue it disenchanted or, as in his case, full of despair.[22] In his mind, medical care was supposed to extinguish his pain, but it did not.

Emotional issues related to "the slings and arrows" of life drive much utilization of primary and some specialty care. Sometimes, patients like Ann are frantic about staying healthy, not recognizing their existential anxiety about the way that their life has been going. On other occasions, people are depressed, like Dalileh, who somaticized and rejected the idea that her symptoms were related to her depression and might respond to treatment for that. Still others, like my patient Olivia, who consulted hundreds of physicians, are panicked and desperate for answers. Yet others, such as Andrew, look for chemical answers to the fading of their years in the context of lives unfulfilled.

Underlying all of these situations is a disconnection from communities, aloofness from relationships, and the lack of a language that articulates their dis-ease in a way that would be amenable to directed approaches. Their physicians respond by pronouncing questionable clinical entities ("nondiseases") to be the culprits because they lack the capacity to delve deeper. Some who otherwise are well-connected in their communities are racially, linguistically, or socioculturally distant from their providers and may insist on more care because they aren't convinced that the doctors have their best interests at heart.

For others, the problem is different. The autonomy that is cherished in American medicine and the larger society can lead to a sense of entitlement:

"Give me the antibiotic or else."

"You can't take my sister off of a ventilator."

"The doctor should be available to answer my questions at a whim."

"Get me home to Paris to die, whatever the consequences for others."

"I shouldn't have to wait in the line of those seeking care."

Sometimes expressed explicitly, sometimes implied, often not even recognized by the individual for what they are, these requests reflect a point of view.

Are these two kinds of issues—longing for care because of an emotional need and demanding or expecting care, whatever the implications for others—distinct problems? I think not. Both bespeak a fractured balance between individualism and communitarianism. The autonomy of many people without meaningful connection to what is good for the community and not just the self[23] disrupts the social equilibrium. Although few patients would regard their own quests in this way, many are simply longing for a heart in a seemingly heartless world. For some, the anguish and unrequited needs are obvious. For others, their behavior is a socially condoned form of acting out. Their actions cannot, in the end, bring them the meaning that comes from connection to a cohesive social whole, in ways that affirm all and harm none.

In this context, policy initiatives to create a more equitable health care system are often met with shock and despair. Those who object are diverse. They include anguished individuals with limitless unmet needs, as well as people with a sense of entitlement who are accustomed to getting what they want. It was diabolically brilliant for opponents of health care reform to label efforts to limit ineffective and futile care as "death panels." They recognized that such policies represented a threat to some, a kind of death knell to their search for meaning in their lives.

What should doctors do? Clearly, they cannot treat all forms of human suffering or meet all kinds of existential needs encountered in clinical contexts. A starting point might be to recognize such needs and suffering for what they are, and to ensure that appropriate services (social workers, community workers, psychologists, psychiatrists, etc.) are available. Some patients will surely resist such interventions. Balint-type groups might identify strategies to set limits on demanding patients, allow clinicians to acknowledge frustrations, and remind them that these phenomena are mediated by larger problems in society. In turn, doctor burnout and tendency to withdraw from patients in need may be reduced. This kind of clinical work is challenging but extremely important. Health systems need to recognize that and reward it appropriately. Medical schools should ensure that doctors with the capacity and inclination for such work are well-prepared.

Policy Makers

Politicians want to please their constituencies. They shy away from health care policy proposals that will offend these constituencies. They prefer to play it safe with crowd-pleasing ideas: moonshots to cure cancer and Alzheimer disease, a "public option" in the same dysfunctional marketplace of health care, incentives to curtail costs that are so modest that no one will notice.

Some politicians advocate radical overhaul of the system, but they have trouble getting such changes across the threshold. The more vocal they are in advocating meaningful change, the more resources that health care-related corporations line up in opposing them. Yet progressives are only addressing issues of access and equity, which, as important as they are, don't get at the other deep pathologies of our health care system: those relating to priorities, our sense of connection, and our shared concern for the common good.

Consciousness, Health Care, and Health

Many, although not all, patients and providers, students and professors, scientists and corporate leaders stand in the way of meaningful transformation of health care because they have untreated conditions. These are the conditions of life in a society that fails to fulfill in ways that could enrich them all without depriving others. Yet the fear of change:

> makes us rather bear those ills we have
> Than fly to others that we know not of.[24]

As contorted, bloated, inequitable, and ineffective as American health care is, it provides the participants with a buffer against the prospect of something even worse. Addressing the problems in health care is a formidable task, and resolving them is perhaps an unattainable goal, unless the many factors contributing to them are addressed. Until that happens, the prescriptive notions that I proffer in this chapter may well improve certain symptoms but are unlikely (in the jargon of molecular biology) to find enough binding sites to achieve their desired full therapeutic effect.

Notes

1. Robert N. Bellah et al., *Habits of the Heart: Individualism and Commitment in American Life* (New York: Harper and Row, Perennial Library, 1986).

2. Bellah, *Habits*, 21.

3. Bellah, *Habits*, 286.

4. Bellah, *Habits*, 47.

5. Bellah, *Habits*, 48.

6. Bellah, *Habits*, 284.

7. Bellah, *Habits*, 252; see also Robert D. Putnam, *Bowling Alone: The Collapse and Revival of American Community* (New York: Simon & Schuster, 2000).

8. Bellah, *Habits*, 285.

9. Bellah, *Habits*, 253–54, emphasis original.

10. Bellah, *Habits*, 286.

11. Bellah, *Habits*, 287.

12. Bellah, *Habits*, 293.

13. Thomas Hobbes, *Leviathan*, 1651, ed. Richard Tuck (Cambridge: Cambridge University Press, 1991), 87–89.

14. Daniel Markovits, *The Meritocracy Trap: How America's Foundational Myth Feeds Inequality, Dismantles the Middle Class, and Devours the Elite* (New York: Penguin Press, 2019), 124–56. See also Gill Crozier, "Race and Education: Meritocracy as White Middle Class Privilege," *British Journal of Sociology of Education* 39, no. 8 (November 2018): 1239–46, https://doi.org/10.1080/01425692.2018.1523354; Natasha Warikoo, *The Diversity Bargain and Other Dilemmas of Race, Admissions, and Meritocracy at Elite Universities* (Chicago: University of Chicago Press, 2016);

Nicholas Lemann, *The Big Test: The Secret History of the American Meritocracy* (New York: Farrar, Straus and Giroux, 1999).

15. Lisa A. Cooper and Neil R. Powe, *Disparities in Patient Experiences, Health Care Processes, and Outcomes: The Role of Patient-Provider Racial, Ethnic, and Language Concordance* (New York, NY: Commonwealth Fund, 2004).

16. Henry Abramovitch, personal communication, October 2020.

17. The structure of the educational institutions and their programs and the composition of their faculties also deflect students from thinking deeper thoughts. If, as Virchow and others held, medicine is a social science, why aren't there more social scientists and humanists in the medical schools to educate the students about vital aspects of their future profession? Most of the teachers are clinicians who derive satisfaction from being generative, in creating more people like themselves in the specialized areas in which they practice. Others are basic scientists who believe in what they do and who see their disciplines as the basis of a good medical education.

18. Lewis Thomas, "Notes of a Biology-Watcher: How to Fix the Premedical Curriculum," *New England Journal of Medicine* 298, no. 21 (May 25, 1978): 1180–81, https://doi.org/10.1056/NEJM197805252982106; Richard B. Gunderman and Steven L. Kanter, "Perspective: 'How to Fix the Premedical Curriculum' Revisited," *Academic Medicine* 83, no. 12 (December 2008): 1158–61, https://doi.org/10.1097/ACM .0b013e31818c6515.

19. Dave Davis et al., "Impact of Formal Continuing Medical Education: Do Workshops, Rounds, and Other Traditional Continuing Education Activities Change Physician Behavior or Health Outcomes?," *JAMA* 282, no. 9 (September 1999): 867–74, https://doi.org/10.1001/jama.282.9.867.

20. Bellah, *Habits*, 290.

21. Christopher Lasch, *Haven in a Heartless World* (New York: Norton, 1995), 134–66.

22. C. Wright Mills, *White Collar* (New York: Oxford University Press, 1951), 259–86.

23. Bellah, *Habits*, 286.

24. Shakespeare, *Hamlet*, Act III, Scene 1.

| Dialogue #11 |

Student: It is infuriating that so many of these groups feel they have too much to lose if we change our dysfunctional health care system.

Professor: Do you feel like our task is complete?

Student: No, but I'm afraid the problem might be unsolvable. Everyone has too much at stake. They are all acting in their perceived self-interest.

Professor: What might help us overcome those limits?

Student: People need to see the bigger picture—how their work relates to everything else in the world of health care.

Professor: Are these problems exclusive to the health care realm?

Student: Of course not.

Professor: A lot of what we've been discussing seems related to the ways that parties interact: how they influence each other, the patterns and nature of their communication, and miscommunication.

Student: I guess I could explore that. But what's the point if it's unfixable?

Professor: Cholera appeared to be unfixable until John Snow figured out that it was infecting London from the contaminated waters of the Broad Street pump, and he removed the handle.

Student: We can't fix American health care so easily. There are too many moving parts.

Professor: Agreed. But we can't conclude a disorder is incurable if we haven't identified its etiology.

Student: OK, I'll take a look. But I remain skeptical.

Professor: Your skepticism is healthy. It will serve you well. But let's see if at least some improvement is possible.

14

Malevolent Messaging

Toxic Interactions in Health Care

It takes two to speak the truth—one to speak and another to hear.
—Henry David Thoreau, "A Week on the Concord and Merrimack Rivers, 1849:
Wednesday"

The preceding chapters have covered the various participants in American health care who contribute to its problems. They do this, in part, through the ways in which they relate to and communicate with each other. They have different circumstances, incentives, predispositions, aptitudes, interests, and needs that shape those interactions (e.g., between health systems and their clinicians, doctors and their patients, or scientists and the government). This chapter synthesizes what we have seen in the patterns of interactions among these groups. I consider the impact of such patterns on behaviors and on often divergent perspectives and priorities. At issue here are all kinds of communication, including mass communication to the public, advertising, lobbying about scientific priorities and health care legislation, discourse among clinicians and researchers about evidence and clinical strategies, interactions between health systems and their clinicians, and conversations between doctors and patients.

In still other situations, it is money that does the talking, metaphorically, to achieve instrumental goals. In many ways, these interactions manage to bring out the worst in all participants by reinforcing behaviors that aggravate the problems. Their patterns of interaction entrench the actors in modes of behaving and relating to each other. They also shape how they think about health care and their expectations from it, in ways that make meaningful change more difficult.

Clinicians and Their Organizations

Physicians and their professional organizations advance an ideology that reflects their economic interests, professional self-image, and preferences in the course of practicing it (see chaps. 3 and 4). Toward these ends, university-educated physicians and their establishment allies strongly supported the successful Flexnerian push to reduce the number of medical schools and to create a more elite profession, whose members have substantial academic preparation prior to medical school. As a result (and as seen in chap. 5), American physicians now receive their medical education in universities and like institutions through programs that follow receipt of at least a bachelor's degree.[1]

Consistent with their elitist goals, physicians were long reluctant to acknowledge the legitimacy of nurse practitioners and other nonphysician clinicians, often characterizing them as "midlevel providers" and "physician extenders."[2] Some critics of that attitude have observed that characterizing these professionals as "extenders" is demeaning and analogous to using the brand name of the food product Hamburger Helper. The available evidence suggests that such practitioners provide care at least comparable to that of physicians.[3]

Opposing Health Care Reform

When not reinforcing their status atop the health care hierarchy, physicians' organizations promote their members' financial interests. The profession that purportedly places patients' well-being above all else has vigorously fought for decades to prevent enactment of government programs that would cover the costs of care for the population as a whole. As I noted in chapter 11, this has included opposition through much of the twentieth century to a range of policy initiatives designed to expand health insurance coverage.

The booming voices of the medical profession continue to make themselves heard in Congress today. By one estimate, some 29,000 visits per year by individual physicians are recorded to the offices of members of Congress and their staffs, amounting to approximately 10 visits per month to each senator's offices and 4 per month to each member of the House of Representatives. The majority of such visits focus upon reimbursement and health policy.[4]

Morris Fishbein, the influential and charismatic editor of the *Journal of the American Medical Association* from 1924 to 1949, was a fervent anti-Communist who viewed social insurance and "government encroachment" on the practice of medicine and other social insurance programs as steps on the road to totalitarianism. Speaking on behalf of the AMA Board of Directors in 1939, Fishbein warned, "all forms of security, compulsory security, even against old age and unemployment, represent a beginning invasion by the state into the personal life of the individual, represent a taking away of individual responsibility, a weakening of national caliber, a definite step toward either communism or totalitarianism."[5]

As reformers advanced proposals to establish group insurance and national health insurance, Fishbein, with the AMA membership behind him, sounded the alarm. When Harry Truman announced his support in late 1945 for a proposal to cover 80% of the US population with government-sponsored health insurance with no deductibles, financed by a 3% payroll tax, the AMA dug in, hiring a public relations firm to campaign against it, a milestone in modern American political propaganda. Truman described the AMA's campaign, which included comic strips in which patients waited in long lines outside of clinics and robots delivered care, as "rabid."[6]

Although preventive medicine was never the AMA's highest priority, the organization has been devoted, consistently and relentlessly, to preventing any outbreaks of meaningful transformation of American health care. The defeat of Truman's proposal provided the AMA with a template to which it would return time and again. A notable weapon in the organization's arsenal was the 1961 recording, *Ronald Reagan Speaks Out against Socialized Medicine*. As we know, the future president could spin a compelling narrative. The album was part of campaign called "Operation Coffee Cup," in which doctors' wives would hold coffee-klatches with friends and neighbors to warn them about the evils of "socialized medicine" and urge them to write to Congress in opposition to proposed legislation to provide government health insurance to the elderly. The Reagan recording was a highlight of those meetings. The actor, who went on to host the television show *Death Valley Days* before entering politics, did not pull his punches in imploring his listeners to act:

> If you don't, this program, I promise you, will pass just as surely as the sun will come up tomorrow; and behind it will come other federal programs that will invade every area of freedom as we have known it in this country. Until, one day . . . we will awake to find that we have socialism.
>
> And if you don't do this and if I don't do it, one of these days you and I are going to spend our sunset years telling our children, and our children's children, what it once was like in America when men were free.[7]

Some other physicians' groups, notably those involved in primary care, have been more amenable to health care reform in recent years.[8] Other medical specialty and subspecialty organizations have been far less attentive to the broad strokes of health reform than to any components of such reforms or other policies that might threaten their income levels. Their concerns in that regard would be a tough sell to the public, but they have been able to effectively communicate their perspectives to the government through their solid voting control on the Relative Value Scale Update Committee convened by the AMA (chap. 3).

Influencing Other Actors in Health Care

Beyond their determination to prevent reform, many practitioners engage in interactions with medical educators, scientists, patients, and the public that serve narrow interests and impede progress toward meeting broader needs. From educators, practitioners seek a continuing flow of appropriately trained practitioners into their fields that is consistent with the priorities of their disciplines and not necessarily with those of society. Their specialty organizations sanction training programs to help accomplish this aim. Their academic departments influence the choices made by scientists about the focus of their scholarship when they hire researchers to do work that enhances their areas of practice. In this way the specialization within medicine comes to be reproduced in the foci of research activity within biomedical science and shapes the research agendas of medical institutions.

To their patients, too many clinicians offer false hopes and futile or ineffective treatments (see chap. 4). They are uncomfortable with ambiguity and so avoid it when speaking to patients. They shun difficult conversations and are reluctant to limit care. In an age when everyone and everything is subject to online ratings and evaluations and corporate employers routinely survey patients about satisfaction with care, knowledge that these ratings can affect their income levels or even their livelihood undermines the clinicians' authority, affects their behavior, and ultimately compromises their integrity.

Advocacy for Their Product Lines

The medical profession has been sadly effective in promoting unnecessary and ineffective care. As we saw in chapter 8, when Deyo and others concluded that back surgery should be performed less frequently in some situations, the North American Spine Society responded furiously, leading Congress to cut the budget of the agency that funded the research. Though his research held up, Deyo was assailed as the devil incarnate. None of his research was found to be lacking in rigor, but the criticism was not attenuated by the facts.[9]

This episode reminds me of a time when I wrote an article for the Los Angeles Times in the 1980s in which I observed that although chemotherapy for many conditions had improved survival remarkably, for some other conditions it had not increased either the quantity and quality of life. This observation aroused the ire of many oncologists. As one faculty member commented to me at the time, "You attacked them in a vital organ: the wallet."

Believing fervently in what they do, many physicians understandably seek to shape discourse about it accordingly. The distinguished British clinical epidemiologist Archie Cochrane tells the story about a famous randomized trial, conducted in the 1960s, that compared home and hospital care for myocardial infarction (heart attack). At the time, little was done in the hospital for heart attack patients beyond strict bed rest for two or three weeks. There were no revascularization procedures, no antiarrhythmic drugs, and no beta-blockers, ACE inhibitors, or angiotensin receptor blockers. Many cardiologists, who believed that the care they provided in hospital was essential, made no secret of their opposition to the study. Cochrane, well aware of the cardiologists' antipathy, presented preliminary results to the committee monitoring the study's safety, showing an advantage for hospital care. The cardiologists called for immediate termination of the study and provision of hospital care to all subjects. Cochrane then revealed that he had reversed the numbers— home care appeared to be more effective. When he then asked them what should be done, the cardiologists no longer wanted to terminate the study. The study's ultimate results showed hospital and home care to be equally effective. And the mischievous Archie Cochrane was memorialized by the Cochrane Organization and Library, the preeminent effort dedicated to advancing evidence-based medicine worldwide.[10]

Cochrane's account particularly resonated with me. My grandfather had a heart attack in 1935, at a time when patients were put on bed rest in the hospital for as long as six weeks. As I have heard the story, that was the extent of his treatment. He died of a pulmonary embolus on the day before he was to be discharged. The embolus was likely caused by the prolonged bed rest. Since then, we have learned that bed rest is not beneficial for heart attack patients, as long as their vital signs are stable. Nowadays, the great majority of hospitalized patients who do require bed rest receive anticoagulants to prevent thromboembolic diseases, including pulmonary embolism. We must always be open to new knowledge that might help us improve care and outcomes. Doctors who stand to benefit, financially or otherwise, should be the last ones to judge the evidence on the usefulness of what they do.

Conflicts of Interest in the Review of Scientific Articles

That raises another consideration. Articles that appear in medical journals are peer-reviewed by experts in the field. In recent decades, journals have increasingly required that reviewers disclose conflicts of interest, such as payments from a drug or device manufacturer whose product is the subject of the study (see chap. 9). Yet reviewers are not asked to disclose what are often far greater conflicts of interest: when they earn all or most of their income from a procedure under review. Are such experts the only ones who can judge the science? Not at all. A statement often attributed to Albert Einstein holds that if you can't explain something to a six-year-old, you don't understand it yourself. A scientific paper can be written with sufficient clarity to enable a researcher who is more distant from that topic (and who has no such conflicts of interest) to judge its merits.

That is not to say that anyone can review a scientific paper, but there are plenty of qualified candidates beyond the limited circle of specialists most invested in its findings. Moreover, the lead and senior authors should be individuals with no direct or indirect financial stake in the outcome, one way or another, without full disclosure of such interests. This also applies to data analysts on such papers. Without such constraints, the potential for distortions and compromised findings remains great. The problem has become clear in recent years, given the overly enthusiastic embrace of studies in personalized, or precision, medicine.[11]

Miscommunicating with Patients

Clinicians' communications with their patients present another potential conflict. Recall the cardiologist who will catheterize anyone with a heartbeat, the oncologist who will continue chemotherapy as long as the patient has a pulse, and the internist who performs pulmonary function tests on the asymptomatic nonsmoker. Such doctors are in "sales"; they do not "lie" as much as they shade the truth. One expects as much from, say, a used car dealer; a patient has the right to expect more from their doctor.

Scientists, Their Organizations, and Their Funders

Science is supposed to proceed with caution, and often replication, based on evidence. As discussed in chapter 8, however, scientists talk up their research, often exaggerating its promise, in the hope of winning government support. The pitch involves trumpeting the alleged value of the science to the public. The media, always eager for headlines about ostensible "breakthroughs," are happy to play their part. One troubling new tactic in this game is the scientific "preprint," a version of a scientific manuscript that is posted on a public server accessible to the media before it has been subject to formal peer review and often without disclosure of authors' conflicts of interest.[12]

Such aggressive sales techniques can reap rewards: gifts, grants, pressure on government to fast-track a product, and so on. Complicating matters is the fact that scientists may hold patents related to the work and may have additional financial incentive to see it move forward. One can easily lose sight of the difference between personal gain and public benefit. More responsible, less self-interested communication would educate the public about skepticism, the common good, and more realistic prospects for breakthroughs.

Organizations such as the Alzheimer's Association, the American Cancer Society, and others raise funds for research with overblown rhetoric, such as "The first survivor of Alzheimer's is out there, but we won't get there without you."[13] Their business model relies on this kind of hype that promises dramatic progress. And when a manufacturer lobbies for approval of a drug, the organizations get on board, notwithstanding a lack of rigorous evidence of effectiveness.[14] Professional organizations representing scientific disciplines encourage a similar suspension of disbelief in their lobbying efforts. At minimum, scientists propagate biological reductionism that is an article of faith in the world of medicine and that obstructs potential progress through other kinds of innovations that might do more to advance health.

Corporate Providers

Corporate providers (chap. 7), including many of the leading academic medical centers, mislead the public about the good things that they do and the bad ones as well. The billions of dollars spent advertising in their local communities and elsewhere emphasize wondrous advances and benefits to ordinary people. Their advertisements fail to mention such niceties as lawsuits against patients for unpaid bills or limits to access for some. They lack transparency about what their care costs and gloss over their barely legal strategies to keep poor, uninsured patients away from their clinics and hospitals. Their required financial reports downplay the accumulation of massive surpluses that add to their enormous net worth and their building programs, often rationalizing such information with sky-is-falling scenarios of financial catastrophe that they suggest are imminent.

These increasingly powerful health care systems are equally circumspect in their communication with government. They accept government money for the care of the poor even when they strive to minimize any such services. They lobby vigorously and effectively for relief from COVID-19-like financial hardships, for better payment rates, and for regulatory laxity in the face of their unprecedented growth and market domination.

They often treat their clinicians, particularly the ones who don't do procedures, as expendable and interchangeable. After all, it is the specialists and their procedures that bring in the big bucks. "America's Best Hospitals" strongly encourage referrals for expensive, elective procedures that are their greatest sources of revenue. They regard diagnosis and management doctors who don't generate surplus as "cost centers" (really as little more than specialist-extenders). Notably, their nonprofessional staff often are paid poorly, even as their procedural practitioners make high salaries, and their senior executives enjoy seven-figure incomes.

Producers

Pharmaceutical and biologic producers communicate in ways that range from prevarication to out-and-out lying (chap. 9). When their advertising was limited to clinicians, they engaged in a range of nefarious practices: peddling their products as useful in populations in whom they had not been studied; bribing clinicians with gifts and trips; hiring prestigious clinicians (with lucrative consultancies sometimes amounting to hundreds of thousands of dollars annually) to pitch their wares; plying medical students and trainees with gifts of medical equipment, dinners, and tickets to sporting events; and including subliminal images in their advertising materials.[15]

When government relaxed regulatory limits on direct-to-consumer advertising in the late 1990s, the floodgates opened.[16] The manufacturers promise wondrous results for those who take their treatments. While they are required to describe adverse effects, including lethal ones, of their products, their television advertisements typically explain the dangers of the drugs in ways that even sophisticated members of the public could not understand or fully grasp.[17]

Studies have found that listing more side effects in drug ads makes patients *more* trusting of the product, even if they don't fully understand implications of those potential harms.[18] Most ads include emotional appeals and emphasize how taking the medicine will enable the patient to participate in more recreational activities.[19] The manufacturers, moreover, have fought successfully to date in Congress and the courts to prevent a requirement for full disclosure of comparative cost information in these ads.[20] Their goal has always been to induce demand. To say that they succeed is an understatement. A colleague at an orthopedic hospital told me that a large proportion of patients who show up with inflammatory arthritis are asking for these new, expensive products they have seen advertised.

The pharmaceutical industry promotes falsehoods about potential legislation and regulatory reform they oppose. It insists that anything that curtails its profits will prevent innovation and product development (even though many of those products emanated directly from government-funded research). It spends enormous sums to defeat ballot initiatives aimed at lowering the cost of its products.[21]

It also spends more than any other sector on lobbying the federal government—about $250 million per year—much of it regarding drug pricing. Its primary goal is to defend rules that allow the industry to extend patents and to charge higher prices in the United States than in other countries. It has succeeded for years in stopping the federal government from negotiating drug prices in Medicare.[22]

Technology manufacturers lobbied successfully to repeal a medical device tax that was part of the Affordable Care Act.[23] The producers of expensive devices work with purchasers to publicize the latter's acquisitions, which puts pressure on competing health systems to add the same products.

The Insurers

Health insurance corporations are great communicators. They know what they want and how to get it. They are not opposed to providing coverage for the entire population. They merely understand that if this were to be accomplished through the government, it would represent an existential threat to their businesses (chaps. 10 and 11). These companies are so enmeshed in people's consciousness in their current incarnations that it is hard for many to remember, for example, that Blue Cross Blue Shield began in the 1930s as two nonprofit entities that were primarily focused upon doing good in society. It was only in the 1990s that the local plans received permission to convert to for-profit status, sometimes in exchange for creating charitable foundations.

When the Clinton administration proposed a substantial health reform to extend health insurance coverage in 1993–94, the proposal was obliterated by organized opposition from the health insurance industry through its lobby, the Health Insurance Association of America. As noted in chapter 11, its yearlong "Harry and Louise" television ad campaign disingenuously argued that the reform would restrict provider choice at a time when existing insurance products imposed substantial limits to "freedom of choice" and were heading toward greater restrictions in the absence of reform. The ads were effective and helped the Republicans in Congress to sink the legislation.[24]

Insurers gave a pass to the Obama reform because it was offering expanded coverage through private entities (notions of a "public option" were quashed). They continue to fund opposition to universal one-payer proposals, still insisting that it would take away the ability of patients and their families to see the providers of their choice.

As noted in chapter 11, Canada, the "socialist Hades" to the north with single-payer health care, allows anyone go to *any* doctor, while in the United States, most people are limited to the choices offered by their health plans. American patients pay substantially more for care if they go to an uncovered physician or facility, or if they encounter a moonlighting uncovered doctor in the emergency room of a covered facility, or an uncovered assistant surgeon helping with a procedure being performed by a covered provider.

One of the insurers' most invidious forms of communication is denial of coverage (chap. 10). Think of it: They calculate that a certain percentage of those so rejected will be unable to cut through the bureaucratic appeal process and insist on their right to insurance payment for vital services. Money in the coffers for the insurer, but risk of financial ruin for those who are denied coverage: the smoker who would benefit from a screening scan of the chest, the woman with severe colitis who needs frequent colonoscopies because of cancer risk, or the man whose knee arthritis prevents him from working but is judged not to merit coverage for surgery.

Medical Schools and the Educators

American medical schools do not do enough to counteract the negative socialization of their students and postgraduate trainees toward values learned in classrooms, clinics, and hospitals that prioritize perceived personal interests over societal needs. They also promulgate biological reductionism (chap. 5), while medical school leaders and faculty members lobby Congress to increase funding for those kinds of scholarly work (chap. 8) rather than for research on health care delivery, preventive services, and unmet needs.

Along with their teaching hospitals, they purport to be committed to population health but really are only interested in the health of the well insured and strategically place their practices to reflect those interests (chaps. 6 and 7). They speak with their investments, shaping the scientific workforce by hiring basic science researchers, from whom they judge that they are likely to see substantial return in the form of federal grants and patents, rather than population and social scientists for whom the health of the population as a whole is a central concern.

Government

Governments at all levels eloquently communicate their priorities and values through laws, regulations, and expenditures, as well as through their absence. By failing to ensure that the numbers of physicians entering various specialties are consistent with society's needs, and by leaving in place a reimbursement scheme that overpays for subspecialized care, they perpetuate a system that is overspecialized, overpriced, and favors procedures over caring. They prioritize biological solutions and "magic bullets" in their clinical programs and research funding rather than devote more resources to improving adoption of healthful behaviors, addressing the social context of illness, and reducing barriers to effective treatments.[25] Lack of universal health insurance and underfunding of many state Medicaid programs unambiguously affirm that not all patients are equally "deserving" (chap. 10). Some fiscal policies, such as subsidizing tobacco growers and polluting industries, promote harm to health.

The Public and the Patients

Patients and members of the public are bombarded with propaganda emanating from corporations, clinicians, disease advocacy organizations, governments, political interest groups, and even religious authorities. Some want to sell them something, whether that's a hospitalization, an insurance policy, an imaging study, or an expensive medication. Others seek to influence their approach to decision-making about their own health care (as at the end of life) or their attitudes to health care policy reform through messaging directed at their fears and perceived needs. The Internet, a potential tool for consumer empowerment, is an unreliable source of objective information accessible to people with varying levels of sophistication, and it only adds to confusion, as it is replete with dangerous misinformation and quackery (as has been abundantly clear regarding COVID-19 remedies and vaccines).

Every medical school does attempt to teach students how to talk to patients, but their efforts fall far short of what is needed. Beyond the propensity of doctors to listen selectively to patients, ignore nonverbal cues, avoid difficult conversations, and even cut off opening statements, communications with medical providers and health care systems are undermined by the sociocultural and linguistic barriers that make it hard for patients and their proxies to impart what they seek to convey, and just as hard for clinicians to comprehend it. The result is often lack of trust and failure to meet the needs of the patients.[26]

As noted in chapters 2 and 13, those who seek more medical care for themselves or their dying relatives, out of longing for something that their lives are not providing, need clearer insights into what may be driving their dis-ease along with unambiguous information on what is medically possible. The absent, inadequate, ineffective, or even counterproductive communication from many of their doctors does nothing to mitigate these demands, address these needs, or counteract confusing messaging from other sources. Politicians' reluctance to offend voters by putting limits on care, and their preference to give constituents something the latter perceive as valuable, doesn't help either.[27]

The Media (General and Political)

Can the modern media provide an oasis of disinterested sanity amid the cacophony of self-promoting stakeholders? Unlikely. Cable news and talk radio stations promote various agendas, as do individuals and groups active on social media. Those not motivated primarily by politics still look to draw audiences with eye-catching headlines. They are always on the lookout for "big" health care stories. A pandemic makes it easy, especially with a rapidly evolving story that offers a new angle every day.

In less turbulent times, the media thrive on sensational stories of breakthrough treatments, technologies, and scientific discoveries. Reports about "the gene that causes Alzheimer's," the "game-changing" drug for pancreatic cancer, or a new kind of transplant operation arouse considerable excitement.[28] Do such breakthroughs matter much to the health of the population? Usually not, and almost never in the short term.

It is much less common for the media to focus on disparities in health and health care. They devote little attention, and certainly rarely with the fervor displayed for more sensational stuff, to the scandalous fact that life expectancy at birth in the United States can vary by 15 years or more between neighborhoods and population subgroups in the same city, or even by as much as 5.7 years between states.[29] Even rarer are stories that dig deeper in trying to explain why the situation is what it is: poorer access to treatment, discriminatory treatment when it is available, unsafe neighborhoods, less access to good nutrition, and so on. The propensity to sensationalize the latest study fails to put it in the context of a larger body of research, information that may well be available at public sites that rarely are accessed by the public, such as that of the Cochrane Organization, discussed above. As one medical journalist wrote, "Instead of trying to translate what the best-available research evidence tells us . . . we report on the latest studies out of context, with little focus on how they were designed, whether they were unduly conflicted by study funders, and whether they agree or disagree with the rest of the research."[30]

The media also misinform the public about the effectiveness and cost of seemingly miraculous treatments. We might be presented with a breathless report about a drug that adds a few months of life for people with prostate cancer, but we're not informed that it costs tens of thousands of dollars a month. Not coincidentally, we may see such a report on media outlets that run advertisements from the drug's manufacturer promoting the product.

It is entirely appropriate for media to investigate problems with quality of care in the community. One such investigation led to closure of a hospital in the Los Angeles area.[31] When this occurs, the journalists should be equally attentive to what the effect is upon people's ability to get the care that they need.[32]

The shortcomings of political media are well known. They polarize the population, promoting an "us versus them" mentality; distort public discourse about the implications of policy choices; and spread misinformation, for example, about the safety and efficacy of vaccines, largely to make political points. It may be unrealistic to expect them to change, but imagine if general media eschewed sensational health stories in favor of attempting to educate people about collective responsibility for the public's health, about being good Samaritans, and about the need to think of each life as equally precious. In all of these respects, media have failed. Economist Uwe Reinhardt once commented that America only cares about the welfare of a child if she falls down a well in Texas. The media can help to change that.

Researchers on Health Care and Medical Educators

Academic medical institutions, their leaders, and many of their faculty have abandoned any pretense of caring about much of anything other than organizational and professional success. Many researchers on health care accept the system's values, tout the effectiveness of managed Medicaid, study minor manipulations to improve efficiency of the existing system, and rarely question separation of care for the poor from that of the "deserving" or the injustice of making people choose between paying for medical care or other basic needs.

Others do study inequality, social factors affecting health, pervasive flaws in the health care system, and the viability of alternatives to it, and they work tirelessly to raise consciousness about these issues. Many are members of the Physicians for a National Health Program and social responsibility, health equity, and anti-racism groups in organizations such as the Society of General Internal Medicine. Some I know well are Arleen Brown and Keith Norris at UCLA, who have devoted great effort to making it possible for diverse populations to be involved in all levels of decision-making in research enterprises; Oliver Fein of Cornell, who is the social conscience of the medical school as well as a vigorous public advocate for a more just health care system; and Steffie Woolhandler and David Himmelstein, whose studies I have cited in previous chapters. A noteworthy exemplar outside of academia is Sidney Wolfe of Public Citizen (chap. 9), a group that documents pharmaceutical company malfeasance, government failure to protect the public from harmful medications, and shortcomings of private insurance products and of the Affordable Care Act.[33] Wolfe's willingness to stand up to powerful forces reminds me of the man facing tanks in Tiananmen Square in 1989. Many more such voices are needed.

Toxic Interactions, Afflicted Communication, and Their Consequences: A Societal Perspective

Given that so much communication among the disparate actors in health care is ineffective, counterproductive, or even harmful, making many of the interactions toxic, the story of the Tower of Babel may come to mind.[34] The tower failed because participants could no longer understand one another. Progress depends on a common understanding of ends and means. Its lack isn't a problem unique to health care. According to German sociologist Jürgen Habermas, such "communicative action" depends upon the nature of interaction and communication across four elements crucial to the functioning of society: those who control capital and produce commodities, those who develop and implement policies, individuals or groups that seek to exert interpersonal influence, and the values and beliefs of members of society.[35] Communication must occur across all of these elements. The forces that control capital effectively communicate their interests to those who formulate and execute policy. They drown out the perspectives of other social actors, leading the entire system to break down and lose legitimacy. This describes the current state of American health care.[36]

The overwhelming power in health care resides with the forces of capital, abetted by governments and professional interest groups. Communicative action becomes difficult, if not impossible, and adversarial situations—such as malpractice suits, insurance denials, collection agencies, and the like—ensue.[37] At the very least, the finances and structure of American health care have made its problems more extreme than those encountered in other affluent countries with more rational systems. Fixing these problems won't be easy. It won't be sufficient to ask, "Can we all get along?"[38]

Too many groups have too much at stake in the current system, and the apocalyptic rhetoric of those opposing change can be mind-numbing. This impasse has far-reaching consequences and calls into question the ways in which health care is conceptualized, financed, researched, taught, delivered, and received. Anyone hoping to remedy this situation needs to keep this context clearly in mind. But the magnitude of the challenge doesn't give us an excuse to shrug our shoulders and lament that nothing meaningful will happen until the world changes. There are things we can and should attempt to accomplish:

- End direct-to-consumer advertising. We have banned tobacco advertising on television and radio because it is dangerous to health. We should do the same with drug ads that oversell indications and downplay potentially dangerous side effects. If we can't ban the ads for constitutional reasons, they need to be far more strictly regulated.

- Advertisements for health systems should also be strictly regulated. Claims about their superior quality are almost always distorted and should be appraised critically. In contrast, such systems could contribute to public service announcements that promote the receipt of health care or preventive services *from any source* or encourage better health-related behaviors.
- Medical societies that organize, promote in any way, or publicize lobbying efforts by their members on behalf of their financial interests should lose tax-exempt status.
- Biomedical scientists, their societies, and the medical schools should also cease and desist from promoting self-interested policies. Let the National Academies of Medicine and Science convene diverse groups to more objectively articulate what is needed in science policy as priority areas for research broadly relevant to health care.
- Pharmaceutical companies and insurers should be impeded from pouring mountains of cash into blocking ballot initiatives they oppose. How can that be done? Perhaps by limiting any expenditure on political advocacy.
- Stop doctors and health systems from selling procedures that people don't need. There has been some improvement in this regard regarding breast cancer and prostate cancer treatments.[39]
- Pay clinicians for their time, not for piecework. In the end, this is the only way to get doctors and the health care corporations for which they work to stop selling stuff to people who don't need it.
- Media should establish and adopt widely standards for communication about new medical research and the health care system as a whole.

There is a lot more that could be done and that deserves attention, sooner rather than later.

Notes
1. In contrast, medical education is an undergraduate program in many European countries.

2. "Use of Such Terms as Mid-Level Provider and Physician Extender," American Association of Nurse Practitioners, accessed July 4, 2020, https://www.aanp.org/advocacy/advocacy-resource/position-statements/use-of-terms-such-as-mid-level-provider-and-physician-extender.

3. Institute of Medicine, *The Future of Nursing: Leading Change, Advancing Health* (Washington, DC: National Academies Press, 2011); Julie Stanik-Hutt et al., "The Quality and Effectiveness of Care Provided by Nurse Practitioners," *Journal for Nurse Practitioners* 9, no. 8 (September 2013): 492–500, https://doi.org/10.1016/j.nurpra.2013.07.004.

4. Steven H. Landers and Ashwini R. Sehgal, "How Do Physicians Lobby Their Members of Congress?," *Archives of Internal Medicine* 160, no. 21 (November 27, 2000): 3248–51, https://doi.org/10.1001/archinte.160.21.3248.

5. "Labeling of Old-Age and Unemployment Insurance as a Step towards Either Communism or Totalitarianism," *Congressional Record* 107, Part 5, Appendix (April 10–27, 1961): A2358.

6. Beatrix Hoffman, *Health Care for Some: Rights and Rationing in the United States since 1930* (Chicago: University of Chicago Press, 2012), 58–61; Sheila Mulrooney Eldred, "When Harry Truman Pushed for Universal Health Care," History.com, November 20, 2019, https://www.history.com/news/harry-truman-universal-health-care.

7. "Ronald Reagan Speaks Out against Socialized Medicine," American Rhetoric, accessed May 3, 2020, https://www.americanrhetoric.com/speeches/ronaldreagan socializedmedicine.htm.

8. Robert Doherty et al., "Envisioning a Better U.S. Health Care System for All: A Call to Action by the American College of Physicians," *Annals of Internal Medicine* 172, no. 2, suppl. (January 2020): S3–S6, https://doi.org/10.7326/M19-2411.

9. Richard A. Deyo et al., "The Messenger under Attack—Intimidation of Researchers by Special-Interest Groups," *New England Journal of Medicine* 336, no. 16 (April 17, 1997): 1177–80, https://doi.org/10.1056/NEJM199704173361611. See also Brian Martin, "Breaking the Siege: Guidelines for Struggle in Science," in *Science under Siege: Zoology under Threat*, ed. Peter Banks, Daniel Lunney, and Chris Dickman (Sydney: Royal Zoological Society of New South Wales, 2012), 164–70, https:// doi.org/10.7882/FS.2012.053.

10. "Cochrane: Trusted Evidence. Informed Decisions. Better Health," Cochrane.org, accessed March 21, 2021, https://www.cochrane.org.

11. In addition to the discussion in chap. 8, see David Clark Aron, "Precision Medicine in an Imprecise and Complex World: Magic Bullets, Hype, and the Fuzzy Line between Health and Disease," *Journal of Evaluation in Clinical Practice* 26, no. 5 (October 2020): 1534–38, https://doi.org/10.1111/jep.13306.

12. May C. I. van Schalkwyk et al., "The Perils of Preprints: Their Use and Platforms Require Greater Scrutiny," *British Medical Journal* 370 (August 17, 2020): m3111, https://doi.org/10.1136/bmj.m3111.

13. "The First Survivor," Alzheimer's Association, accessed July 4, 2020, http://alz.org/firstsurvivor/overview.asp.

14. Michael Grecius and G. Caleb Alexander, "People Want an Alzheimer's Drug. This Isn't the One," *New York Times*, May 28, 2021, https://www.nytimes.com/2021/05/28/opinion/alzheimer-treatment-FDA-aducanumab.html?searchResultPosition=1.

15. Michael S. Wilkes, Bruce H. Doblin, and Martin F. Shapiro, "Pharmaceutical Advertisements in Leading Medical Journals: Experts' Assessments," *Annals of Internal Medicine* 116, no. 11 (June 1, 1992): 912–19, https://doi.org/10.7326/0003-4819-116-11-912; David A. Kessler, "Addressing the Problem of Misleading Advertising," *Annals of Internal Medicine* 116, no. 11 (June 1, 1992): 950–51, https://doi.org/10.7326/0003-4819-116-11-950.

16. Notably, New Zealand is the only other advanced industrial society that allows such advertising.

17. The ads typically describe the potential harms of the drugs without text on screen, while showing positive images, such as a man helping his son repair a car, a woman watching the sunset in a beautiful locale, or a grandfather fishing with his progeny.

18. Niro Sivanthan and Hermant Kakkar, "How Drug Company Ads Downplay Risks," *Scientific American*, February 20, 2019, https://www.scientificamerican.com/article/how-drug-company-ads-downplay-risks/; Julia Belluz, "Why Prescription Drug Ads Always Have That Absurd List of Side Effects at the End," Vox, September 29, 2015, https://www.vox.com/2015/9/29/9414145/direct-consumer-advertising-pharmaceutical-regulation.

19. Janelle Applequist and Jennifer Gerard Ball, "An Updated Analysis of Direct-to-Consumer Television Advertisements for Prescription Drugs," *Annals of Family Medicine* 16, no. 3 (May 2018): 211–16, https://doi.org/10.1370/afm.2220.

20. Kelsey Waddill, "Federal Judge Strikes Down New Drug Pricing Transparency Rule," Health Payer Intelligence, July 10, 2019, https://healthpayerintelligence.com/news/federal-judge-strikes-down-new-drug-price-transparency-rule; "Another Battle in the Political Fight over How to Address High Drug Prices," *National Law Review* 11, no. 299 (August 16, 2021): https://www.natlawreview.com/article/another-battle-political-fight-over-how-to-address-high-drug-prices.

21. "Drug Companies Funnel $108 Million to Defeat California Drug-Price Ballot Question," Modern Healthcare, October 20, 2016, https://www.modernhealthcare.com/article/20161020/NEWS/161029987/drug-companies-funnel-108-million-to-defeat-california-drug-price-ballot-question.

22. In nine months in 2017, 153 companies were involved in lobbying related to drug pricing, four times the number of corporations so engaged four years earlier. "A Bitter Pill: How Big Pharma Lobbies to Keep Prescription Drug Prices High," Citizens for Responsibility and Ethics in Washington (CREW), June 18, 2018, https://www.citizensforethics.org/reports-investigations/crew-reports/a-bitter-pill-how-big-pharma-lobbies-to-keep-prescription-drug-prices-high/.

23. Bruce Japsen, "Medical Device Tax Is History after Trump Signs Repeal," *Forbes*, December 21, 2019, https://www.forbes.com/sites/brucejapsen/2019/12/21/medical-device-tax-is-history-after-trump-signs-repeal/?sh=1afa2d364ed4.

24. Theda Skocpol, *Boomerang: Clinton's Health Security Effort and the Turn against Government in U.S. Politics* (New York: W. W. Norton, 1996).

25. Eric B. Larson, "Prevention of Late-Life Dementia: No Magic Bullet," *Annals of Internal Medicine* 168, no. 1 (January 2, 2018): 77–79, https://doi.org/10.7326/M17 -3026.

26. See chap. 4. See also Aaron D. Baugh, Allison A. Vanderbilt, and Reginald F. Baugh, "Communication Training Is Inadequate: The Role of Deception, Non-verbal Communication, and Cultural Proficiency," *Medical Education Online* 25, no. 1 (December 2020): https://doi.org/10.1080/10872981.2020.1820228.

27. An additional influence that can complicate the picture is that an individual's personal religious advisor may express views at variance with the formal perspectives of their denominations. They might, for example, maintain that life must be pre-served at all costs, including by keeping someone alive by artificial means when there is no hope of recovery, even though most religions do recognize some acceptable limits to efforts to extend the life of someone who is terminally ill. "Religious Groups' Views on End-of-Life Issues," Pew Research Center, November 21, 2013, https://www .pewforum.org/2013/11/21/religious-groups-views-on-end-of-life-issues/.

28. See, e.g., Benjamin Heigle et al., "Use of Exaggerated Language in News Stories to Describe Drugs for Treatment of Alzheimer's Disease," *Alzheimer's and Dementia Journal* 6, no. 1 (August 13, 2020): e12062, https://doi.org/10.1002/trc2.12062.

29. Laura Dwyer-Lindgren et al., "Variation in Life Expectancy and Mortality by Cause among Neighborhoods in King County, WA, USA, 1990–2014: A Census Tract-Level Analysis for the Global Burden of Disease Study 2015," *Lancet Public Health* 2, no. 9 (September 5, 2017): e400–410, https://doi.org/10.1016/S2468 -2667(17)30165-2; Antonio Fernando Boing et al., "Quantifying and Explaining Variation in Life Expectancy at Census Tract, County, and State Levels in the United States," *Proceedings of the National Academy of Sciences of the United States of America* 117, no. 30 (July 28, 2020): 17,688–94, https://doi.org/10.1073/pnas.2003719117; "Life Expectancy at Birth (in Years): Timeframe: 2018," Kaiser Family Foundation State Health Facts, accessed September 26, 2021, https://www.kff.org/other/state -indicator/life-expectancy/?currentTimeframe=0&sortModel=%7B%22colId%22:%2 2Location%22,%22sort%22:%22asc%22%7D.

30. Julia Belluz, "Health Journalism Has a Serious Evidence Problem. Here's a Plan to Save It," Vox, June 21, 2016, https://www.vox.com/2016/6/21/11962568/health -journalism-evidence-based-medicine.

31. "The 2005 Pulitzer Prize Winner in Public Service: *Los Angeles Times*," The Pulitzer Prizes, accessed July 11, 2020, https://www.pulitzer.org/winners/los-angeles -times-3.

32. Kara Odom Walker et al., "Increased Patient Delays in Care after the Closure of Martin Luther King Hospital: Implications for Monitoring Health System Changes," *Ethnicity and Disease* 21, no. 3 (Summer 2011): 356–60, PMID 21942170.

33. "Health Research Group Publications," Public Citizen, accessed July 10, 2021, https://www.citizen.org/article/health-research-group-publications/.

34. Genesis 11:1–9.

35. Jürgen Habermas, *The Theory of Communicative Action*, vol. 2: *Lifeworld and System*, trans. Thomas McCarthy (Boston: Beacon Press, 1985). Policy and influence occur in the public arena, while money/accumulation of capital and values/commitments are primarily private sector phenomena. Habermas uses slightly different terminology. He refers to the sphere of money and accumulation of capital as "adaptation." He calls the political power sphere "goal attainment." He calls the values sphere "latency or value commitments." The effects of groups or individuals on each other are "influence." In addition, he characterizes the money/capital and power/policy spheres as "system," and the values and influence spheres as "lifeworld."

36. Habermas characterizes such communication as "colonized" and the situation as a "legitimation crisis." Jürgen Habermas, *Legitimation Crisis*, trans. Thomas McCarthy (Boston, MA: Beacon Press, 1975).

37. Arthur W. Frank, "Notes on Habermas: Lifeworld and System," University of Calgary People, accessed February 27, 2012, https://people.ucalgary.ca/~frank /habermas.html.

38. After Rodney King; see also Paula D. McClain and Jessica D. Johnson Carew, *Can We All Get Along? Racial and Ethnic Minorities in American Politics*, 7th ed. (New York: Hachette, 2018).

39. It took a lot of effort by activists to get surgeons and other clinicians involved in the care of persons with breast cancer to provide comprehensible information on options for its treatment. There also has been some progress in improving communication about alternatives to prostatectomy. Rather than lobbying, specialty societies should collaborate with those lacking vested interests to develop materials and recommended forms of communication about a vast array of clinical situations and what should and should not be communicated: about the need for colonoscopy, chemotherapy, expensive drugs, dermatologic procedures, and so on.

Dialogue #12

Professor (looking up from the document): Well, things sure are tangled up.

Student: I agree. Every participant, at least to some degree, seems to be affecting the perspectives and actions of every other one in negative ways and impeding the changes that we need.

Professor: What is your most important takeaway from our consideration of toxic interactions?

Student: I think it would be that progress requires a common understanding of how to proceed, and all of these messed-up relationships make communicative action so much more difficult.

Professor: Very good.

Student: I know that we proposed a number of reforms, but working on this chapter on toxic relationships and communication makes me feel that they won't accomplish much. Trying to eradicate these problems is like trying to swim across a vast sea of molasses.

Professor: Interesting image! We've laid out a lot of the problems. Why can't we find a way to address them effectively?

Student: There are three colossal issues. The world of health care is highly commodified, and everyone wants their piece of the action. Beyond that, there are all these other obstacles: values, interests, capabilities, limitations, unmet needs, and on and on. Then there's the relationships and communication, which are a mess and make everyone do their very worst.

Professor: That is all true, but look how much we have learned. When we started this project, you identified cost, equity, and outcomes as the issues to address. Now we can see some "colossal" ones, as you say, standing astride of those.

Student: That's hardly encouraging. There are so many different participants whose needs, expectations, and actions would need to be addressed. Easier to turn back the tide than to fix this, it seems to me.

Professor: Let's try a thought experiment.

Student: OK.

Professor: Consider HIV. Childhood leukemia. Hodgkin disease.

Student: All very serious illnesses.

Professor: And?

Student: There are pretty good treatments for them now.

Professor: And how did we get to that point?

Student: Well, someone found treatments that worked.

Professor: It is a bit more complicated than that. In each case, we found a treatment that we thought might work, but it only made things a little better. Then the disease came roaring back.

Student: How did we overcome that?

Professor: By learning to combine a number of treatments to attack the disease at different points in its path of doing harm. Over time, we found the right combinations to get the job done.

Student: I'm not convinced by the analogy. We're not talking about biology. There are competing interests involved.

Professor: You're right. But if we don't think about the problem this way, we may miss something crucial.

Student: We can't fix the world.

Professor: That's not our job. But perhaps we can figure out which paths might be fruitful, which ones not, and what it is that we're looking for. Can we proceed incrementally or selectively in addressing the issues? Or is a more global solution needed? Or can we do both?

15

Healing American Health Care

To Palliate, to Cure, or Both?

Healing is a matter of time, but it is sometimes also a matter of opportunity.
—Hippocrates

Never believe that a few caring people can't change the world. For, indeed, that's all who ever have.
—Margaret Mead

How are we to make sense of all the issues that we have covered? I will try to do so by bringing together the themes of the last three chapters: the consequences of health care in the United States being treated more as a commodity than as an act of healing and promotion of well-being, the consciousness and internal life of the participants, and the toxic relationships and problematic communication in and about health care. In so doing, it is possible to glean some understanding of the range of problems that need to be addressed, as well as whether there is a magic bullet, in the form of a piece of legislation or some more comprehensive strategy, that can deal effectively with all, or even most, of the problems that we have encountered. To begin to sort through them, let's quickly recap how these three themes manifest and interact for each of the groups of participants.

The Impact of Commodification, Consciousness, and Communication on Actors in Health Care

Practicing physicians are caught up in a world of commodities that is antithetical to the central tenets of their profession. They mostly earn a fee for each service provided. Even in systems where they are salaried, their relative incomes generally reflect the going rate for those services in the fee-for-service world (in which "invasive" cardiologists and orthopedic surgeons earn much more than psychiatrists, endocrinologists, and generalists). The medical profession has been able to advance practitioners' incomes over the past century far beyond the gains in other professions, and even more so relative to society as a whole. The relative incomes in different medical fields have enormous influence on specialty choices of medical students and residents. Specialty societies fight fiercely to protect members' income levels. Taking care of people with insurance that does not pay well is an affliction that many clinicians fervently avoid. In private practices, clinicians have bills to pay. In institutional practices, they have relative value units to generate. So, they run the till with well-insured patients, avoiding lengthy visits, and accumulating their relative value units (RVUs): lub, dub.

In addition to the distortion of their work by financial considerations, doctors have limitations, experiences, and characteristics that shape the way they practice. Far too many don't have great interpersonal skills. They commonly care for populations from whom they are socioculturally distant. Some are much more comfortable performing their procedures than building relationships with patients. Furthermore, these procedural physicians live in a society that values what they do (discrete technical acts leading to a diagnosis or a cure) more than what "diagnosis and management" (nonprocedural) physicians spend their time doing (ideally, the long haul of developing empathic, humane relationships with patients, guiding them through hard times, including chronic illnesses, and knowing them well enough to be able to recognize disease and dis-ease before it is disabling).

In the sphere of relationships and communication, some practitioners misrepresent to patients the need for procedures that command higher costs than diagnosis and management services. Many devote little if any time to counseling patients that they don't need procedures. Often as not, they leave it to their "extenders" (nonprocedural doctors, nurse practitioners, and others) to share bad news. Still others may offer hope to their patients even when the clinical situation and the evidence don't warrant it, because that is easier than the hard truth (and may be associated with better remuneration for their work). In relation to the scientists and educators, few physicians resist the biological reductionism of much of clinical ideology, notwithstanding what they may have seen in their practices. To government, many professional organizations forcefully defend their interests, opposing health care and reimbursement reform, while their members engage in the ethically problematic practice of conveying the profession's policy messages to legislators who are their patients.

Is there a policy intervention, or a series of measures, that could address how physicians act, what they want, and the capabilities that they possess? Changing the financial incentives in clinical practice might bring a modicum of success, but the problems are likely to persist unless attitudes, values, perceived needs, capabilities, and expectations change along with the incentives. These factors can and should be addressed, but many reflect broader issues in society rather than isolated phenomena in health care.

Stepping back from the practicing clinicians, can any of this be fixed in medical schools? Thinking first about the students, the vast majority come from relatively advantaged backgrounds economically, and the expectations of their families (and themselves) are not that they will be downwardly mobile. It is true that many students carry enormous debt burdens when they graduate, but physicians almost all emerge from their student debt and lead comfortable lives. That longer view apparently is not part of the calculus of students who point to debt as a major influence on their specialty choice. On some level, that is a rationalization. Why else would 15% of one medical school's class show up the first day aspiring to be orthopedic surgeons, one of the highest-paying specialties? This may reflect both familial expectations and societal norms. Furthermore, being selected on the basis of academic performance can lead students to believe that they deserve the rewards that they have "earned."

The social commitment and altruism that populate their carefully crafted applications are little more than the rote checking of boxes for some applicants. For others, the professed values are genuine, but they wane rapidly as medical training progresses. We might think of values-related actions over time as the pertinent variable. In that regard, among the most relevant actions are the choices that physicians make about whether to care for the disadvantaged. For many of those who choose not to do so, altruistic items on their applications are decorative artifacts.

For those whose idealism is genuine but wanes, educational experiences must bear some responsibility. In the course of their training, they are exposed to other students, residents, and professors who buy into commodification and extremely high incomes for people like them. They do receive some instruction about societal needs and ethics, and some professors care deeply about these issues. For the most part, however, this exposure seems insufficient to immunize many of them against an ethos of acquisition and status. Once those viruses have disseminated and been established in the organism, immunization can't do much.

Could medical schools select different students, with genuine social commitment, relative indifference to acquisition and greater capacity for empathy? They certainly could try harder, probably with somewhat greater success. It wouldn't hurt to abandon the standardized test and the propensity for selecting students with backgrounds in the sciences who have never explored the world enough to deviate far from a perfect grade point average. Still, if the rewards system remains unchanged, improved student selection might not do much. I laid out some prescriptions earlier in the book that are directed at different aspects of the problem. One can envision a kind of triple therapy for this problem: radical change in how students are selected; making values, ethics, and social responsibilities a dominant component of the medical school and postgraduate curriculum; and changing the financial incentives in medical practice. Combined, they might have an impact, but it is hard to see how such "treatments" would be consistently implemented—or be effective enough to move the needle substantially—other than in a broad transformation of medicine and beyond.

In chapter 5, I talked about a fateful encounter with my uncle as I began medical school. He observed that the choices that I made regarding maximizing my income versus serving the needs of society would invite judgments of my worth as a human being. I reflect on that frequently, wondering if I am doing enough. Every medical student needs and deserves such a jolt to their system. Sadly, cloning my late uncle is not an option. But medical schools ought to make this a central component of what they convey to their students.

Easier said than done. Addressing the needs of society, in the broadest sense, is not a high priority for medical educators, whose perspectives, like those of most clinicians and scientists, are narrowly focused. They gladly take on the training of a highly specialized workforce, meeting institutional rather than social needs. This makes their academic practices economically productive and fulfills the desire to produce a new generation in their own image, one that learns to maximize RVUs and incomes.

The emphasis on biological reductionism shields medical schools from the catastrophic consequences of medical care that fails society. Schools tout their technological advances and obscure their abrogation of meaningful social commitment. That must change. When I think about what my uncle might say now about my worth, I conclude that he would say the matter is not yet settled. That is certainly true of medical schools today.

Scientists and their societies also pursue their economic interests in the commodified terrain of health care. They have a large workforce, and they need to maintain the flow of funds to stay in business. They therefore "go where the money is," studying the problems of greatest interest to the funders. When they have opportunities to produce patents, the potential rewards are irresistible. Quite apart from their economic interests, scientists, much like medical proceduralists, love what they do, and they get to where they are by staying singularly focused upon it. Once you have won your Nobel Prize, you can talk about socially responsible science, but it is not something that most scientists spend time thinking about. To the contrary, their communications often accomplish the opposite: inflating the implications of their findings, lobbying for more resources in their particular niche, and perpetuating the notion that the answers to problems in health reside overwhelmingly in biology.

Is this just a matter of taking pride in what you do? Socially responsible science can be compatible with such sentiments. But it has to go beyond such narrowly focused passions as well. It is not clear what policies would bring about such change, but rebalancing the funding scales in favor of public health and the medical social sciences would be a good start. Rethinking the education of scientists—broadening their view with the social context of their work—would also be a plus. Changing the incentives in science would help even more.

Corporate clinical providers (including the ones affiliated with medical schools) reek of commodification, whether their businesses are nominally for-profit or for-surplus/"nonprofit." And they wreak much harm as a consequence. They covet, and invest in, revenue-generating product lines that make health care more expensive for everyone. They negotiate fiercely for maximum payments from insurers. Many avoid Medicaid insurance with its suboptimal reimbursement. They place their practices to attract high-revenue patients. They pursue payment vigorously, even from patients facing financial ruin. They continually crank up their assembly lines, trying to turn cost centers into profit centers.

Executives are rewarded for these behaviors. It is what they have been trained to do. Besides, they compete with other like-minded systems, so what choice do they have? Their communication is contaminated with lies: "population health," "service to our community," and so on. They advertise blithely to their target populations, touting the great things they do, while passing in silence over reprehensible business practices that they must hope will be interred, unnoticed, with their bones.[1] "Medicare for All" might lead them to sue fewer of their patients, and turn away fewer of the poor, but they would look for ways to run their businesses much as they currently do. Is there no hope of changing their behavior?

Changing the financial incentives would seem essential. In a single-payer system like Canada's, hospitals have global budgets to provide care and no incentive to maximize product sales, to compete with other hospitals for market share, or to preferentially admit the well-off. Leaders of American health systems, whether academic or not, are unlikely to embrace such change. But wouldn't it be nice?

Other corporations behave similarly. Absent meaningful regulation, pharmaceutical and biologics manufacturers seek to maximize profits, even for older products and those developed with government grants. They extend their patents whenever possible. "Price points" are often out of reach for some sectors of society, or for whole nations, even when access to products can mean the difference between life and death. They are occasionally shamed into providing a product to someone who cannot afford it. In the corner suites, there is little discussion of social responsibility. The executives' main constituents are the shareholders, not their customers. "The common good" is of no interest when they are convinced that they have "uncommon goods" to sell.

The communications emanating from these corporations are likely the most afflicted (and afflicting) in health care. They spend billions on influencing government to extend patents, on fighting legislation or regulations that would reduce prices, on bribing and recruiting physicians to peddle and use their products, on advertising to providers, and on inducing demand among patients for increasingly expensive and profitable treatments. Manufacturers of medical equipment operate in a somewhat different world, but inducing demand is also their core activity. Universal health insurance alone would not change all of that. But the combined effect of price transparency, less distorted advertising, and the ability to negotiate prices for these products on behalf of society would make at least some difference.

Insurers are deeply invested in the status quo. To extract profit, they have built wasteful bureaucracies. As successful as they are, they cannot help but strive for more, marketing to enroll clients least likely to generate high costs while denying coverage of needed services. Their advertising is deceptive. Even more so is their misrepresentation of possible alternatives, such as exist in countries with single-payer approaches. Not surprisingly, they lobby to avoid any competition from public options and to secure shares of public programs that do exist by "cherry-picking" from the most profitable slices of the populations served, as happened with Medicare Advantage. We cannot expect them to go off quietly into the sunset. Winning the battle for universal health insurance won't be easy precisely because there is so much at stake.

Employers and employees throughout the American economy have disparate perspectives on America's employer-based insurance market. Many employers are focused upon containing the mounting costs of their contributions to health insurance and have found provisions to cap employer contributions to be appealing. Some provide generous insurance as a benefit to attract and retain skilled workers. Those with largely unskilled workforces have tended not to provide generous benefits and have been less than enthusiastic about mandates to cover their employees.[2] The introduction of the Affordable Care Act reversed the decline in the proportion of employers offering health care coverage, but some restrict hours (particularly of low-wage workers) or reduce the number of employees they are obliged to cover, and many lower-income workers do not choose to enroll because of the cost. As a result, the majority of full-time workers earning less than 250% of the federal poverty level do not have employer-based insurance (see chap. 10).

Employees who receive health benefits in the workplace often see them as a two-edged sword: a hard-won asset they are reluctant to forego but also something that anchors them to their current jobs. A government program funded through a payroll tax makes sense, but it leaves employers and employees alike suspicious that they are paying more than their fair share. Fear of economic loss thwarts rational discussion of alternatives. Both groups express this loudly and clearly to policy makers. Overcoming this deterrent to change might well be accomplished more readily than some of the others that we are considering here.

Governments regard health care as a commodity no less than these other groups. They bear substantial costs and seek to rein them in. Many politicians are reluctant to invest in new programs to expand coverage.

Even the Affordable Care Act retained Medicaid, which is less generous than Medicare or most private insurance, and failed to cover all of the uninsured. Many state Medicaid programs are extremely stingy. Governments at every level are reluctant to confront difficult questions of redistributing health care funds in ways that mean less for some in order to provide more for others. Confronted by such epithets as "death panels," governments are even less prepared to entertain diversion of health care funding to other societal needs. Political leaders might find the courage to address health care issues more forthrightly if they regarded current arrangements as a serious risk to society.

The challenge of dealing with these constituencies underlines the need to change public discourse about health care in the United States. We should forego happy talk about "the greatest system in the world" and emphasize instead the idea of health care and health as rights, the need to address the common good, and the importance of limiting futile care. Our public discourse should be honest about how we measure up against the superior effectiveness, greater efficiency, and better outcomes of health care systems elsewhere—systems that are not all privately administered, not based on employment, and not shockingly unequal for different sectors of society. This will require determined engagement on the part of media, public intellectuals, and courageous politicians.

Patients, their families, and the general public behave in ways that reflect their experiences and values. To many of them, health care is a dear commodity. Health insurance is expensive, and millions cannot afford it. Copayments and deductibles keep people away from care even if they have insurance and may lead to serious financial problems, including bankruptcy. It is entirely understandable that such patients want to get their fair share of the goods: visits, procedures, medicines, days in the hospital, and so on. Many find themselves having to choose between their money or their life, so the latter becomes a commodity as well, and they bargain with their doctors to extend it, even when treatment is futile. Others simply want to consume luxury items, for example, by having a concierge doctor respond to their every whim. Some patients apply to their medical encounters the negotiating techniques that have served them well in all of their market transactions in maximizing their take of the goods: insisting on the more expensive imaging study or even threatening the doctor who won't do the test or prescribe the antibiotic or pain medicine that they want.

Patients' motives can be as varied as their lives. We have witnessed the lonely soul, looking for a heart in a heartless world; the spiritually unfulfilled person longing for more from life; the adversarial stance of those used to getting what they want; and the individual who does not trust a medical authority who is racially and socioculturally too remote, unconsciously biased, or overtly hostile. Many of these patient stories bespeak an atomized society in which self-interest blinds us to the common good and overweening material acquisitiveness produces a deficit in connection to our shared humanity. It also reflects a health care system that epitomizes these distorted values.

What patients hear gives voice to these distortions: the sensationalizing of the medical advance, the overselling of new research and new products, the pervasive failure to acknowledge and analyze disparities in health care and health, and the misleading advertisements that promote expensive drugs and procedures. They hear a policy discourse that is politicized and highly polarized, misrepresenting the implications of policy choices and leaving little room for calm reflection.

We can address some of the problems that patients face through effective policies pertaining to other actors, such as restrictions on pharmaceutical advertising and improved physician training to increase their ability to recognize and help patients grapple with emotional and interpersonal challenges. But many of the issues that affect patients reflect problems beyond the health care domain.

Philosophical Musings on the Task of Societal Change

Addressing the afflictions of health care in the United States is frustratingly hard because almost everyone feels they have something to lose if the system is changed. Consider these two famous episodes, one historical and one literary. In a momentous historical event, when Julius Caesar went to the Curia of Pompey's Theater on March 15, 44 BC, almost everyone there wanted him dead: Cassius and Brutus, perhaps more than others, but many more were complicit and participated in his murder. In the realm of literary fiction, when Inspector Poirot investigates the murder of Ratchett in Agatha Christie's *Murder on the Orient Express*,[3] he deduces that all of the other passengers had motives to kill the victim and participated in his murder. Analogously, many efforts at reform of American health care have failed because so many parties—doctors, patients, clinical corporations, insurers, manufacturers, medical educators, and biomedical scientists—want those efforts to die.

Transforming health care is an urgent necessity, but the breadth of needed change is substantial. Many of those involved regard such change as a threat. Economic relations, the inner life of the participants, and the contorted communication among them make it seemingly impossible to arrive at a common understanding about how to proceed. Everyone is afraid of what change will mean, so, like the senators at the Curia, they all would rather kill it.

Can policy effect change in the face of substantial reluctance? The United Kingdom was able to create a National Health Service, and Canada adopted a single-payer system of health insurance, notwithstanding substantial opposition in each instance. As momentous as these changes were, there was much that they could not change. The United States seems incapable of doing even that much.

How is progress possible when consensus is absent? This is an important question. How can we solve any social problems without tackling problems of values, perspectives, and individual experience—what I have referred to here as "consciousness"?

Philosophers including Plato, Immanuel Kant, G. W. F. Hegel, and Karl Marx have long pondered the relationship between consciousness and the world—and how, if at all, we can bring the former to bear upon the latter. Their writings shed some light on the challenges to realizing concrete change.[4]

Writing separately in the 1920s, Hungarian Georg Lukács and German Karl Korsch both argued that social transformation requires solving problems *simultaneously* at two levels: the world outside of the individual (political economy) and the world within, which Lukács called class consciousness, meaning the perspective of a group within society, and Korsch referred to as both philosophy and consciousness.[5] Italian Antonio Gramsci, who also was concerned with the role of consciousness in affecting the prospects for radical social change, identified a need to confront society's "ideological and cultural hegemony" by addressing education, media, law, and mass culture, including such elements as myths, values, beliefs, and cultural traditions.[6]

Theorists associated with the Institute for Social Research (later known as the Frankfurt School), led by Max Horkheimer and Theodor Adorno, built their critical theory—a neo-Marxist and anti-Leninist critique of advanced capitalism—around the centrality of consciousness to understanding societal problems and the prospects for their resolution. They judged that many aspects of experience in such domains as culture, psychology, social organization, and the ways in which we reason about the world can impair our ability to transform society in positive ways, and even can lead to catastrophes, such as the rise of totalitarian movements and states.[7] For example, Herbert Marcuse asked why advanced capitalism, which is so constraining and limiting to human development and freedom, has not been transcended. He judged that the individuals have been dominated ideologically in advanced, industrial societies, which do a better job than their predecessors of meeting material needs. Through technology and transformation of culture, they render people "one-dimensional" and incapable of action to change things.[8]

According to this line of thinking, the best hope for a path to meaningful change requires successfully addressing both consciousness (the inner life) and existence (the external world). Short of that, capitalist economies deliver just enough of the goods to quell upheaval. Plied with the dominant (or "hegemonic") culture and ideology, blasted with afflicted communication (as Habermas points out) about what is wrong and what is possible to fix it, and fraught with trepidation about major transformation, people don't comprehend in what kind of society they would feel more fulfilled and are thus incapable of acting to achieve change.[9]

Transforming Health Care

Can all of this help us understand, and even solve, the problems facing health care today? Long term, I believe so. But that is not to say that we should refrain from pursuing more immediate reforms.

Health care is a prism through which we can view much of society because health care's afflictions are manifestations of societal problems. We can see inequality, obscene profits, economic hardship, and commodified relationships throughout the realm of health care. There also are people with vast unmet needs. Others are incapable of meaningful, empathic human relations. Some lack not only any sense of the common good, but also a conscience for the direct and indirect consequence of their treatment of others, or for other actions. The media, the profiteers, and the general culture glorify the dominant vision of health care profits over people, while inducing demand for what is not vital and obliterating that which is far more important.

Is meaningful change possible? Only if we take into account the economic forces that oppose it, the problems of consciousness that obscure it, and the vast apparatus of toxic relationships and afflicted communication that reinforce the status quo and incapacitate those who might be inclined to do something about it. Is this too pessimistic a view?

Health care can be improved in ways that can have important effects on people's lives. We must do all we can to address each of the health care system's problems, and we should pursue such efforts vigorously and unambivalently. But we should not lose sight of the fact that curing the overall condition of health care—transforming the economic relations and their consequences, the attitudes and values, the capacities and proclivities, the communication and the behaviors, as well as the perceived needs of recipients and providers—will take much more. We can address these problems with varying degrees of effectiveness, and in health care we have an obligation to do that, but we cannot eradicate them in one sector of society when society as a whole is on a different trajectory.

The criticism of health care, in this sense, is the criticism of the conditions that give rise to these sorts of arrangements, experiences, needs, and consequences. To address them satisfactorily, society will have to change. As the philosophers I cited suggest, bringing about that change will be a struggle: in our economic and political systems, in our culture and values, in the broadest sense, and in the processes that mediate and perpetuate these infuriatingly destructive arrangements.

The goals and ideals of medicine are compelling, but too often they are neglected. Yet the values inherent in them can be weapons in the struggle to make medicine more humane. They can serve as a moral compass to help guide us when our efforts to transform health care and society as a whole fall short. If we continue to insist, with Donne, that every avoidable death diminishes each of us, then we will keep trying. Addressing the afflictions of health care as part of a struggle to create a better society is a daunting task. Success is neither easy nor assured. But we must continue to pursue it. In the words of first- and second-century rabbi and scholar Tarfon, "It is not your duty to finish the work, but neither are you at liberty to neglect it."

Notes

1. Adapted from William Shakespeare, *Julius Caesar*, act 3, scene 2.

2. Paul Starr, *Remedy and Reaction: The Peculiar American Struggle over Health Care Reform* (New Haven, CT: Yale University Press 2013), 114–17, 217–20.

3. Agatha Christie, *Murder on the Orient Express* (New York: Dodd Mead, 1934).

4. For example, Plato explored concepts like justice, which he saw as fixed and external to humans, using dialogues between Socrates and others, who present a proposition that Socrates contradicts. An extended "dialectical" exchange ensues, leading to a resolution that differs from the original proposition. Plato, *The Republic* (London: Global Classics, 2017). (The dialogues that appear between the chapters of this book borrow shamelessly from the dynamic in Plato's *Republic*). Immanuel Kant contended that we know the world through our ability to reason, but he did not account for the possibility of knowing what is actually out in the world independently of how we think about it (the "thing-in-itself"). Immanuel Kant, *Critique of*

Pure Reason, ed. and trans. Paul Guyer and Allen W. Wood (Cambridge: Cambridge University Press, 1998). G. W. F. Hegel argued that the rationality in our heads also exists in the world, so we can see that concepts like justice are part of an imperfect world and hence amenable to change or resolution through interaction between the mind and the thing-in-itself. Georg Wilhelm Friedrich Hegel, *Elements of the Philosophy of Right*, ed. Allen W. Wood, trans. H. B. Nisbet (Cambridge: Cambridge University Press, 1991).

Karl Marx complained that "philosophers have hitherto only interpreted the world in various ways. The point is to *change* it." Karl Marx, "Theses on Feuerbach," in Karl Marx and Frederick Engels, *The German Ideology*, ed. C. J. Arthur (New York: International Publishers, 1970), 123. But Marx's writings send mixed messages about how to reorder society while navigating the relationship between human perception and the external world. He asserts that "It is not the consciousness of men that determines their existence, but their social existence that determines their consciousness." Karl Marx, "Preface," in *A Contribution to the Critique of Political Economy*, ed. Maurice Dobb (New York: International Publishers, 1970), 22. At other times he articulates a far more nuanced relationship between the two and dwells at length on the inner life of society's members. Karl Marx, *The Economic and Philosophical Manuscripts of 1844*, ed. Dirk J. Struik (New York: International Publishers, 1973); *Grundrisse: Foundations of the Critique of Political Economy*, trans. Martin Nicolaus (Harmondsworth, UK: Penguin, 1973); David McLellan, *Marx before Marxism* (London: MacMillan, 1980), 207–20.

5. Lukács judged that Marx broke with Hegel because Hegel failed "to overcome the duality of thought and being, of theory and practice, of subject and object." Georg Lukács, *History and Class Consciousness: Studies in Marxist Dialectics*, trans. Rodney Livingstone (Cambridge: Massachusetts Institute of Technology Press, 1972), 16. For Lukács, "society becomes the reality for man" (Lukács, *History*, 19), and it is the totality of society that is at play. Social existence *and* consciousness both are crucial, and the relationship between them is not static (Lukács, *History*, 1). Korsch made a similar argument the same year, insisting that "Philosophy cannot be abolished without being realized. . . . This struggle will only end when the whole of existing society and its economic basis have been totally overthrown in practice, and the consciousness has been totally surpassed and abolished in theory." Karl Korsch, *Marxism and Philosophy*, trans. Fred Halliday (London: New Left Books, 1970), 93. For attempting to recapture the Hegelian elements in Marx, Korsch was expelled from the Communist movement for apostasy, while Lukács was required to suppress publication of his book for many years. Nonetheless, their ideas were picked up by other theorists.

6. Writing in the context of a failed revolution, Gramsci saw such transformation as a difficult, organic process involving the interplay of all of these—the totality—with economics and politics. Carl Boggs, *Gramsci's Marxism* (London: Pluto Press, 1976), 11–20; Walter L. Adamson, *Hegemony and Revolution: A Study of Antonio Gramsci's Political and Cultural Theory* (Berkeley: University of California Press, 1980), 169–79; Antonio Gramsci, *Selections from the Prison Notebooks*, ed. and trans. Quintin

Hoare and Geoffrey Nowell Smith (New York: International Publishers, 1971), 55–60, 104–6, 206–8, 210, 275–76.

7. See, e.g., Max Horkheimer, *Eclipse of Reason* (New York: Seabury Press, 1974), which explores in this way the rise of fascism. Horkheimer and Adorno contended that the Enlightenment, which opened the possibility for freedom of thought, also created the tools for its repression. Max Horkheimer and Theodor W. Adorno, *Dialectic of Enlightenment*, trans. Edmund Jephcott (Stanford, CA: Stanford University Press, 2002). Another major interest was in the psychological dimensions that made people susceptible to authoritarian ideologies and fearful of transformative change. Erich Fromm, *Escape from Freedom* (New York: Farrar & Rinehart, 1941).

8. Herbert Marcuse, *One-Dimensional Man* (Boston: Beacon Press, 1966), x, 7, 252.

9. Toward this end, Horkheimer and Adorno suggest an approach that explores fully the ways in which the tensions in the relationship of consciousness to existence manifests throughout the culture, illuminating phenomena (including those in the realm of consciousness) that worsen societal problems, obstruct their resolution, or both. They contend that doing so is more valuable than offering prescriptive solutions and is essential to the effort to identify the way forward. Max Horkheimer, *Critical Theory: Selected Essays* (New York: Seabury Press, 1968); Theodor W. Adorno, *Negative Dialectics* (New York: Seabury Press, 1973). Russell Jacoby explained the rationale thus: "It is better to see the situation for what it is than to pretend it is something else. The insistence that all criticism should end with ten bullet points of recommendations is part of the problem." *On Diversity: The Eclipse of the Individual in a Global Era* (New York: Seven Stories Press, 2020), 180.

Lessons Learned

Professor: This is a nice piece of work.

Student: It feels in some ways like a waste of time.

Professor: Why do you say that?

Student: Beyond telling a tale of sound and fury, we didn't accomplish anything.

Professor: It seems to me that we laid out the problem and much of its complexity.

Student: But we didn't resolve the problem. We didn't even get close to resolving it.

Professor: Well, lots of people have been trying for some time. I think we brought some useful clarity to the situation.

Student: So what? We just interpreted the world one more way. The point is to change it!

Professor: I think that we all can agree with that. Figuring out how to effect change is the challenge.

Student: Aren't we just throwing in the towel?

Professor: If we proceed down the wrong road, what will we accomplish?

Student: There is so much wrong in health care. Why not fix a little bit of it?

Professor: We absolutely can and should. That's not inconsistent with the journey we've been on. We've laid out quite a few steps that can be taken without broader change. Is that at all reassuring?

Student: I guess it's somewhat reassuring. But now I'm confused about what that journey has been.

Professor: What would you say it has been? Don't say it's been an effort to fix health care. We didn't. What else?

Student: To understand complexity?

Professor: In part, what else?

Student: To see where things get off track?

Professor: Yes. What else?

Student: How much more can there be?

Professor: Think about this like a clinical problem.

Student: We ruled out certain diagnoses and treatments.

Professor: Yes, we did, and . . .

Student: Achieved a bit of clarity.

Professor: By?

Student: Excluding some mistaken notions of what's needed.

Professor: Exactly. We've informed the situation by discounting certain illusions of what needs to transpire. We also have identified both the need for "combination therapy" and at least some of the "sites" at which each of the "treatments" need to work.

Student: Well, that's something, I suppose. I understand that solving all the problems in medicine is going to require broader changes in society. But shouldn't we at least assemble a list of some of the important steps we've identified that we need to at least try to implement in American health care, even while we wait for the revolution?

Professor: That's a good idea. That would make a nice appendix for the book.

Student: I'll get to work on that. Do you have any more projects in mind that I could be involved in?

Professor: There's definitely more work that we can do. For one thing, we might explore in greater depth various attempts to address the problems we have highlighted. A thorough look at how the factors afflicting health care played out in the face of the COVID-19 pandemic would also be useful. Finally, I have been considering delving more deeply into philosophical arguments about what might be required to achieve broad transformation of consciousness and policy. This may well lead to consideration of critiques of classical liberalism and of neoliberal notions of deregulation and of limiting the role of government in the economy. Are you in?

Student: Yes, I'm interested. Those are important questions. Let's hope we get the COVID-19 study done in time to influence thinking before the next pandemic shows up.

Professor: I certainly agree with you about that. Since it appears we're going to be doing more work together, let's go discuss next steps over a nice lunch at the Bendidea.[1]

Student: But please, professor, not too much more Hegel! He's really hard to understand.

Professor: Don't worry. I'll do what I can to limit your pain.

The method of negation, the denunciation of everything that mutilates mankind and impedes its free development, rests on confidence in man.
—Max Horkheimer, *Eclipse of Reason*

Note

1. Bendidea was a Thracian festival held in honor of Bendis, the goddess of healing. The Athenians Hellenized Bendis and celebrated this festival annually on the 20th day of the month of Thargelion. This festival was occurring at the time of the exchange between Socrates and Thrasymachus in Book I of Plato's *The Republic*.

It takes a rather large village. I owe a great debt to those who stimulated my interest in and taught me to think critically about sociology, history, and social theory, including Donald Bates, Joseph Lella, and Immanuel Wallerstein at McGill; and Edward Alpers, Russell Jacoby, Peter Loewenberg, and Peter Reill at UCLA. My uncle Sam Abramovitch introduced me to writings of the Frankfurt School and challenged me to apply my medical training to bettering society. I learned to think boldly about what is possible in health care with much help from mentors, teachers and colleagues such as Ted Tulchinsky, who worked to improve health care in Saskatchewan, Manitoba, and Israel; John Beck, Robert Fletcher, Suzanne Fletcher, and Robert Oseasohn at McGill, who encouraged me to pursue training in health services research; and physician health services researchers Robert Brook, Sheldon Greenfield, and Charles Lewis, and sociologists Ronald Andersen, Howard Freeman, and Lawrence Linn, with all of whom I worked at UCLA. Many wonderful clinicians taught me how to think about medical problems, how to be there for patients, and what is important in the practice of medicine. Some of my best teachers have been my patients and my students. I cherish the relationships that I have had with them.

I also very much appreciate the encouragement that I received to push forward with this book project from Ivan Berend, Keith Norris, Monika Safford, and especially from my wife, Barbara Vickrey, and my sons Matthew and Daniel. Colleagues at UCLA's and Cornell's medical schools provided me with helpful comments on talks that I gave early on as I was developing the themes in the book. My cousin, author/editor Ilana Abramovitch, offered thoughtful insights about what I was doing right and wrong in an early draft and how to order and structure the book. Her brother, Henry Abramovitch, who has taught behavioral medicine and studied medical education throughout his career at Tel Aviv University, offered detailed criticisms and suggestions, effectively challenging many of my assumptions and assertions about what is right and wrong and how it can be fixed in medical education and health care. William Hackman, who edited a later version, did not pull his punches in letting me know what needed to be done substantively and stylistically to make the book accessible, consistent, and intellectually defensible.

Dana Baran, Ivan Berend, Philip Boche, Robert Charrow, Russell Jacoby, Robert Kaplan, Katalin Radics, David Scales, Harry Schachter, Matthew Shapiro, Barbara Vickrey, Elaine Wethington, and Sidney Wolfe all provided valuable feedback on all or parts of the manuscript. Robin Coleman, my acquisitions editor at Johns Hopkins University Press, recognized its promise and guided me expertly through revisions with many wise recommendations. Two anonymous reviewers at the press made excellent suggestions for improving the manuscript. My copy editor, Ashleigh McKown, did a great job of getting it in final form. All these individuals made recommendations that allowed me to improve the book, but none of them are responsible for any deficiencies, inaccuracies, misconceptions, or erroneous conclusions that remain herein.

Finally, my dear parents, Myer and Tillie Shapiro, bore witness to what is wrong with health care and what needs to be done to fix it. I hope that this book fairly represents what they came to understand.

Quixotic Proposals for Treating
American Health Care's Afflictions

Below I offer potential components of combination therapy, all of which are essential, to address the afflictions of commodification, consciousness, and communication in health care, while anticipating the need for analogous changes in society.

Medical Education

- Develop mechanisms to identify medical school applicants driven by altruism, rather than prestige and potential income.
- Select students based on empathic capacity, psychological openness, moral and ethical outlook, and evidence of sustained commitment to societal well-being.
- Allow underserved communities to nominate medical school matriculants.
- Eliminate premedical science requirements and replace them with courses in humanities, ethics, and social sciences.
- Dramatically reduce reliance on grades and abandon test scores for evaluating medical school applicants.
- Clinical training should consistently encourage psychological openness. It should also give more weight to social context of illness and less to biological reductionism.
- Ethics, morality, social responsibility, and communication skills should comprise half of the first two years of medical school curriculum and be integrated into clinical training.
- Undergraduate and postgraduate training programs should develop interventions to counteract negative socialization and burgeoning materialism among trainees at the expense of responsibilities to individual patients and to society.
- Residency recommendations should reflect these educational priorities.

Medical Practitioners

- Pay doctors for their time, not for piecework.
- Hourly pay across specialties should not differ, except for modest adjustments to account for the impact of differences in length of training

on expected lifetime earnings and augmentation of rates for clinicians who work in communities with health personnel shortages.
- Require procedural specialists and hospital administrators to attend regular sessions in which they discuss strategies and set targets to reduce use of costly interventions that do not contribute meaningfully to outcomes.
- Health systems, medical schools, and the government should identify mechanisms to incentivize clinicians to seek insight-oriented or cognitive behavioral therapy to help them better understand and relate to patients, their needs, and their values.
- Promote Balint-type groups for clinicians to discuss challenges in doctor-patient relationships and stresses in practice.
- Require all clinicians to participate in periodic small group sessions to improve skills in communication and negotiation with patients.
- Require all clinicians to participate in periodic sessions on ethics, morals, and social responsibilities tied to discussions of caregiving experiences.
- Include simulated interviews with behaviorally challenging patients in recertification requirements.

Clinical Corporations and Their Executives

- Limit the total compensation of voluntary (nonprofit) health system CEOs and other executives to the level of pay for public hospital executives in each state.[1]
- Don't pay executives for their winnings: no bonus payments for surplus revenue that reflects antisocial business practices.
- Require training of health system executives in social responsibility and ethics.
- Require full participation in Medicaid of all their clinicians for health systems to maintain nonprofit status.
- Prohibit lucrative funding by industry to health systems that occurs in exchange for clinical specimens or use of their products.

Scientists

- Training in social responsibility in science should be a core and substantial feature of scientific education.
- Prioritize National Institutes of Health (NIH) and other governmental research on bringing effective care to populations, and deemphasize biological reductionism by requiring each institute to commit a specified percentage of its budget to research on such care.
- A multidisciplinary group with no major financial or intellectual conflicts of interest should be convened by the National Academy of

Medicine to propose a revised set of budget priorities for the NIH and other federal health-related research agencies that emphasizes population health and defines the level of allocation to research on population health for each institute and agency.
- Half of the members of the council of each NIH institute should be nominated by members of diverse communities affected by conditions in their areas of clinical focus.
- Revenue from inventions funded by federal grants should accrue largely to the government; participation of scientists and research institutions in such revenue should be limited.

Manufacturers

- Allow the government to negotiate prices of all pharmaceuticals and other products.
- Do not allow patent extensions for variations on existing products ("evergreening").
- Reduce pharmaceutical industry influence on the FDA's drug approval process by ending industry funding of those FDA activities; instead, fund drug approval regulatory activity entirely with government funds.
- The federal government should receive most of the revenue from products emanating from federal grants and use it to fund additional research, including studies of the relative cost-effectiveness of these products, and of ways to ensure that they benefit all populations.

Government and Financing

- Provide the same insurance coverage to everyone (with the government as the single payer); separate is never equal.
- End or severely curtail copayments and deductibles.
- A group of experts with a broad range of expertise about health care costs, access, outcomes, administration, clinical medicine, patient behavior, and competing social needs, but who personally do not have major conflicts of interests in the areas of focus, should make annual recommendations to the government about the magnitude of the overall budget for care and about how to allocate it.
- Decisions about the magnitude of health care expenditures and their allocation should be based on the principle that any approved procedure or treatment be available to all and that sufficient resources be arrayed to eliminate any delays in care that harm population health.
- The government should fund studies that assess the marginal benefit and cost of all new treatments and procedures relative to existing ones prior to authorizing their coverage.

- The government should fund on an ongoing basis studies of access and barriers to care and of interventions to address them at a sufficient level to mitigate such problems across all populations and conditions in a timely manner.

Communication

- End direct-to-consumer advertising by pharmaceutical companies that promotes their products; limit it to general information about diseases and their treatment and to public health promotion.
- Regulate advertising by health systems more strictly; limit it to public health promotion.
- Doctors and health systems should stop selling procedures to people who don't need them. They should also be required to provide objective data to patients on how much more income they earn by doing any proposed procedures and on what evidence says about alternatives.
- Medical societies that promote their members' financial interests in any way, including through guidelines and the Relative Value Unit Update Committee, should lose tax-exempt status and be required to register as lobbyists.
- End overselling of implications of biomedical science and lobbying for the current priorities of the NIH by scientists and scientific organizations.
- Disease advocacy organizations should be required to report any funding from pharmaceutical and biologic companies in all of their advertising and solicitations.
- Health care provider organizations need to exhibit greater transparency by providing easily comprehensible information about all medical prices and alternative approaches to treatment.
- Change laws to limit funding for opposition to ballot initiatives that seek to reform health care.
- Media should establish communication standards for reporting on new research and its implications.
- Medical journals should list in their print editions all financial relationships of the authors of editorials, reviews, and commentaries to entities with interests potentially relevant to the topic discussed.

Patients and the Public

- Ensure that patients have access to all the mental health care, social services, financial support, and other government programs (such as housing, nutrition, and transportation) that they require. Failure to meet these needs may result in demands on primary care providers that they cannot easily address, as well as in requests for more tests and treatment.

- Give patients and communities meaningful roles at all levels of research organizations and health care systems, so that their voices are heard and they can affect decision-making in those organizations about their priorities and programs.
- Medical schools and residency programs should train clinicians who can relate to the diverse communities in need of caring.
- Clinicians, government agencies, and community organizations should educate patients and the public about the common good and fair distribution of limited medical resources.
- All actors in health care should offer clearer communication about the limits of what medicine can accomplish.
- Limit patient and family autonomy when it places the health of others at risk.

Note

1. In 2019 the president of New York City's public system, New York City Health and Hospitals, earned about $670,000. The CEOs of some of the voluntary hospital systems received compensation of five to ten times that amount, or even more. "Mitchell Katz Overview," GovSalaries, accessed May 5, 2022, https://govsalaries .com/katz-mitchell-92389503; "Health Pulse 2019 Compensation Database," Crain's New York Business, January 8, 2020, https://www.crainsnewyork.com/health-pulse -compensation-database-2019.

abortion, 335, 339
Accountable Care Organizations, 396
Accreditation Council for Graduate
    Medical Education (ACGME), 195
adalimumab (Humira), 297–98
administrators, 194, 220–21, 225, 411–12,
    451, 468
Adorno, Theodor, 457
aducanumab, 307
advance directives, 13, 33, 34
Advanced Research Projects Agency for
    Health (ARPA-H), 283n41
advertising and marketing: direct-to-
    consumer, 296, 304, 392, 430–31, 438,
    455, 470; of drugs, 290, 294–96, 392,
    438, 452, 455, 470; by hospitals, 190,
    218, 222–23, 232–33, 304, 388, 392, 429,
    439, 451, 470; by insurers, 452; of
    medical technology, 304; and opposi-
    tion to national strategies, 361–62,
    432; regulating, 295, 296, 438–39, 470
Affordable Care Act (ACA): challenges
    to, 362; and colon cancer screening,
    58; and employers, 362, 366, 453;
    fines, 362; and insurers, 323, 432; and
    labor, 365, 366; marketplaces, 362;
    and Medicaid, 327, 333, 362, 454;
    medical device tax, 431; as national
    strategy, 362–63; public option, 362,
    363, 453; and risk to providers, 396
AFL-CIO, 364, 365
Agency for Health Care Policy and
    Research (AHCPR), 258
Agency for Healthcare Research and
    Quality (AHRQ), 65–66, 258–59, 336
AIDS/HIV, 114–15, 253, 322, 327
allergists, 54, 69, 234

All of Us Research Project, 264
ambiguity: about prognosis, 163;
    tolerance of, 107–8, 163, 404, 425
American Board of Internal Medicine,
    54, 67, 173
American Board of Medical Specialties,
    54, 174
American College of Physicians, 65, 173,
    198, 296
American College of Surgeons, 173
American Medical Association (AMA),
    74–75, 133, 195, 304, 359–60, 423–24
America's Health Insurance Plans
    (AHIP), 337
anesthesiology, 62–65, 70, 173, 292,
    304, 325
antibiotics, 32–33, 293
anti-dumping laws, 328
apprenticeships, 131, 132
architecture, hospital, 226–27
Arrow, Kenneth, 395
Asian Americans, 5n3
Association of American Medical
    Colleges, 175, 254
authoritarianism, 38, 159, 461n7
autonomy: patient, 13–14, 33–38, 43, 401,
    416, 455, 470; physician, 83, 153

Balint groups, 104–5, 410, 417, 468
bankruptcy, 225, 321, 454
Banting, Frederick, 293
Bayh, Birch, 266, 267
Bayh-Dole Act, 266–69
Beeson, Paul, 102
behavioral medicine courses, 157, 158
behavioral science and NIH, 260–61
Bellah, Robert, 400–402, 403, 412

beneficence, ethic of, 395
Bethune, Norman, 150
Bevan, Aneurin, 356
Beveridge, William, 355
bias: and grants, 251; and journals, 297; and medical school, 139, 141
Biden, Joe, 283n41, 301
Bill and Melinda Gates Foundation, 277
biological reductionism, 101–2, 160–62, 407, 429, 433, 448, 450, 467, 468
Biologics Control Act, 248
Bismarck, Otto von, 352
Blacks: as faculty, 143; health metrics, 3, 5n3, 5n5; and inequities in care, 2, 226–28; and transplants, 328; and trust, 38–39
bladder cancer, 284n47
breast cancer, 66, 107, 264, 439
Brown, Arleen, 437
burnout, 82, 103, 306, 417

Callahan, Daniel, 395
Camus, Albert, 163
Canada: administrative costs in, 323–24; copayments research in, 319; cost barriers in, 375; drug costs in, 294; general practitioners in, 175; health metrics in, 5nn5–6; hospital budgets in, 367, 452; inequities in care, 371, 375; spending on health care, 2; universal coverage in, 356–58, 367–69, 456; wait times in, 370–71, 372, 375
cancer: and advertising, 296; and conflicts of interest, 68, 71, 106, 298, 425–26, 439; launch prices, 298; and precision medicine, 263–64; research priorities, 256, 261; in stories, 13, 41–42, 104, 113–14, 117, 120. See also oncology
capital and surplus, 386–87
capital investments by hospitals, 216–17, 226–27
cardiology, 60, 70, 77, 82, 154, 173, 176, 383
Carnegie Foundation for the Advancement of Teaching, 133, 134, 135
Centers for Disease Control, 300
Chadwick, Edwin, 350

Children's Health Insurance Program (CHIP), 219
Choosing Wisely Campaign, 67–69
circumcision, 335–36
clinical networks. See hospitals, corporatization of
clinical practice and medical schools, 172, 182–84, 188–99. See also hospitals, academic
Clinton, Bill, 361–62, 365, 432
COBRA (Consolidated Omnibus Reconciliation Act), 338
Cochrane, Archie, 61, 426
Cochrane Organization and Library, 426, 435
cognitive specialties: and compensation, 15, 53, 55–57, 69–71, 75–78, 154–55, 176, 408, 447; and gender, 149–50
Cohn, Ferdinand, 291
coinsurance, defined, 324
Collins, Francis, 253, 263
colonoscopies, 57–59, 62–63, 64
Colwell, Nathan, 133
Committee for National Health Insurance, 364–65
Committee on the Costs of Medical Care, 359–60
commodification: and consolidation of markets, 215–23, 225, 242, 451; definition of commodities, 383–84; in dialogues, 383, 399, 444–45; and efficiency reforms, 395–96; and end-of-life care, 392–93; and ethics, 383–85, 411–12; and financial incentives, 42, 55–57, 59–61, 68–69, 80–81, 199, 383–85, 439, 448, 470; and free markets, 386, 393–97; of health and health care, overview, 16; and idealism, 82–85; and inequities in care, 218–23, 387, 389–90, 393–97, 429; and insurance, 317–26, 339, 383, 390–91, 452–54; and investors, 233–35, 391; of medical acts, 77–78; and medical schools, 135, 390, 391, 447–49; and patient attitudes, 44, 322, 454–55; and patient-doctor relationship, 99, 394–95, 447–48; of patients, 190–91, 392–93, 394–95; of physicians, 190–91, 389–90, 394–95, 429–30;

and procedures, 77–78, 388–89, 408; of research, 390–91, 450–51; summary of challenges, 447–55; vs. value, 387, 389. *See also* hospitals, corporatization of; manufacturers; patents and royalties
common good, 402, 452, 454, 471
commons, tragedy of the, 139
communalism, 246–47, 273
communication: challenges in patient-doctor relationship, 100–108, 425, 427–28, 434–35, 447–48, 468; and end-of-life care, 105–7, 409, 442n27, 448; in ethos of science, 246–47, 273; evaluating trainees, 195–97; faculty skills in, 196; and medical school admissions, 103; and medical school instruction, 105–7, 152, 158, 407, 434, 467; proposals for, 108, 410, 437–39, 467–68, 470; types of, 421–22
communication, distortions in: by government, 433–34, 453–54; by health care systems, 429–30; by insurers, 431–32, 452–53; by manufacturers, 430–31, 452; by media, 435–36; by medical schools, 433; overview of, 16, 421–22; and patient-doctor relationship, 427–28; by patients, 454–55; by physician organizations, 422–28; proposals for, 437–39; and research, 427, 428–29, 451
community: vs. individualism, 401–2, 416, 455; involvement in research, 469; lack of, 401, 415; service and hospitals, 230, 451
compassion fatigue, 103
compensation and income: and academic hospitals, 192–94; administrators, 194, 225, 451, 468; basing on time spent, 411, 439, 467; and clinical work by faculty, 192–94; and commodification, 221, 384–85, 447; comparison by specialty, 70; comparison by the hour, 77–78; comparison with other countries, 53, 354; and concierge medicine, 79; and diversity efforts, 87–88; financial incentives for procedures and products, 42, 55–57, 59–61, 68–69, 80–81, 199, 383–85, 439, 448,

470; grant restrictions on, 192, 252; history of, 51–53; increases in, 52–53, 70, 447; and job satisfaction, 169n54; and lifetime earnings, 154, 468; from manufacturers, 304; and Medicaid, 2, 186; and Medicare, 55–57, 75, 327; vs. other professions, 52–53, 70, 447; and patient-doctor relationship, 114, 119–20, 408–10; as percentage of health care costs, 56, 57; of primary care physicians, 154–55, 221, 389; procedural vs. cognitive care, 15, 53, 55–57, 69–71, 75–78, 154–55, 176, 408, 447; proposals for, 439, 467–68; and relative value scale, 73–75, 447; and researchers, 192, 200–202, 252–53, 391; specialists vs. generalists, 15, 52–57, 69–71, 74–77, 154–55, 176, 385, 387–88, 389–90, 447; and students' career choices, 14–15, 75–76, 142, 152–55, 447, 448–49; and value, 385
comprehensive care physicians, 182
concierge medicine, 41, 79, 454
conflicts of interest: in cancer treatment, 68, 71, 106, 298, 425–26, 439; in dialogues, 289; disclosure of, 270, 272–73, 427; and drugs, 66–67, 71, 72, 269, 271, 298, 302; and faculty, 192, 269–70; and FDA, 271, 301, 469; and guidelines, 66–69; and journals, 270, 274, 427, 428, 470; and manufacturers, 66–67, 232, 269–73, 303, 304, 425–27; and medical devices, 66, 304; and medical schools, 229, 232, 269–70; and patents, 271–72, 428; and patients' decision-making ability, 72–73; and researchers, 269–73, 427, 428; and specialists, 178, 392; and technology, 303
Congress of Neurological Surgeons, 67
Connaught Laboratories, 293
consciousness: and health and health care, 16, 22, 219, 402–18, 466, 467; and societal change, 456–58
continuity of care, 84–85, 179–80, 185–87, 329
copayments, 317–22, 324, 332, 339, 383, 454, 469

corporations: communication distortions by, 429–30; corporate responsibility, 412; and definition of health care, 9; opposition to national strategies, 358–59, 364, 366; proposals for, 412–13, 468–69; specialty service providers, 233. *See also* hospitals, corporatization of; manufacturers

costs: add-on costs of procedures, 56–59, 62–65, 234, 304; administrative costs of insurance, 323–24, 363, 452; and capital investments, 216–17; and components of prices, 386; and consolidation of health care markets, 218, 451; cost-conscious care, 189; in dialogues, 1–2; disclosure of, 430, 436; distribution of, 57; of electronic medical records, 306; and facility fees, 57, 64, 304; and health outcomes, 1–2, 8, 387; and in-/out-of-network care, 324–25, 432; and investors, 234, 235; of medicalization, 32; and medical technology, 55–56, 303, 304–5; of mental health care, 25, 78–79; and national strategy efforts, 359–60; in other countries, 367–68; of precision medicine, 265–66; of procedures, 55–59, 62–65, 77, 234, 322, 388–89, 429, 470; proposals for, 468; and relative value scale, 73–75; research infrastructure costs, 192, 251–52; research on cost-effectiveness, 260, 336; rise in, 2, 8, 57; of tests, 42, 57–59; and upcoding, 59, 73; vs. value, 231–32, 387. *See also* copayments; prices

Council on Medical Education, 133

covered lives term, 218–19. *See also* inequities in care

COVID-19: pandemic, 4n1, 225, 232, 242, 331, 335, 338, 374–75, 463; vaccine, 335, 374

critical care, 160, 176

culture: cultural competency and students, 136, 138–40, 405, 406; idioms of distress, 25–26; and patient-doctor relationship, 25–26, 38–39, 44, 86–87, 103, 107, 159, 403, 415, 447–48, 455, 471; and societal change, 457–58

Dally, J. F. Hallis, 29

death and dying: conversation about, 118, 163; education on, 148–49, 164. *See also* end-of-life care

death panels, 260, 454

debt: hospital, 216–17; medical, 225, 321–22, 451, 454; student, 143, 155, 448–49

deductibles, 324, 339, 454, 469

dementia, 115–16, 307

dental care, 57, 64–65

dermatology, 68–69, 71, 82, 169n55, 234

Deyo, Richard A., 425

diabetes, 271, 292–93

disinterestedness, 247, 273–74

doctoring courses, 157, 158, 198

Dole, Bob, 266

Douglas, Tommy, 356–57, 358

drugs and drug makers: advertising of, 290, 294–96, 392, 438, 452, 455, 470; and conflicts of interest, 66–67, 71, 72, 269, 271, 298, 302; drug prices, 293–94, 297–98, 299, 431; history of, 292–93; and innovation, 298, 299, 302, 452, 469; lobbying by, 299, 428–29, 431, 439, 452; and mollifying patients, 28, 32–33, 455; as percentage of health care costs, 57; proposals for, 469; regulation of, 299–302, 469; and revenue, 294, 299, 452; warnings on packaging, 301–2

Eastman, Richard, 271

education: and common good, 403; conferences, 102; continuing education, 409–10, 468; history of medical education, 131–35, 215; postgraduate medical education, 172–88, 450. *See also* faculty, medical school; medical school; residents and residency; students, medical

Einthoven, Willem, 303

electronic medical records, 217, 305–6

Eli Lilly, 292, 293, 310n34

Emanuel, Ezekiel J. and Linda L., 171n72

emergency medicine: and copayments, 319; inequities in care, 328, 330; and physician income, 70 emotions, 108, 111, 148–49, 407–9

empathy, 103, 138–39, 146, 149, 152, 404, 406, 467

employees: and ACA, 362, 366, 453; and employer-based insurance, 336–39, 352, 354, 355, 358–59, 363–64, 453; and labor movement, 360–61, 363–66; and race, 227. See also faculty, medical school; physicians; researchers

endocrinology, 54, 70, 176

end-of-life care: advance directives, 13, 33, 34; and autonomy, 13–14, 33–38, 470; and commodification, 392–93; and communication, 105–7, 409, 442n27, 448; effect on physician, 118; and emotions, 111, 148–49; ethics of futile care, 13–14, 34–35, 43, 80, 454, 470; and family, 14, 33–35, 43; goals of care, 118; and medical school, 148, 163–64; and race, 106; and religion, 14, 33, 43, 442n27; and rituals, 163–64; stories, 110–11, 117–18; and trust, 39

entitlement, 39–42, 44, 150, 408

entrepreneurial ideology, 99

ethics: and autonomy, 34–38; and commodification, 383–85, 411–12; and common good, 402, 452, 454; and corporatization of hospitals, 218–23, 229–32, 235–36, 411–12, 429–30, 468; and cultural differences, 107; and end-of-life care, 13–14, 34–35, 43, 80, 454, 470; and financial incentives, 42, 55–57, 59–61, 68–69, 80–81, 199, 383–85, 439, 448, 470; and insurance, 328–31, 412–13; and lobbying, 254, 428–29; and medical school, 136, 139, 197–99, 279, 403, 404, 405–7, 449–50, 467; of non-malfeasance vs. beneficence, 395; and overtesting, 42, 50, 59–60, 199; physician proposals, 407–11, 468; and reimbursement variations, 328–31; and researchers, 277–79, 413–14, 450–51, 468; and research fund-raising, 428; and teaching hospitals, 184–86, 329. See also communication, distortions in; conflicts of interest; inequities in care; social responsibility; values and medical school

ethos of science, 246–47, 273–74, 414

Europe: medical school model, 131–32, 144, 422; price controls in, 353; public health in, 348–50, 352; universal coverage in, 351–56, 359, 364

executive health programs, 194

existential distress, 26–31, 42–43, 415–17, 455

facility fees, 57, 64, 304

faculty, medical school: and academic freedom, 193; communication skills of, 196; and conflicts of interest, 192, 269–70; and diversity in research, 200–204; evaluation of residents by, 194–97; productivity of, 182–84, 202–3; and race, 143; reviews of, 193; royalties sharing by, 271, 391; salaries and clinical work, 192–94; salaries and research, 192, 200–202; teaching vs. clinical practice, 182–84; teaching vs. research, 202–4

family medicine, 54, 70, 71, 82, 104, 153

Federally Qualified Health Centers (FQHCs), 186–87

Fein, Oliver, 437

Fishbein, Morris, 423

Fleming, Alexander, 293

Flexner, Abraham, 133, 134–35

Flexner Report, 133–34

Fogelman, Alan, 191

follow-up care, inequities in, 184, 185–86, 231, 328, 329, 393

Food and Drug Administration (FDA), 271, 285n53, 295, 296, 299–302, 469

framework/proposals for change: and communication, 108, 410, 437–39, 467–68, 470; for government, 417, 469–70; for health care systems, 411–12, 468; and individualism, 401–2; for insurers, 412–13, 469; for manufacturers, 412–13, 469; for medical schools, 402–7, 449–50, 467; and patient-doctor relationship, 108, 408–10, 468; for patients, 414–17; for physicians, 407–11, 467–68, 470; for procedures, 410, 470; for research, 413–14, 468–69; and theories of societal change, 455–58

France: life expectancy in, 5n5; and public health, 348–49; spending on health care, 4n2; universal coverage in, 349, 354

free clinics. See hospitals and clinics, public

free markets, 386, 393–97

Freidson, Eliot, 35

funerals, 117, 122–23

Galen, 51, 152

gastroenterology: and colonoscopies, 58, 62–63; growth of specialty, 54, 76; guidelines, 68; and income, 71, 154, 176; and investors, 234; and job satisfaction, 82; and patient-doctor relationship, 60–61; training, 154

GDP (gross domestic product): and COVID-19 pandemic spending, 4n1; health care spending as percentage of, 2, 265; incomes ratio to, 53

gender: and communication, 107, 149; and declining care, 63; and empathy, 149; in medical school, 142; and procedural focus, 149–50

Genentech, 304

generalists: and academic hospitals, 191; competition for resources, 408; income vs. specialists, 15, 52–57, 69–71, 74–77, 154–55, 176, 385, 387–88, 389–90, 447; and job satisfaction, 82, 180–81; and postgraduate education, 175–76

genomics and genetic medicine, 253, 261–66, 275–76, 277, 427

Germany: life expectancy in, 5n5; and public health, 349–50; spending on health care, 4n2; universal coverage in, 352–53, 364; wait times in, 370

goals of care, 118, 163

Gompers, Samuel, 364

government: and communication distortions, 429, 433–34, 453–54; and definition of health care, 9; in dialogues, 315–16; funding of medical school, 188; proposals for, 417, 469–70; and public health, 348–52; role in inequities in care, 373–75, 433–34; role in insurance,

347; role in research funding, 191–92, 372–73; summary of challenges, 453–54

grades and medical school admissions, 137–40, 403–4, 449, 467

Gramsci, Antonio, 457

grants: bias in, 251; and drug prices, 298; for implementation research, 277; and infrastructure costs, 192, 251–52; and medical school funding, 188, 191–92; by NIH, 192, 248–49, 250–53, 277, 298, 391; in non-medical academia, 200–201; peer review system for, 249, 250–51, 253; and researcher salaries, 192, 200–202, 252–53, 391; and research priorities, 253, 254–55; and revenue, 469

guidelines, 57–58, 65–69, 259, 266, 370

gynecology, 54, 66, 70, 98, 101, 102, 169n55, 173

Habermas, Jürgen, 437–38, 458

Hatch, Orrin, 255

health care: actors as interconnected, 400, 424–25, 455–56; as basic right, 318, 373–75, 396, 454; challenges of changing, 9, 346–47, 438, 455–59; definitions of, 9; delusions about, 1–2, 454; factors overview, 16–17; interest in delivery research, 244–45

health care systems: administrator salaries, 194, 451, 468; communication distortions by, 429–30; and cost-conscious care, 189; economic competition, 189–91, 219–20, 223; executive health programs, 194; and manufacturers, 303; and physician autonomy, 83; and physician productivity, 81–82; procedures focus, 388; proposals for, 411–12, 468; revenue focus, 224–25, 230, 231–32, 235–36, 386–87, 429, 451; summary of challenges, 451–52. See also hospitals, corporatization of

Health Information Technology for Economic and Clinical Health Act, 305

Health Insurance Association of America, 432

health outcomes: and copayments, 319–21, 332, 383, 454; and costs, 1–2, 8, 387; in other countries, 8; US metrics, 3

hedge funds, 233–35

Hegel, Georg Wilhelm Friedrich, 140, 456

hematology, 54, 70

Himmelstein, David, 323–24, 437

Hippocratic Oath, 99

Hispanic Americans, 5n3, 143

Horkheimer, Max, 457

hospice care, 71–72, 150

hospitalists, 181–82, 191

hospitals: administrators, 194, 220–21, 225, 411–12, 451, 468; advertising and marketing of, 190, 218, 222–23, 232–33, 304, 388, 392, 429, 439, 451, 470; architecture, 226–27; budgets and universal coverage, 367, 452; capital investments by, 216–17, 226–27; and clinical networks, 215–16; and consolidation of markets, 215–23, 242; in dialogues, 211–12; economic competition among, 189–91, 219–20, 223; and electronic medical records, 305–6; funding of, 214–15, 216; history of, 214–17; and hospitalists, 181–82, 191; increases in hospitalization, 319; and inequities in care, 11–13, 184–86, 218–23, 226–31, 329, 388, 429; and in-/out-of-network care, 325, 388–89, 432; and insurance-related administrative costs, 323–24; mission statements, 230; and percentage of health care costs, 57; procedures focus, 77–78, 231, 234, 388; surplus revenue, 224–25, 230, 386–87, 429; upcoding by, 59. See also health care systems

hospitals, academic: advertising and marketing of, 190, 222–23; and community service, 230; corporatization of, 220, 221–23, 230–31; and economic competition, 189–91, 219–20, 223; executive health programs, 194; executive salaries, 194; faculty salaries, 192–94; funding of, 184; and inequities in care, 184–86, 329; and postgraduate education, 184–86; revenue focus, 230; rise of, 215. See also health care systems

hospitals, corporatization of: and advertising and marketing, 232–33, 388, 429, 451; and community service, 230, 451; and consolidation of markets, 215–23, 242; and cost-effectiveness, 231; in dialogues, 211–12, 242; and ethics, 218–23, 229–32, 235–36, 411–12, 429–30, 468; and idealism, 82–85; and inequities in care, 11–13, 218–23, 226–31, 388, 429; and investors, 234–35; and revenue, 77, 224–25, 230, 231–32, 235–36, 386–87, 390, 429, 451; and sales language, 213, 383; value vs. costs of, 231–32

hospitals and clinics, public, 41, 84–85, 185–87, 221, 330–31

Human Genome Project, 253

humanities, 145–46, 152, 164, 467

hyper/hypotension, 28–29, 275, 277

idealism: and admissions to medical school, 99, 130, 150, 152, 390, 404, 449; and corporatization of hospitals, 82–85; examples of physicians, 85–89; and free clinics, 186–87; nurturing, 405–6; and residents, 187; squashing of, 142, 150–51, 152, 155, 156, 390, 404, 449

immigrants, 12–13, 86, 187, 353, 354, 373, 375

income. See compensation and income

individualism vs. community, 401–2, 416, 455

inequities in care: at academic hospitals, 184–86, 329; in Canada, 371, 375; and commodification, 218–23, 387, 389–90, 393–97, 429; and concierge medicine, 41, 79, 454; and continuity of care, 84–85, 179–80, 185–87, 329; and cost controls, 332; and COVID-19 pandemic, 331, 335, 374–75; in dialogues, 1–2, 242; and emergency medicine, 328, 330; and entitlement, 39–42, 44; and evaluating trainees, 197; and follow-up care, 184, 185–86, 231, 328,

inequities in care (*cont.*)
329, 393; government's role and, 373–75, 433–34; and hospitals, 11–13, 184–86, 218–23, 226–31, 329, 388, 429; and insurance type, 326–31, 339, 469; and media, 435–36; and Medicaid, 2, 327; and medical schools, 228–29, 433; and race, 2, 226–28; and regional variations in resources, 334–35; research interest in, 436–37; and state program variations, 333–35, 373; and technology, 335; and transplants, 12–13, 327–28
infant mortality, 3
infectious disease, 54, 70, 154, 176
Institute of Medicine, 305
insulin, discovery of, 292–93
insurance: and administrative costs, 323–24, 363, 452; COBRA, 338; coinsurance, 324; and commodification, 317–26, 339, 383, 390–91, 452–54; and communication distortions, 431–32, 452–53; complexity of policies, 324–25; and consolidation of markets, 217–18, 223, 388, 451; cost of, 322–26, 336–37; denial of coverage, 298, 326, 390, 432, 452; in dialogues, 2, 3; and drug prices, 297–98; as employer-based, 336–39, 358–59, 363–64, 453; in Europe, 352–56; for-profit conversion, 431; government's role in, 347; and hospital development, 216–17; inequities in, 326–31, 339, 469; in-/out-of-network care, 324–25, 388–89, 432; and investors, 234; limits, 324; and lobbying, 363, 432, 453; marketplaces, 362; and mental health coverage, 25, 78–79; and national efforts in US, 358–66, 432; proposals for, 412–13, 469; and race, 5n3; RAND study of, 320–21; and revenue, 323, 363; summary of challenges, 452–53; taxes on, 338; upcoding, 59, 73; value of, 322–23. *See also* Affordable Care Act (ACA); Medicaid; Medicare; universal coverage
intensive care, 14, 34, 35, 41, 160
interest groups, 255, 428, 470

internal medicine: attitudes toward, 76–77, 105, 408; as career choice, 15, 76, 107, 153–54, 180; and diversity, 88; general internists in health systems, 190–91, 244, 389; growth of specialty, 51, 54, 173; and income, 53, 70; and research, 201; residencies, 153, 175–76, 195; satisfaction of, 82
International Committee of Medical Journal Editors, 270
interviews, 141, 167n38
investors, 233–35, 299, 391, 412–13

Japan: health outcomes, 5nn5–6; spending on health care, 4n2
job lock, 337, 453
Johnson, Lyndon B., 331, 361, 364
journals, medical, 270, 274, 295, 297, 427, 428
justice, 17, 87–88, 142, 401, 403, 404, 459n4. *See also* inequities in care

Kaiser Permanente, 215–16, 221
Kant, Immanuel, 456
Kaplan, Stanley, and test prep, 138
Katz, Mitch, 84
Kelsey, Frances, 299–300
kickbacks, 392
Koch, Robert, 291, 350
Korsch, Barbara, 100
Korsch, Karl, 457

labor movement, 360–61, 363–66
Laënnec, René, 291
launch prices, 298
Lawrence, John, 82
Leblond, Charles, 147
lectures, 146, 151, 157, 272–73, 405
life expectancy, 3, 5n5, 8, 175, 373
lifestyle treatments, 31–32
Lilly, Eli, 292
lobbying: by drug makers, 299, 428–29, 431, 439, 452; by insurers, 363, 432, 453; by interest groups, 255, 428; by medical schools, 254, 433; and NIH, 253–55, 470; by physician organizations, 253–55, 259, 423, 439, 449, 470

loneliness and social isolation, 22–23, 42–43, 401, 451, 455
Lukács, Georg, 457

MacLean, Lloyd, 162
Macleod, J. J. R., 293
mammogram guidelines, 66
manufacturers: communication distortions by, 430–31, 452; and conflicts of interest, 66–67, 232, 269–73, 303, 304, 425–27; in dialogues, 289, 315; and electronic medical records, 217, 305–6; focus on revenue, 306–7, 386–87, 391, 452; history of, 291–93, 302–3; and lifestyle treatments, 31–32; proposals for, 412–13, 469; and technology marketing, 302–5. See also drugs and drug makers
"march-in" provisions, 267–68
Marcuse, Herbert, 140, 457
marketing. See advertising and marketing
MCAT (Medical College Admission Test), 136–39, 167n38
media: distortions by, 435–36; interest in research, 428, 435; medical journals, 270, 274, 295, 297, 427, 428; and medical school ratings, 138–39; proposals for, 439, 470
Medicaid: and ACA, 327, 333, 362, 454; and access to care, 2, 185, 186, 327; and AIDS/HIV, 327; budget, 331; copayments, 319–20; and drug prices, 298; eligibility, 333; and hospital corporatization, 219, 220, 231, 451, 468; limits on services, 333, 335–36, 454; and market consolidation, 217–18; and public hospitals and clinics, 330; reimbursements, 2, 186, 327, 328–29, 333, 387, 451; rise in costs, 331–32; and specialty care, 185, 186; spending per enrollee, 334; state program variations, 333–35, 373; state vs. federal share of costs, 333–34; and teaching hospitals, 184–86; and transplants, 12–13, 328
medical devices, 66, 304, 431
medical histories, 183, 196–97

medicalization of life, 31–32
medical school: accreditation of, 195; as anti-intellectual, 406; biological reductionism in, 101–2, 407, 433, 450, 467; and clinical practice, 172, 182–84, 188–99; and commodification, 135, 390, 391, 447–49; communication instruction in, 105–7, 152, 158, 407, 434, 467; and conflicts of interest, 229, 232, 269–70; and corporatization of hospitals, 222, 228–29; and cost-conscious care, 189; cost of, 143, 155; and critical thinking, 157; decision-making in, 157, 158, 159; in dialogues, 211; diversity efforts in, 87, 88; doctoring and behavioral medicine courses, 157, 158, 198; dropout rates, 136; and end-of-life care, 148–49, 163–64; and entrepreneurial ideology, 99; ethics instruction in, 279, 403, 405–7, 449–50, 467; focus on unusual cases, 101, 162–63; funding for, 188, 191–92, 229; and gender, 142; hidden curriculum, 197–99; history of medical education, 131–35, 215; humanities in, 145–46, 152, 164, 467; and inequities in care, 228–29, 433; lobbying by, 254, 433; mission statements, 172, 189, 204, 230; and patient-doctor relationship, 30, 98, 146–47, 152, 156–59, 161–64; and patient values and experiences, 147–49; physicians' influence on, 424–25; and postgraduate education, 172–88, 450; and precision medicine, 264; proposals for, 402–7, 449–50, 467; and race, 143; ratings, 138–39; science focus of, 145–46; social science in, 152, 419n17, 467; structure of, 157–59; summary of challenges, 448–50; US vs. European model, 131–32, 144, 422; and white coat ceremonies, 99, 140–41. See also faculty, medical school; hospitals, academic; research and medical schools; residents and residency; students, medical; values and medical school
medical school admissions: bias in, 139, 141; and communication skills, 103; costs of, 143; diversity in, 141–43;

medical school admissions (*cont.*)
essays and applications, 138, 141–42; and ethics, 136, 139, 404, 406, 449–50; and grades, 137–40, 403–4, 449, 467; interviews, 141, 167n38; narrow focus of, 133, 134, 135–40, 144–45, 162, 164, 406, 467; proposals for, 404–5, 449–50, 467; and résumés, 404; social responsibility in, 142, 407–8, 449; and socioeconomic status, 137–38, 139, 403, 448; and tests, 135–39, 143, 145, 403–4, 449, 467; and values, 136, 138–39, 203–4, 405, 467

Medicare: administrative costs, 363; and colonoscopies, 63–64; and drug prices, 294, 299, 431; and facility fees, 64; fee schedule, 55, 73–74; funding for, 332; and hospital development, 216–17; and market consolidation, 217–18; Medicare Advantage, 453; Medicare for All, 363, 365, 366, 451; reimbursements and compensation, 55–57, 73–74, 75, 327; and relative value scale, 73–75; rise in costs, 331–32; and unions, 364, 366; and upcoding, 73

mental health: care, 25, 78–79, 375; of physicians, 103, 105, 109, 411, 468; and research priorities, 256, 257, 258; of students, 404, 405, 406, 407, 467; and use of medical care, 20–32, 42–43, 415–17, 455

Merton, Robert, 246–47, 273–74, 414

Miller, Saul, 346

mission statements, 172, 204, 230, 249, 256, 451

moonshots, 261–62, 417

mortality: child, 277; infant, 3

Moser, Willy, 403

Moss Test, 135–36

mutual-aid societies, 352, 354, 355

Nader, Ralph, 300

National Academies of Medicine and Science, 439

National Academy of Medicine, 305, 468–69

National Cancer Institute (NCI), 248, 250, 256, 261, 280n7

National Center for Advancing Translational Sciences (NCATS), 250, 280n7

National Center for Complementary and Integrative Health (NCCAH), 250, 280n7

National Center for Health Services Research, 258. *See also* Agency for Healthcare Research and Quality (AHRQ)

National Eye Institute (NEI), 250, 280n7

National Guidelines Clearinghouse, 65–66, 259

National Health Service (UK), 355–56, 367, 369, 456

National Heart, Lung, and Blood Institute (NHLBI), 250, 261, 280n7, 282n29

National Human Genome Research Institute (NHGRI), 250, 280n7

National Institute of Allergy and Infectious Disease (NIAID), 250, 253, 257–58, 280n7, 282n29

National Institute of Arthritis and Musculoskeletal and Skin Diseases (NIAMS), 250, 280n7

National Institute of Biomedical Imaging and Bioengineering (NIBIB), 250, 280n7

National Institute of Child Health and Human Development (NICHD), 250, 280n7

National Institute of Dental and Craniofacial Research (NIDCR), 250, 280n7

National Institute of Diabetes and Digestive and Kidney Diseases (NIDDK), 250, 271, 280n7, 282n29

National Institute of Environmental Health Sciences (NIEHS), 250, 280n7

National Institute of General Medical Sciences (NIGMS), 250, 280n7

National Institute of Mental Health (NIMH), 250, 256, 257, 258, 280n7

National Institute of Neurological Disorders and Stroke (NINDS), 250, 280n7, 282n29

National Institute of Nursing Research (NINR), 250, 256, 280n7

National Institute on Aging (NIA), 250, 280n7, 282n29
National Institute on Alcohol Abuse and Alcoholism (NIAAA), 250, 280n7
National Institute on Deafness and Other Communication Disorders (NIDCD), 250, 280n7
National Institute on Drug Abuse (NIDA), 250, 256, 280n7
National Institute on Minority Health and Disparities (NIMHD), 250, 257, 280n7
National Institutes of Health (NIH): budget, 254, 255, 259, 276, 279, 469; grants, 192, 248–49, 250–53, 277, 298, 391; history of, 247–50; and infrastructure costs, 192, 251–52; list of institutes, 249–50; and lobbying, 253–55, 470; mission statement, 249, 256; peer review system, 249, 250–51, 253; salary restrictions, 192, 252; and scientific workforce, 251–53. See also research and NIH
National Library of Medicine (NLM), 250, 280n7, 282n29
National Physicians' Practice Costs and Income Survey, 70
National Quality Measures Clearinghouse, 259
National Science Foundation, 255
nephrology, 54, 176
neurology, 54, 67, 70, 76, 169n55
Nobel Prizes, 245–46, 292, 293, 303
nondisease, 28–32
non-malfeasance, ethic of, 395
Norris, Keith, 437
North American Spine Society, 259, 425
nursing homes, 57, 233, 323

Obama, Barack, 361–63, 365, 432
objective structured clinical examinations (OSCEs), 158, 197
Office of the National Coordinator, 305
oncology, 68, 71, 82, 106–7, 176, 408, 425–26
ophthalmology, 54, 70, 82, 174, 234

organizations: disease-specific, 255, 428, 470; physician, 253–55, 259, 422–28, 439, 449, 470
organized skepticism, 247, 274
orthopedics: device makers, 312n59; growth of specialty, 54; guidelines, 67; and income, 70, 76, 447, 449; and job satisfaction, 82; and Medicaid, 185, 198; and patient-doctor relationship, 182–83; and residency slots, 169n55; wait times for, 372
Osler, William, 51–52, 142, 203
otolaryngology, 54, 70, 82, 169n55, 234

Park, Ed, 177–78
Parke-Davis, 271
Pasteur, Louis, 291, 349
patents and royalties, 266–69, 271–72, 299, 302, 391, 442, 452, 469
pathology, 54, 56, 57, 64, 234, 263, 304, 325
Patient-Centered Outcomes Research Institute (PCORI), 259–60
patient-doctor relationship: and commodification, 99, 394–95, 447–48; communication challenges, 100–108, 425, 427–28, 434–35, 447–48, 468; communication distortions in, 427–28; and cultural differences, 25–26, 38–39, 44, 86–87, 103, 107, 159, 403, 415, 447–48, 455, 471; and definition of health care, 9; examples of, 10–11, 60–61, 77, 109–23, 182–83; and medical school, 30, 98, 146–47, 152, 156–59, 161–64; and nondisease, 28–32; and patient distress, 20–32, 42–43, 415–17, 455; and physician stress, 103–5; proposals for, 108, 407, 408–10, 468; and race, 38–39, 403, 455; and residents, 178–82, 195–97; and risk, 163; and trust, 38–39, 86–87, 455
patients: autonomy of, 13–14, 33–38, 43, 401, 416, 455, 470; commodification of, 190–91, 392–93, 394–95; communication obstacles, 434–35, 454–55; decision-making ability, 72–73; and definition of health care, 9; in dialogues, 18–19, 48; and entitlement,

patients (*cont.*)

39–42, 44; influences on, 21–23, 424–25; mollifying, 24, 28, 32–33, 42, 101–2, 455; proposals for, 414–17, 470–71; psychological distress of, 20–32, 42–43, 415–17, 455; summary of challenges, 454–55; as term, 21. *See also* patient-doctor relationship

pediatrics, 54, 70, 71, 100, 150, 169n55

peer review: grants, 249, 250–51, 253; journals, 270, 427

Pellegrino, Edmund, 394–95, 396

penicillin, discovery of, 293

Permanente Medical Group, 216

personalized medicine. *See* precision medicine

Pfizer, 292, 293, 310n34

Physician Payment Review Commission, 74

physicians: advertising to, 295, 430; autonomy of, 83, 153; burnout, 82, 103, 306, 417; commodification of, 190–91, 389–90, 394–95, 429–30; and definition of health care, 9; in dialogues, 48–49, 97; diversity of, 87–88, 107, 143; elitism of, 422; and funerals, 117, 122–23; historical education of, 131–35; influence of, 424–25; and in-/out-of-network care, 324–25, 432; job satisfaction, 82, 169n54, 180–81, 306; lobbying by, 253–55, 423, 439, 449, 470; mental health of, 103, 105, 109, 411, 468; productivity of, 81–82, 182–84, 202–3; proposals for, 407–11, 467–68; ratings, 425; resistance to universal coverage, 356, 357, 358–60, 361, 364, 422–24; stress of, 82, 103–5; work hours, 78. *See also* compensation and income; faculty, medical school; generalists; researchers; specialists

Physicians for a National Health Program, 437

plastic surgery, 54, 70, 82, 169n55

Plato, 17, 390, 396–97, 456, 464n1

politics: campaign contributions, 310n34, 363; and definition of health care, 9; and moonshots, 261–62, 417; and NHS (UK), 369; and NIH, 253–55,

470; proposals for policy makers, 417, 470; restrictions on public programs, 335–36; restrictions on research, 259–60, 335–36. *See also* government; lobbying

postgraduate medical education, 172–88, 450. *See also* residents and residency

poverty and care for poor: and corporatization, 82–85, 221; government role in, 349, 374–75; and health outcomes, 3; and hospitals, 214–15; and life expectancy, 3; in other countries, 349, 367; and rationing, 266; and teaching hospitals, 184–86. *See also* inequities in care; Medicaid; socioeconomic status

Precision Health Economics, 297

precision medicine, 262–66, 277, 278, 427

Precision Medicine Initiative, 264–66

Prescription Drug User Fee Act (PDUFA), 301–2

prices: components of, 386; drug prices, 293–94, 297–98, 299, 431; government controls of, 353; lack of transparency on, 63–64, 322, 388–89, 429, 452, 470; and market consolidation, 218, 223; price elasticity, 340n6; vs. value, 387. *See also* costs

primary care physicians: and academic hospitals, 190–91; in Canada, 175; duration of visits to, 182; income, 154–55, 221, 389; and life expectancy metrics, 175; and Medicaid, 327; and Medicare, 75; mental health care by, 78–79; satisfaction of, 180–81; shortage of, 154, 175

Pritchett, Henry S., 134, 143

private equity corporations, 233–35, 299, 391

procedures: by academic faculty, 192, 194; and compensation, 15, 53, 55–57, 69–71, 75–78, 154–55, 176, 408, 447; control of by specialists, 102–3, 160; costs of, 55–59, 62–65, 77, 234, 322, 388–89, 429, 470; data on, 177–78; and facility fees, 57, 64, 304; financial incentives for, 55–57, 59–61, 80–81,

439, 448, 470; focus on and commodification of health care, 77–78, 231, 234, 388–89, 408; focus on and gender, 149–50; focus on and reductionism, 160–62; guidelines on, 57–58, 65–69, 259; and job satisfaction, 180–81; proposals for, 410, 470; and relative value scale, 73–75; and residency slots, 153–54; unnecessary, 65, 67–69

productivity metrics, 81–82, 182–84, 202–3

prostate cancer, 158, 439

psychiatry, 25, 54, 70, 71, 78–79, 169n55

psychology and psychologists: access to, 25, 78; and mental health of physicians, 103, 105, 109, 411, 468; and mental health of students, 404, 405, 406, 407, 467; and nondisease, 28–32; psychological distress and use of medical care, 20–32, 42–43, 415, 455; rejection of psychiatric diagnoses, 25–27, 30

Public Citizen Health Research Group, 300–301, 437

public health, 274–79, 348–52, 360, 374

Public Health Service Act, 249, 285n53

public option, 362, 363, 453

pulmonary specialists, 54, 160, 176

race: and end-of-life care, 106; and health outcomes, 3; and hospital employees, 227; and inequities in care, 2, 226–28; and infant mortality, 3; and insurance coverage, 5n3; and life expectancy, 5n5; and medical school, 143; and patient-doctor relationship, 38–39, 403, 455; of physicians, 107, 143; and transplants, 328

radiology: as add-on cost, 234; growth of specialty, 54; guidelines, 68; and income, 69, 70; and in-/out-of-network care, 325; and job satisfaction, 82; and patient-doctor relationship, 105; and redundant tests, 61; and residency slots, 169n55; and training, 154

Ramsdell Act, 248

rationality, 460n4

RBRVS (resource-based relative value scale), 73–75

Reagan, Ronald, 40, 347, 361, 424

reason, 459n4

recertification, 410, 468

reimbursements: and academic hospitals, 190; ethics of variations in, 328–31; in Europe, 354; and hospital networks, 216, 217–18, 451; and in-/out-of-network care, 324–25, 388–89; and investors, 234; Medicaid, 2, 186, 327, 328–29, 333, 387, 451; Medicare, 55–57, 73–74, 75, 327

Reinhardt, Uwe, 297, 436

Relative Value Scale Update Committee (RUC), 74–75

relative value units (RVUs), 81–82, 182–84, 202–3, 387, 447

religion, 14, 33, 43, 442n27

research: commodification of, 390–91, 450–51; distorted communication about, 428–29, 451; and federal agencies, 258–61; on health care delivery, 244–45, 468; on inequities in care, 436–37; lack of innovation in drug research, 298, 299; media interest in, 428, 435; and moonshots, 261–62, 417; patents and royalties, 266–69, 271, 391, 428; priorities, 253–58, 260–69, 274–78, 336; proposals for, 413–14, 468–69; restrictions on, 259–60, 335–36; summary of challenges, 450–51

research and medical schools: clinical practice as subsidizing cost of, 191–92; commodification of, 391; impact on education, 200–204; infrastructure costs, 192, 251–52; intellectual diversity in, 200–204; patents and royalties, 266–69, 271, 391; and precision medicine, 264; and revenue, 200; and tripartite mission, 172, 200

research and NIH: grants, 192, 248–49, 250–53, 277, 298, 391; history of, 247–50; and patents, 268; and precision medicine, 263–66, 277; researchers' salaries, 192, 252–53; research priorities, 253, 254–58, 260–64, 274, 276–78; and scientific workforce, 251–53 researchers: and biological reductionism, 429, 468; commodification of, 390–91; communication distortions by, 428–29, 451; and conflicts of interest, 269–73, 427, 428; contributions of US, 245–46; and definition of health care, 9; in dialogues, 243, 289; effect of funding on research topics, 253, 254–55; and ethics, 277–79, 413–14, 450–51, 468; and ethos of science, 246–47, 273–74, 414; and health system shortcomings, 436–37; influence of physicians on, 424–25; and NIH workforce, 251–53; and patents and royalties, 268–69, 271, 391, 428; proposals for, 468–69; salaries, 192, 200–202, 252–53, 391

Residency Review Committees, 174, 195

residents and residency: and continuity of care, 179–80, 185–87, 329; and end-of-life care, 106, 409; evaluation of, 194–97; and free clinics, 187; internal medicine, 153, 175–76, 195; numbers by specialty, 153–54; and patient-doctor relationship, 178–82, 195–97; proposals for, 407, 467

resource-based relative value scale (RBRVS), 73–75

retirement and insurance, 337–38, 364, 366

Reuther, Walter, 364–65

revenue: and commodification, 386–87; and corporatization of hospitals, 77, 224–25, 230, 231–32, 235–36, 386–87, 390, 429, 451; and drug makers, 294, 299, 452; and grants, 469; and insurers, 323, 363; and investors, 233–35; and manufacturers, 306–7, 386–87, 391, 452; and medical schools, 188–92, 200

rheumatology, 54, 70, 154, 176

rituals, 163–64

Rockefeller Foundation, 134, 135

Romanow, Roy, 368

Romanow Commission, 368–69, 370

Romney, Mitt, 329

Röntgen, Wilhelm, 302

salaries. *See* compensation and income

Sanders, Bernie, 365

satisfaction: patient, 218; physician, 82, 169n54, 180–81, 306

Schwabe, Art, 60–61, 71, 384

science: ethos of, 246–47, 273–74, 414; falsification in, 247; focus on in medical school, 133, 134, 135, 136, 137, 139–40, 144–46, 406, 467; theory of scientific revolutions, 274

Shattuck, Lemuel, 351

Shine, Ken, 220

sickness funds, 352–53, 358, 364

skepticism, organized, 247, 274

social responsibility: and continuing education, 410, 468; and corporate responsibility, 412; and manufacturers, 452; and medical school, 142, 152, 407–8, 449, 467; proposals for, 467, 468; and researchers, 277–79, 413–14, 450–51, 468

social science and scientists, 9, 152, 200–202, 260–61, 391, 419n17, 467

societal change theories, 455–58

socioeconomic status: and corporatization of hospitals, 219–21; and entitlement, 39–42, 44; and medical school admission, 137–38, 139, 141–43, 403; of medical students, 137–38, 139, 402–3, 448, 467; and patient-doctor relationship, 38–39, 44, 86–87, 107, 159, 447–48, 455; and prestige, 52–53, 134–35, 140–41, 153, 155, 176

sociology, salaries in, 201–2

specialists: and additional costs in procedures, 56–59, 62–65, 234, 304; autonomy of, 153; and biological reductionism, 102, 160–62; communication skills of, 410; competition for resources, 408; and conflicts of interest, 178, 392; control of procedures by, 102–3, 160; and corporatization of hospitals, 231, 232–33; costs of training to society, 174–75, 177; and definition of health care, 9; duration of visits to, 182; growth of specialization, 54–55, 173–74; guidelines by, 57–58, 65–69; incomes by specialty, 70; income vs. generalists, 15,

52–57, 59, 69–71, 74–77, 154–55, 176, 385, 387–88, 389–90, 447, 448–49; influence on research, 425; job satisfaction of, 82; kickbacks, 392; limiting, 177–78, 368, 372; and Medicaid, 185, 186; numbers of, 174–75, 177–78, 204, 390; and patient-doctor relationship, 10–11; postgraduate education, 154, 172–88, 450; pressure to declare, 180–81; proposals for, 467–68; and relative value scale, 73–75; residency slots, 153–54; status and prestige of, 153, 155, 176; wait times for, 370, 372

spinal fusion, 259, 336, 425

Squibb, 292, 293

stress, physician, 82, 103–5

students, medical: and ambiguity, 163; cultural competency of, 136, 138–40, 405, 406; and debt, 143, 155, 448–49; and entitlement, 150; focus on income, 14–15, 75–76, 142, 152–55, 447, 448–49; focus on unusual cases, 162–63; and longitudinal care, 156–57; mental health of, 404, 405, 406, 407, 467; and patient values and experiences, 147–49; and pressure for specialty decisions, 180–81; proposals for, 402–7; socialization of, 140–41, 150–52, 467; socioeconomic status of, 137–38, 139, 402–3, 448, 467. See also idealism; medical school admissions

sulfanilamide, 299

surgeons and surgery: and facility fees, 64; growth of specialty, 54, 131, 173, 174; guidelines, 67, 69, 336, 425; and hospital revenue, 77; and income, 70, 76, 78, 80, 385; and inequities in care, 2, 39, 40, 227–28, 328; and in-/out-of-network care, 325; and job satisfaction, 82; and Medicaid, 185, 328; and patient-doctor relationship, 76–77, 159, 162, 177–78, 182–83, 196, 408; and residency slots, 169n55; and technology, 303; and tolerance for ambiguity, 107; wait times for, 370, 371, 372, 375

Sweden: life expectancy in, 5n5; public health in, 349; sickness funds, 355; spending on health care, 4n2, 294

taxes, 332, 338, 367, 431, 453

teaching hospitals. See hospitals, academic

technology: and conflicts of interest, 303; and costs, 55–56, 303, 304–5; electronic medical records, 217, 305–6; marketing of, 190, 218, 232–33, 302–5; and societal change, 457

testing: costs of periodic, 57–59; and ethics, 42, 50, 59–61, 199; and mollifying patients, 24, 42, 455

test prep courses, 137–38, 167n38

tests, medical school admission, 135–39, 143, 145, 403–4, 449, 467

thalidomide, 299–300

Thomas, Lewis, 52, 140

transplants, 12–13, 106, 327–28

Traven, B., 385, 396

Treasure of the Sierra Madre, The (1948), 385, 396

treatment: and additional testing, 61; halting, 119–20; lifestyle treatments, 31–32; research on dissemination of, 258, 262–63, 265, 274–79; resistance to, 113–14

troglitazone (Rezulin), 271

Truman, Harry, 360–61, 423

Trump, Donald J., 259, 362

trust, 38–39, 86–87, 455

Tulchinsky, Ted, 346, 357

unions, 360–61, 363–66

United Kingdom: cost barriers in, 375; health metrics in, 5nn5–6; private insurance in, 356; public health in, 350; universal coverage in, 355–56, 367, 369, 456; wait times in, 370, 371

United States: government's role in public health, 350–51; health metrics, 3; national insurance strategy efforts, 358–66, 432; research contributions, 245–46; spending on health care, 2, 265; wait times in, 370

universal coverage: challenges in other countries, 366–72, 375; insurer resistance to, 453; lack of in US, 8, 10, 456, 469; physicians' resistance to, 356,

universal coverage (cont.)
  357, 358–60, 361, 364, 422–24; rise of in
  other countries, 349, 351–58, 364, 456;
  and taxes, 367, 453; and wait times,
  370–71
universalism, 246, 273
upcoding, 59, 73
Uppsala Code, 278
urology, 54, 70, 173–74, 234
US Department of Health and Human
  Services, 267, 302
U.S. News and World Report, 138–39
uterine cancer, 110, 284n47

value: vs. commodification, 387, 389;
  and compensation, 385; vs. costs,
  231–32, 387; of insurance, 322–23;
  public value of patents, 268. See also
  relative value units (RVUs)
values: in employer-based insurance,
  339; and end-of-life care, 118; and
  societal change, 457–58
values and medical school: and admissions, 136, 138–39, 203–4, 405, 467;
  in curriculum, 146–47, 150–52, 390,
  406–7; and hidden curriculum, 197–99;
  patient values and experiences in,
  147–49; problems with, 98, 158–59,
  161–63, 204, 390, 433, 449–50
Veterans Affairs, 305, 306
Virchow, Rudolf, 151, 349–50, 419n17
visits: duration of, 182–84; junk visits,
  81; reduction in with copayments,
  319, 321, 454
von Behring, Emil, 292

wait times, 370–71, 372, 375
Weiner, Herb, 104, 105
Welch, William H., 135
white coat ceremonies, 99, 140–41
whites, health metrics, 3, 5n3, 5n5
Wilkes, Michael, 290
Wilson, Harold, 356
Wilson, Woodrow, 360
Winthrop, John, 131, 402
Wolfe, Sidney, 300, 437
women. See gender
Woolhandler, Steffie, 323–24, 437
World Health Organization, 373
World War II, 249, 293, 353

x-rays, development of, 302–3

Zulman, Donna, 108